Endocrinology: Pediatric and Geriatric (Case Studies)

Endocrinology: Pediatric and Geriatric (Case Studies)

Editor: Harley Lloyd

AMERICAN
MEDICAL PUBLISHERS
www.americanmedicalpublishers.com

AMERICAN
MEDICAL PUBLISHERS
www.americanmedicalpublishers.com

Cataloging-in-Publication Data

Endocrinology: pediatric and geriatric (case studies) / edited by Harley Lloyd.
p. cm.
Includes bibliographical references and index.
ISBN 979-8-88740-637-4
1. Endocrinology. 2. Endocrine glands--Diseases. I. Lloyd, Harley.
RC648 .C55 2023
6164--dc23

American Medical Publishers,
41 Flatbush Avenue,
1st Floor, New York,
NY 11217, USA

ISBN 979-8-88740-637-4 (Hardback)

Contents

Preface

Pediatric and geriatric endocrinology are two specialized branches of endocrinology that focus on the unique hormonal challenges and disorders experienced by children and older adults. Pediatric endocrinology primarily deals with hormonal disorders in children and adolescents. Hormonal imbalances during growth and development can have a significant impact on a child's overall health, growth and sexual development. Some of the conditions which are studied and treated under pediatric endocrinology are growth disorders, childhood diabetes (Type 1 and Type 2), thyroid disorders, puberty disorders, adrenal gland disorders and disorders of sexual development. Geriatric endocrinology, on the other hand, focuses on the hormonal changes and disorders that occur in older adults. It involves managing conditions such as menopause and osteoporosis. It also involves diabetes management in older adults, thyroid disorders, adrenal disorders, and hormone-related issues affecting cognitive function and mood. This book provides comprehensive insights into the field of pediatric and geriatric endocrinology. It will serve as a valuable source of reference for graduate and postgraduate students.

All of the data presented henceforth, was collaborated in the wake of recent advancements in the field. The aim of this book is to present the diversified developments from across the globe in a comprehensible manner. The opinions expressed in each chapter belong solely to the contributing authors. Their interpretations of the topics are the integral part of this book, which I have carefully compiled for a better understanding of the readers.

At the end, I would like to thank all those who dedicated their time and efforts for the successful completion of this book. I also wish to convey my gratitude towards my friends and family who supported me at every step.

Editor

1

Graves' Thyrotoxicosis Leading to Adrenal Decompensation and Hyperandrogenemia in a Pediatric Patient with Salt-Wasting Congenital Adrenal Hyperplasia

Meghan E. Fredette and Lisa Swartz Topor

Pediatric Endocrinology, Rhode Island Hospital/The Warren Alpert Medical School of Brown University, 111 Plain Street, 3rd Floor, Providence, RI 02903, USA

Correspondence should be addressed to Meghan E. Fredette; meghan_fredette@brown.edu

Academic Editor: Wayne V. Moore

Introduction. Thyroid hormone is known to accelerate glucocorticoid turnover. In a thyrotoxic state, individuals with adrenal insufficiency are unable to increase endogenous cortisol production to compensate for increased turnover, placing them at risk for symptoms of glucocorticoid deficiency and adrenal crisis. In patients with salt-wasting congenital adrenal hyperplasia (SW-CAH), hyperandrogenemia is a measurable reflection of relative glucocorticoid insufficiency. *Case Presentation*. A 12-year-old girl with SW-CAH reported 3 recent episodes of vomiting without diarrhea, and accompanying tachycardia, responsive to stress dose steroids. In the previous 9 months, she unintentionally lost 2.6 kg. She had tachycardia and new thyromegaly. Labs showed suppressed TSH, elevated free T4 and total T3, and elevated thyroid stimulating immunoglobulin (TSI) consistent with Graves' disease. Adrenal androgens were markedly elevated. Maintenance hydrocortisone dose was 25 mg/m^2/day and was not changed. Methimazole was initiated. Four weeks later, free T4 and adrenal androgens normalized. She had no further vomiting episodes. *Conclusions*. Thyrotoxicosis must be included in the differential diagnosis of individuals with SW-CAH who present with episodes concerning for adrenal crises, escalating hydrocortisone requirements, and/or inadequate suppression of adrenal hormones.

1. Introduction

Salt-wasting congenital adrenal hyperplasia (SW-CAH) is the most common cause of primary adrenal insufficiency in pediatric patients, and in over 95% of cases it is caused by a mutation in the *CYP21A2* gene, which causes a deficiency of the enzyme 21-hydroxylase [1]. Deficiency in 21-hydroxylase causes both gluco- and mineralocorticoid deficiency as well as hyperandrogenism due to the diversion of adrenal steroid precursors to adrenal androgens. Treatment consists of mineralocorticoid supplementation, as well as supraphysiologic glucocorticoid doses to suppress ACTH and minimize formation of adrenal androgens.

Management of glucocorticoid dosing in the growing child with SW-CAH is challenging. Typical dosing of hydrocortisone ranges from 10 to 15 mg/m^2 daily in 3 divided doses [1]. Cortisol clearance increases in puberty, and glucocorticoid dose requirements often increase [2]. Glucocorticoid overtreatment can compromise height and result in symptoms of glucocorticoid excess. Undertreatment can also compromise height due to accelerated epiphyseal maturation and can result in bothersome virilization and prompt adrenal crises. Close monitoring of growth and biochemical measurement of androgens are essential for the care of the pediatric patient with SW-CAH.

In this case report, we describe a 12-year-old female with previously well-controlled SW-CAH, who presented to a pediatric emergency department with multiple episodes concerning for adrenal crises, responsive to stress dose steroids. She was found to have poorly suppressed androgens on supraphysiologic glucocorticoid doses. Ultimately, she was diagnosed with Graves' disease.

2. Case Presentation

A 12-year-old female with SW-CAH presented to the pediatric endocrinology clinic for routine follow-up. She

TABLE 1: Androgens and thyroid studies at baseline, diagnosis, and after 4 and 12 weeks of treatment.

Lab Value	Reference Range	15 Weeks prior	Diagnosis	4 weeks	12 weeks
TSH (uIU/ml)	0.35-5.5		0.019	0.021	4.345
Total T3 (ng/dl)	82-213		331	150	99
Free T4 (ng/dl)	0.8-1.8		2.82	1.42	0.89
17-Hydroxyprogesterone (ng/dl)	11-155	639	11,600	717	33
Androstenedione (ng/dl)	50-170	28	257	74	89
Testosterone (ng/dl)	15-35	8	67	18	15

was diagnosed with SW-CAH in the newborn period after presenting with ambiguous genitalia and was treated with supraphysiologic hydrocortisone divided three times daily throughout her life (prepubertal dosing range 10-15 mg/m^2/day, pubertal dosing range 15-25 mg/m^2/day), as well as fludrocortisone (0.1 mg daily). She was monitored every 3-4 months with clinical examinations, growth parameters, and serum measurements of 17-hydroxyprogesterone (17-OHP), androstenedione, and testosterone (Esoterix Laboratory, Calabasas Hills, CA), which together guided her medication dosing. She had no evidence of glucocorticoid excess and her growth velocity was normal, without evidence of acceleration or suppression. She and her parents reported continued excellent compliance with her medication regimen.

At age 12 3/12 years, she reported 3 recent emergency department visits for persistent vomiting without diarrhea, abdominal pain, inability to tolerate oral steroids, and tachycardia. One of the episodes was accompanied by fever >39°C. There was no hypotension during any of these episodes, but heart rates were elevated ranging from 124 to 154 beats per minute. Sodium and potassium were normal: Na 137-140 meq/L (reference range, 133-143 meq/L) and K 3.6-4.1 meq/L (reference range 3.4-4.7 meq/L). Each episode was treated with normal saline boluses and intravenous stress dose steroids, and treatment led to immediate improvement in symptoms. She was discharged from the emergency department with recommendations for stress dose steroids by mouth. Over the prior 9 months, she had also unintentionally lost 2.6 kg and had an accelerated annualized growth velocity of 10.6 centimeters per year. BMI was 15.4 kg/m^2 (Z-score -1.38). She denied any heat intolerance, jitteriness, palpitations, sweating, diarrhea, or vision complaints. While in clinic, her resting pulse was elevated at 136 beats per minute and blood pressure was normal. She was noted to have new symmetric thyromegaly without nodules. She had no lid lag or stare. She was in mid-puberty, with tanner 3 breasts. There was no family history of autoimmune disease or thyroid disease. Labs (Table 1) showed a suppressed TSH, and an elevated free T4 and Total T3. Thyroid antibodies were consistent with Graves' disease, with a thyroid stimulating immunoglobulin (TSI) of 652% (reference range <140%). She had no prior thyroid studies for comparison. Adrenal androgens were markedly elevated with 17-OHP 11,600 ng/dl (reference range 11-155 ng/dl, target <1000 ng/dl in SW-CAH). At a clinic visit 15 weeks prior to this evaluation, her 17-OHP on the same dose of hydrocortisone (25 mg/m^2/day) was improved at 639 ng/dl. She was initiated on methimazole 0.5 mg/kg/day. Her hydrocortisone dose was not changed and remained at 25 mg/m^2/day. Four weeks later, repeat labs demonstrated normal free T4 with mildly suppressed TSH and normal total T3. 17-OHP was stable at 717 ng/dl (Figure 1). She had no further vomiting episodes after initiation of methimazole, and her tachycardia resolved.

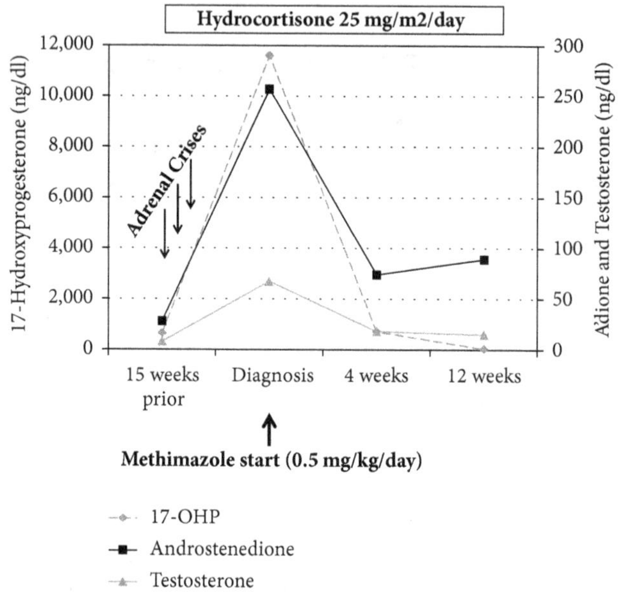

FIGURE 1: Graphic demonstration of adrenal androgen levels over time.

Three months after treatment began for Graves' disease, her TSH and free T4 were in the reference range, and methimazole was decreased to 0.3 mg/kg/day. Repeat 17-OHP was low at 33 ng/dl, indicating suppression on the unchanged hydrocortisone dose of 25 mg/m^2/day. Her hydrocortisone dose was decreased to 21 mg/m^2/day.

3. Discussion

Thyroid hormone is well-known to accelerate the metabolism of cortisol. In the adrenally sufficient individual, the thyrotoxic state both increases the production of cortisol, and shortens the half-life of cortisol due to an increased turnover rate, with a net effect of normal circulating cortisol levels [3]. Cortisol requirements are increased due to the stress and increased metabolic demands of thyrotoxicosis. The mechanism of increased cortisol clearance appears to be due to thyroid hormone effects on the activity of 11βHSD and 5-α reductase enzymes [4].

Patients with adrenal insufficiency are unable to mount an adrenal response by increasing cortisol levels in the setting of excess thyroid hormone, placing them at risk for adrenal crises. Recurrent adrenal crises have been reported in individuals with autoimmune primary adrenal insufficiency upon development of autoimmune thyrotoxicosis [5]. Similarly, it is well documented that hypothyroid patients initiated on thyroid hormone repletion with undiagnosed primary or secondary adrenal insufficiency can present with adrenal crisis [6, 7]. In the hypothyroid state, cortisol clearance is slowed, protecting the hypothyroid, adrenally insufficient patient from symptoms of adrenal insufficiency. With thyroid hormone initiation, cortisol clearance increases, and adrenal crisis may occur, similar to the thyrotoxic patient with adrenal insufficiency.

The literature includes only 2 cases of adult patients with congenital adrenal hyperplasia who experienced symptomatic adrenal insufficiency and/or adrenal crisis associated with thyrotoxicosis. Takasu et al. described a 75-year-old female who was admitted for treatment of Graves' thyrotoxicosis and was found unconscious due to adrenal crisis during her hospitalization [8]. She was ultimately diagnosed with nonclassical 21-hydroxylase deficiency. Kim et al. reported the case of a 23-year-old male with Graves' thyrotoxicosis who was diagnosed with nonclassic 11-beta hydroxylase deficiency after he presented with hypokalemia and hypertension and was found to have adrenal hyperplasia on imaging [9]. Our report is the first case describing a pediatric patient with CAH, who experienced repeated episodes concerning for adrenal crises and hyperandrogenemia secondary to the onset of Graves' thyrotoxicosis, demonstrating the impact of thyroid hormone excess on the metabolism of glucocorticoids *in vivo*.

4. Conclusions

This unusual case demonstrates the unique findings of thyrotoxicosis in a pediatric patient with SW-CAH on glucocorticoid supplementation. She presented with classic signs and symptoms of Graves' disease including thyromegaly, weight loss, and tachycardia, as well as SW-CAH specific symptoms reflecting cortisol deficiency including biochemical hyperandrogenemia and repeated episodes concerning for adrenal crises. Increased clearance of cortisol in the setting of thyrotoxicosis resulted in recurrent adrenal decompensations due to insufficient cortisol, though 1 episode was accompanied by fever and thus may have been triggered by illness. Hyperandrogenemia and episodes concerning for adrenal crises resolved with normalization of thyroid levels, without any change in glucocorticoid dose. Thyrotoxicosis must be included in the differential diagnosis of individuals with any form of adrenal insufficiency, including CAH, who present with escalating glucocorticoid requirements, or recurrent adrenal crises despite appropriate glucocorticoid adherence and dosing.

Disclosure

This case was presented as a poster at the 99th Annual Meeting of the Endocrine Society.

References

[1] P. W. Speiser, R. Azziz, L. S. Baskin et al., "Congenital adrenal hyperplasia due to steroid 21-hydroxylase deficiency: an endocrine society clinical practice guideline," *The Journal of Clinical Endocrinology & Metabolism*, vol. 95, no. 9, pp. 4133–4160, 2010.

[2] E. Charmandari, C. G. D. Brook, and P. C. Hindmarsh, "Why is management of patients with classical congenital adrenal hyperplasia more difficult at puberty?" *Archives of Disease in Childhood*, vol. 86, no. 4, pp. 266–269, 2002.

[3] T. F. Gallagher, L. Hellman, J. Finkelstein et al., "Hyperthyroidism and cortisol secretion in man," *The Journal of Clinical Endocrinology & Metabolism*, vol. 34, no. 6, pp. 919–927, 1972.

[4] M. Hoshiro, Y. Ohno, H. Masaki, H. Iwase, and N. Aoki, "Comprehensive study of urinary cortisol metabolites in hyperthyroid and hypothyroid patients," *Clinical Endocrinology*, vol. 64, no. 1, pp. 37–45, 2006.

[5] D. Naik, K. Felix Jebasingh, and N. Thomas, "Delayed diagnosis of Graves' thyrotoxicoisis presenting as recurrent adrenal crisis in primary adrenal insufficiency," *Journal of Clinical and Diagnostic Research*, vol. 10, no. 4, pp. OD20–OD22, 2016.

[6] L. Graves III, R. M. Klein, and A. D. Walling, "Addisonian Crisis precipitated by thyroxine therapy: a complication of type 2 autoimmune polyglandular syndrome," *Southern Medical Journal*, vol. 96, no. 8, pp. 824–827, 2003.

[7] C. E. Higham, G. Johannsson, and S. M. Shalet, "Hypopituitarism," *The Lancet*, vol. 388, no. 10058, pp. 2403–2415, 2016.

[8] N. Takasu, K. Nakachi, and H. Higa, "Development of Graves' hyperthyroidism caused an adrenal crisis in a patient with previously unrecognized non-classical 21-hydroxylase deficiency," *Internal Medicine*, vol. 49, no. 14, pp. 1395–1400, 2010.

[9] J. H. Kim, G. Park, S. Y. Kim, and H. Y. Bae, "Thyrotoxic periodic paralysis with graves' disease leading to the discovery of a hidden nonclassic 11β hydroxylase deficiency," *Internal Medicine*, vol. 52, no. 1, pp. 85–88, 2013.

2

Growth Hormone Deficiency in a Patient with Becker Muscular Dystrophy: A Pediatric Case Report

Valeria Calcaterra,[1,2] **Annachiara Malvezzi,**[2] **Rossana Toglia,**[2] **Angela Berardinelli,**[3] **Elena Bozzola,**[4] **Mauro Bozzola,**[1,2] **and Daniela Larizza**[1,2]

[1] *Department of Internal Medicine, University of Pavia, 27100 Pavia, Italy*
[2] *Department of Pediatrics, IRCCS Policlinico S. Matteo Foundation, 27100 Pavia, Italy*
[3] *IRCCS C. Mondino Foundation and University of Pavia, 27100 Pavia, Italy*
[4] *Pediatric and Infectious Disease Unit, Department of Pediatrics, Bambino Gesù Children's Hospital, 00165 Rome, Italy*

Correspondence should be addressed to Valeria Calcaterra; v.calcaterra@smatteo.pv.it

Academic Editors: G. Aimaretti, M. A. Boyanov, and H. Ikeda

Objective. To describe a biochemical growth hormone (GH) deficiency and to evaluate therapeutic result in a six-year-old male with Becker muscular dystrophy (BMD). *Methods.* GH peak was evaluated after response to arginine and insulin. Bone age was evaluated according to Greulich and Pyle method. *Results.* The GH-supplementary therapy was very effective in terms of growth gain. *Conclusion.* The possibility of a growth hormone deficiency and treatment with GH in patients with BMD cannot be excluded, especially considering the good therapeutic response.

1. Introduction

Becker muscular dystrophy (BMD) is a condition due to mutations in the gene that expresses the dystrophin protein, located in X chromosome. Dystrophin is present in the muscle cytoskeleton and its failure causes sarcolemma instability and disruption. This seems to be the main factor of myopathy occurring in DMB, resulting in progressive muscle weakness, especially of the upper districts and dilated cardiomyopathy [1, 2].

A gradual slowing down of growth is described in muscular dystrophies, particularly in Duchenne's; however, this does not seem related to growth hormone deficiency [3–6].

We report a case of BMD with GH-deficient short stature who showed a good growth response to recombinant human GH therapy.

2. Case Presentation

D. R. was born at 40 weeks' gestation with a birth weight of 3000 g. At 18 months of age, Becker muscular dystrophy was diagnosed (deletion of exons 45–47 in the locus of dystrophin).

At the age of six yr the patient was referred to our Endocrinology Unit for short stature and delayed bone age in relation to chronological age (bone age according to Greulich and Pyle method: 42 months).

At first evaluation D. R. showed the following: height 99.4 cm (−3.1 SDS) with height genetic target of 165.7 cm (10th centile); weight 17.6 kg (3th–10th centile); BMI 17.9 kg/m^2 (75th–90th centile); pubertal stage 1 according to Tanner [7, 8].

Initial laboratory studies revealed the following: IGF 53 ng/mL (25th percentile for age and gender), normal thyroid function with absence of autoantibodies, negativity of anti-endomisium and anti-tissue tranglutaminase, normal adrenal function. The evaluation of GH secretion showed a partial GH deficiency (GH peak response to arginine: 4.0 ng/mL; GH peak response to insulin: 8.7 ng/mL). After oral glucose test a normal tolerance was found. Magnetic resonance imaging of the hypothalamic-pituitary region was normal.

TABLE 1: Clinical, hormonal, and radiological parameters of the patient during GH therapy.

Parameters	Time of therapy				
	Start	1 year	2 years	3 years	4 years
Age	6 yr and 4 m	7 yr and 7 m	8 yr and 6 m	9 yr and 5 m	10 yr and 5 m
Height					
(cm)	100	108.5	115	122	128.5
(SDS)	−3.66	−3.01	−2.72	−2.34	−2.07
Weight (Kg)	17.5	20.4	22.4	25.8	29.3
BMI					
(kg/m^2)	17.9	17.3	16.9	17.3	17.7
(SDS)	0.62	0.38	−0.03	−0.11	−0.21
Height velocity					
(cm/yr)	Unknown	6.65	7.52	7.22	6.59
(SDS)		1.53	2.56	2.53	2.12
Bone age	42 months	4–6 yr	6 yr	8-9 yr	11 yr
IGF 1					
(ng/dL)	53	68.4	174.0	267.0	221
(centile*)	25th	25th–50th	50th–95th	50th–95th	50th–95th

*Centile for age and sex [7].

At the age of six yr and four months, GH replacement therapy was started at the dose of 0.027 mg/kg/day. The GH-supplementary therapy was very effective in terms of growth gain (Table 1).

At the last evaluation, at the age of 11, the patient showed the following: height 131.4 cm (5th centile; 1.9 SDS); height velocity 1.8 SDS; weight 29.9 kg (25th centile), BMI 17.4 kg/m^2 (25th–50th centile), pubertal stage 2 according to Tanner.

During followup the child maintained stability of the clinical frame (characterized by mild weakness, fatigue, myalgias, and hypertrophy of the calves), neuro- and cardio-respiratory functions, and metabolic parameters.

3. Conclusion

Becker muscular dystrophy is a neuromuscular recessive disease related to X chromosome caused by qualitative and quantitative alterations of the dystrophin. BMD affects about 5/100,000 newborns; however, the high premature mortality explains why the disease has such a low incidence (2.4/100,000) [1, 2]. From a clinical point of view, affected patients present a progressive loss of strength, which is more marked in charge of proximal districts, particularly in the proximal pelvic girdle, and dilated cardiomyopathy, which often plays a decisive role in the evolution of the disease. Clinical evolution shows sural triceps pseudohypertrophy; femoral quadriceps can occur to be both hypo- and hypertrophied. Compared to the Duchenne muscular dystrophy, the BMD hardly presents respiratory compromisation.

In muscular dystrophies, especially in DMD, a peculiar pattern of growth has been described, which is characterized by regular weight and length at birth and a slow progressive statural slowdown in the first years of life [3, 4]. Short stature does not seem to be related to GH deficiency or GH-IGF axis alterations [5]; instead, it might be related to several other factors such as reduced physical activity [4], abnormal response to GH [5], SHOX (short stature homeobox-containing) gene alterations, which is mapped to chromosome Xq22, therefore potentially involved in the anomalies of the nearly region Xq21, which contains the coding gene for the dystrophin [3, 4, 6].

In our report, short stature is related to GH deficiency. GH deficiency may be total or partial, isolated, or associated with other abnormalities of pituitary hormones. In childhood the disease is usually idiopathic but may be secondary to morphological abnormalities, malformations, or brain tumors. Our patient presents a partial GH secretion deficiency, which is not associated with other secretory anomalies and is not secondary to alterations of the hypothalamic-pituitary region. The growth hormone therapy had a beneficial effect in terms of growth gain, with stability of the neuromuscular disease, but we cannot define any specific positive effects on muscle. In the literature, the association between BMD and GH-deficiency has not been previously reported; other studies will help to determine if this association is casual or if in BMD growth hormone secretion and response to treatment are different from Duchenne Muscular Dystrophy.

In conclusion, the possibility of growth hormone deficiency and treatment with GH in patients with BMD cannot be excluded, also considering the beneficial effect of the therapy.

References

[1] K. M. D. Bushby, M. Thambyayah, and D. Gardner-Medwin, "Prevalence and incidence of Becker muscular dystrophy," *The Lancet*, vol. 337, no. 8748, pp. 1022–1024, 1991.

[2] K. M. D. Bushby and D. Gardner-Medwin, "The clinical, genetic and dystrophin characteristics of Becker muscular dystrophy.

I. Natural history," *Journal of Neurology*, vol. 240, no. 2, pp. 98–104, 1993.

[3] U. Eiholzer, E. Boltshauser, D. Frey, L. Molinari, and M. Zachmann, "Short stature: a common feature in Duchenne muscular dystrophy," *European Journal of Pediatrics*, vol. 147, no. 6, pp. 602–605, 1988.

[4] D. Rapaport, G. M. Colletto, M. Vainzof, M. C. Duaik, and M. Zatz, "Short stature in Duchenne muscular dystrophy," *Growth Regulation*, vol. 1, no. 1, pp. 11–15, 1991.

[5] M. Zatz, D. Rapaport, R. C. M. Pavanello, J. M. L. Rocha, M. Vainzof, and W. Nicolau, "Nocturnal rhythm of growth hormone in Duchenne patients: effect of different doses of mazindol and/or cyproheptadine," *American Journal of Medical Genetics*, vol. 33, no. 4, pp. 457–467, 1989.

[6] B. H. P. Nagel, W. Mortier, M. Elmlinger, H. A. Wollmann, K. Schmitt, and M. B. Ranke, "Short stature in Duchenne muscular dystrophy: a study of 34 patients," *Acta Paediatrica*, vol. 88, no. 1, pp. 62–65, 1999.

[7] M. W. Elmlinger, W. Kühnel, M. M. Weber, and M. B. Ranke, "Reference ranges for two automated chemiluminiscent assays for serum insulin-like growth factor I (IGF-1) and IGF-binding protein 3 (IGFBP-3)," *Clinical Chemistry and Laboratory Medicine*, vol. 42, no. 6, pp. 654–664, 2004.

[8] E. Cacciari, S. Milani, A. Balsamo et al., "Italian cross-sectional growth charts for height, weight and BMI (2 to 20 yr)," *Journal of Endocrinological Investigation*, vol. 29, no. 7, pp. 581–593, 2006.

3

Pediatric Cushing's Disease and Pituitary Incidentaloma: Is this a Real Challenge?

Rosa Maria Paragliola, Pietro Locantore, Alfredo Pontecorvi, and Salvatore Maria Corsello

Endocrinology Unit, Catholic University School of Medicine, Largo Gemelli No. 8, 00168 Rome, Italy

Correspondence should be addressed to Salvatore Maria Corsello; corsello.sm@mclink.it

Academic Editor: Michael P. Kane

Cushing's disease (CD) is the most common cause of endogenous Cushing's syndrome in children and adolescents and represents a rare cause of short stature. A 14-year-old boy came to our attention for progressive weight gain and short stature. At examination, height was 140 cm (3rd centile) and weight was 37.7 kg (10th centile). Tanner stage was G2, PH 3, testis 3 mL. Hypothyroidism and growth hormone deficiency were excluded. A marked increase of urinary free cortisol, a nonsuppressible serum cortisol after Liddle 1 test, and an elevated ACTH value confirmed the diagnosis of ACTH dependent Cushing's syndrome. Pituitary magnetic resonance imaging (MRI) showed a left microadenoma and a right focal area of lesser enhancement. Therefore, bilateral inferior petrosal sinus sampling (BIPSS) with CRH stimulation was performed to obtain an accurate preoperative localization of the adenoma: the interpetrosal sinus ACTH gradient indicated lateralization of ACTH secretion to the left side. The patient underwent transsphenoidal surgery with selective microadenomectomy, with an immediate ACTH decline in the postoperative phase. Histology confirmed the diagnosis of corticotrophic pituitary adenoma. Glucocorticoid replacement therapy was instituted. Clinical examination demonstrated a rapid catch-up growth (10th centile), with a normalization of body mass index and an adequate pubertal development.

1. Introduction

Cushing's disease (CD) is the most common cause of endogenous hypercortisolism in children and adolescents and represents a rare cause of short stature. Growth failure and weight gain are frequently observed in subjects with ACTH-dependent hypercortisolism, while in ACTH-independent Cushing's syndrome the secretion of adrenal androgens may lead to an acceleration of bone age and eventually compromise growth potential [1, 2]. The most important factor causing growth failure in pediatric CD is the prolonged overexposure to glucocorticoids, although the decrease in free IGF1 and the resistance to IGF1 and other growth factors can also contribute; moreover, concomitant GH deficiency, both before and after surgery, has been described [3]. Early diagnosis and adequate treatment are important prerequisites to assure a catch-up growth after remission, avoiding compromising the final adult height: however, diagnosis and treatment of pediatric CD often represent a challenge for the clinicians.

2. Case Report

A 14-year-old boy came to our attention for progressive weight gain and short stature. Family history was negative for endocrine diseases, and his final estimated target height was 175 cm (~50th centile).

Birth length (53 cm) and weight (3100 gr) were normal and clinical history was negative for use of glucocorticoids. Patient had regularly played soccer up to 5-6 months before, but he had to stop because of the onset of severe fatigue.

At physical examination, height was 140 cm (3rd centile) and weight was 37.7 kg (10th centile). His weight increased by 5 kg in the last three months. Blood pressure was normal and there were not striae rubrae, acanthosis, facial plethora, hirsutism, and dorsocervical or supraclavicular fat pad. Tanner stage was G2, PH 3, testes 3 mL. Bone age was consistent with chronological age. Routine blood text exams did not show abnormalities and in particular hypokaliemia was not detected. Hypothyroidism and growth hormone deficiency were excluded. There was a marked increase of urinary free cortisol, with a nonsuppressible serum cortisol after low-dose dexamethasone suppression test and detectable ACTH value which confirmed the diagnosis of ACTH-dependent Cushing's syndrome. Hormonal laboratory evaluations are as follows:

FT_3: 3.07 pmol/L (n.v. 3.53–6.45),

FT_4: 12.98 pmol/L (n.v. 11.03–20.12),

TSH: 0.66 μU/mL (n.v. 0.35–2.8),

FSH: 0.5 mU/mL,

LH: 0.1 mU/mL,

testosterone: 0.92 nmol/L,

IGF_1: 74.67 nmol/L (n.v. for age 42–103),

serum cortisol (morning): 872 nmol/L (n.v. 221–607),

ACTH: 21.77 pmol/L (n.v. 2.22–12.22),

urinary free cortisol: 173 μg/die (n.v. 36.5–137),

serum cortisol after low dose dexamethasone suppression test (dexamethasone 0.5 mg every 6 hours for 48 hours): 317.28 nmol/L,

serum cortisol after high dose dexamethasone suppression test (dexamethasone 2 mg every 6 hours for 48 hours): 87.18 nmol/L

(n.v.: normal values).

The MRI of the pituitary gland showed a left microadenoma (9 mm) and another right focal area of lesser enhancement of about 5-6 mm. Therefore, bilateral inferior petrosal sinus sampling (BIPSS) with CRH stimulation was performed to obtain an accurate preoperative localization of the adenoma: the interpetrosal sinus ACTH gradient indicated lateralization of ACTH secretion to the left side (Table 1).

The patient underwent transsphenoidal surgery with selective microadenomectomy, followed by an immediate ACTH and serum cortisol decline (<1.1 pmol/L and 28 nmol/L, resp.) in the postoperative phase. Histology confirmed the diagnosis of "corticotrophic left pituitary microadenoma." Glucocorticoid replacement therapy was instituted and progressively reduced over a 12–14-month period and eventually discontinued. Clinical examination showed a rapid catch-up growth (10th centile), with a normalization of body mass index and an adequate pubertal development (G5, P5, testes 15 mL). Biochemical evaluation did not show any deficiency of pituitary function and, after 5 years of follow-up, the patient can be considered free of disease. At the age of 19 height is 174 cm (~50th centile) according to patient's estimated target height.

3. Discussion

Pediatric Cushing's syndrome (CS), caused by prolonged exposure to excessive exogenous or endogenous glucocorticoids, is a rare condition in childhood and adolescence. The incidence of CS in the general population is about 2–5 cases per million per years, and only in 10% of cases this condition is diagnosed in children or adolescents [4].

The most frequent cause of CS is the iatrogenic administration of supraphysiological doses of glucocorticoids, for example, for the treatment of pulmonary, dermatologic, autoimmune, and neoplastic diseases.

Similar to what is observed in adults [5], the most frequent cause of endogenous CS in children and adolescents is Cushing's disease, which consists in ACTH overproduction from a pituitary adenoma, and represents approximately 75% of all cases of CS in children over 7 years. This condition shows a higher prevalence in males than in females in prepubertal age. Under 7 years, adrenal causes of CS are most frequent (adenoma, carcinoma, bilateral hyperplasia, and McCune Albright syndrome). Ectopic ACTH syndrome or CRH-dependent CS is very rare in children and adolescents [5].

The most common presentation of CS in children is growth retardation and weight increases [6] although patients with virilizing adrenal tumors can present with a growth acceleration induced by androgens [7]. Thus, CS should always be considered in the evaluation of short stature in children. Pubertal disorders may be encountered: younger children may present virilization with pseudoprecocious puberty while older children and adolescents may have delayed puberty as a consequence of glucocorticoid-induced hypogonadism [1]. Bone age in children and adolescent with CS is consistent with the chronological age in 81% of cases, while it is accelerated in 8% and delayed in 11%, correlating with early and delayed sexual development, respectively [1]. Other signs such as moon face, acne, hirsutism, hypertension, and striae rubrae may be seen in about half of patients with inappropriate cortisol overproduction [8]. Moreover, hypercortisolism can cause alterations in body composition with increase in visceral adiposity, increased fasting insulin, and decreased bone mass [9]. An increased risk of infections related to immunosuppression can occur.

The most important clinical feature seen in our patient, as well as growth failure and weight gain, was fatigue that had a sudden onset and led to the impossibility to play sport. However, muscle weakness was not present at physical examination: in fact this sign, which has high specificity in adult patients, may be less common in pediatric and adolescent patients [1]. The investigation protocols used for pediatric CS are the same used in adult practice. An appropriate therapeutic approach depends on an accurate diagnosis of the disease. Detailed medical history and clinical evaluation, including review of growth data, are important to make the initial diagnosis of CS, even if variable clinical presentation with subtle signs and symptoms can make the diagnosis difficult. Moreover, rare cases of human glucocorticoid receptor gene mutation have been described both in germline and somatic state in CD. In these cases, a partial glucocorticoid resistance can lead to the relative absence of characteristic signs and symptoms of cortisol overproduction [10]. Briassoulis et al. recently described a pediatric patient with a pituitary ACTH secreting adenoma confirmed by histology, with little clinical evidence of CD. However, in this case, no mutation in glucocorticoid receptor gene was detected [11].

Since the majority of these pediatric patients come to medical evaluation for height failure, other causes of

Table 1: Bilateral inferior petrosal sinus sampling after CRH stimulation.

	0′	5′	10′	15′	30′	60′
Serum cortisol (nmol/L) (brachial vein)	910	1021	1132	1230	1297	1109
ACTH (pmol/L) (brachial vein)	23	33	55	67	66	53
ACTH (pmol/L) (right petrosal sinus)	22	19	20	24	27	23
ACTH (pmol/L) (left petrosal sinus)	58	124	203	253	220	201

short stature (such as GH deficiency, hypothyroidism, and malabsorption) should be considered and excluded. Upon suspicion of CS, co confirmatory laboratory and imaging tests are necessary. Guidelines for the diagnosis of pediatric CS have been published [12]: the first step is to confirm or rule out the presence of CS and secondly to determine the etiology. A reasonable approach to confirm the inappropriate cortisol secretion is based on urinary free cortisol, midnight serum or salivary cortisol levels, and serum cortisol levels after low dose dexamethasone suppression test. Elevated urinary free cortisol, better if corrected for body surface area [12], should be confirmed on three consecutive 24-hour urinary collections. This test represents the first line investigation and has high sensitivity but low specificity. Midnight serum cortisol greater than 18 ng/mL is considered by some authors [5], the best discriminator in the diagnosis of CS, even if in some cases cortisol nadir is reached earlier than midnight. Late salivary cortisol measurement can have logistical benefits in children [13]. A dexamethasone dosage of 0.5 mg 6 hourly is generally used to perform low dose dexamethasone suppression test in children weighing ≥40 kg, while, in patients <40 kg, a dosage of 30 mcg/kg/day is recommended by guidelines [12]. A serum cortisol below 50 nmol/L after suppression test is considered normal.

In our patient first line tests confirmed an inappropriate cortisol secretion, and the detectable ACTH levels were suggestive for ACTH-dependent CS. While in adult patient a "detectable" ACTH value (>2.22 pmol/L) is suggestive of an ACTH-dependent CS, in children a cut-off value of 6.44 pmol/L has been reported to have a sensitivity of 70% in identifying an ACTH-dependent form of CS [14]. In our case an ACTH value of 21.7 pmol/L was clearly suggestive of an ACTH-dependent CS, thus leading to perform the high-dose dexamethasone suppression test to exclude an ectopic ACTH secretion. This test, performed by administering 2 mg of dexamethasone every 6 hours over a 48-hour period, showed an adequate serum cortisol suppression, hence excluding the clinical suspicion of ectopic ACTH syndrome, which indeed is an extremely rare condition among the pediatric population, in contrast with adults where it accounts for about 15% of ACTH-dependent CS [15]. The vast majority of pediatric CD is caused by ACTH-producing pituitary microadenomas, while macroadenomas are extremely rare [16]. Localization of CD by pituitary MRI represents an important tool for the clinicians and should be performed with high resolution method and always with gadolinium to allow detection of microadenomas (only macroadenoma will be detected without contrast). Following administration of gadolinium, more than 90% of ACTH-secreting tumors appear as hypoenhanced lesions. It should be noted that classic spin echo MRI is able to detect only approximately 50% of pituitary lesions [1]. A greater sensitivity seems to be obtained using a post-contrast spoiled gradient-recalled MRI [17]. In our patient the pituitary MRI showed both left and right lesions of 9 mm and 6 mm, respectively: although the radiological finding of the left lesion was suggestive of an ACTH-secreting adenoma, we still preferred to perform bilateral inferior petrosal sinus sampling (BIPSS) [18]: according to the methodology described in the literature, we measured ACTH at baseline and at 3, 5, and 10 minutes after CRH administration. Patients with an ACTH-secreting pituitary adenoma have at least a 2-to-1 central-to-peripheral gradient at baseline or a 3-to-1 central-to-peripheral gradient after stimulation with CRH. In our patient, there were a clear central-to-peripheral gradient and a left-to-right gradient, confirming the suspicion of a left ACTH-secreting microadenoma, with a concomitant right pituitary "incidentaloma," which can occur in 6% of pediatric population [19]. Some authors report limitations of BPISS in determining the lateralization of ACTH secreting adenoma in pediatric CD, stating that the integration of MRI findings and BPISS cannot predict the location of the tumor more frequently than MRI alone [20]. Moreover, false negative sampling results can occur in presence of a unilateral hypoplastic or plexiform inferior petrosal sinus which results in anomalous venous drainage from the pituitary gland [21]. In our case the patient underwent successfully transsphenoidal surgery which represents the treatment of choice in pediatric CD and which has a similar remission rate as in adults [22]. The pathology report confirmed the diagnosis of pituitary ACTH secreting tumor, and the success of the surgery was established by the reduction in ACTH and serum cortisol levels in the postoperative period and the patient's requirement for hydrocortisone replacement therapy. The patient's pituitary function was periodically monitored to exclude deficiencies of other pituitary hormones. Indeed, during the postsurgical period, a GH hyposecretion induced by supraphysiological glucocorticoid secretion can be observed for at least one year after surgery, with a return to normal GH secretion in about 18 months after successful treatment. There is no agreement about the auxological outcome of children successfully cured: in fact, in the majority of studies the catch-up growth is

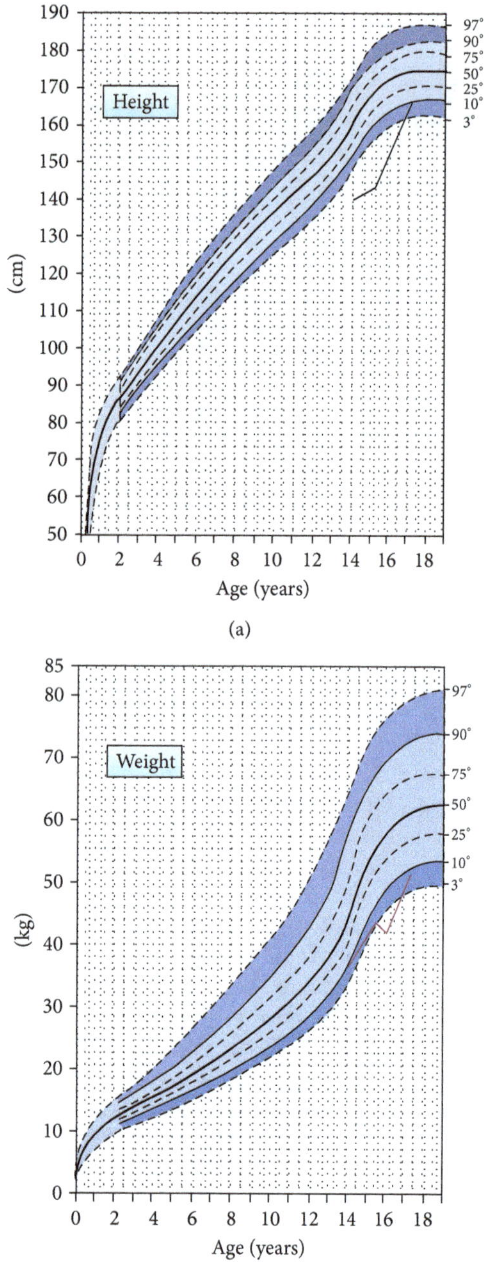

(a)

(b)

FIGURE 1: After the remission of hypercortisolism, a rapid catch-up growth was documented during three years of follow-up. Body mass index normalized and pubertal development was adequate.

not achieved even after an adequate treatment, and the final height remains compromised [23], underscoring the significance of early detection and treatment. On the other hand, other authors have reported that a long-term catch-up growth and a satisfactory final height can be obtained in these patients [24]. In our patient, a rapid catch-up growth was documented after about 3 years of follow-up, with a normalization of body mass index and an adequate pubertal development (Figure 1).

4. Conclusions

We described a rare case of pediatric Cushing's disease, characterized by the association between ACTH-secreting pituitary adenoma and pituitary incidentaloma: one of the most reliable indicators of hypercortisolism in these patients is growth failure associated with weight gain. Laboratory data and pituitary MRI are very important tools to confirm the clinical suspicion. In our case, BIPSS was necessary to lateralize the site of ACTH production, because of the coexistence of an ACTH-secreting microadenoma and a pituitary "incidentaloma." Transsphenoidal surgery led to a successful remission of the hypercortisolism, followed by a dramatic improvement in the patient's auxological parameters.

References

[1] M. A. Magiakou, G. Mastorakos, E. H. Oldfield et al., "Cushing's syndrome in children and adolescents: presentation, diagnosis, and therapy," *The New England Journal of Medicine*, vol. 331, no. 10, pp. 629–636, 1994.

[2] A. B. Hayles, H. B. Hahn Jr., R. G. Sprague, R. C. Bahn, and J. T. Priestley, "Hormone-secreting tumors of the adrenal cortex in children," *Pediatrics*, vol. 37, no. 1, pp. 19–25, 1966.

[3] M. A. Magiakou, G. Mastorakos, M. T. Gomez, S. R. Rose, and G. P. Chrousos, "Suppressed spontaneous and stimulated growth hormone secretion in patients with Cushing's disease before and after surgical cure," *The Journal of Clinical Endocrinology and Metabolism*, vol. 78, no. 1, pp. 131–137, 1994.

[4] C. A. Stratakis, "Cushing syndrome in pediatrics," *Endocrinology & Metabolism Clinics of North America*, vol. 41, no. 4, pp. 793–803, 2012.

[5] L. F. Chan, H. L. Storr, A. B. Grossman, and M. O. Savage, "Pediatric Cushing's syndrome: clinical features, diagnosis, and treatment," *Arquivos Brasileiros de Endocrinologia e Metabologia*, vol. 51, no. 8, pp. 1261–1271, 2007.

[6] A. Weber, P. J. Trainer, A. B. Grossman et al., "Investigation, management and therapeutic outcome in 12 cases of childhood and adolescent Cushing's syndrome," *Clinical Endocrinology*, vol. 43, no. 1, pp. 19–28, 1995.

[7] P. D. K. Lee, R. J. Winter, and O. C. Green, "Virilizing adrenocortical tumors in childhood: eight cases and a review of the literature," *Pediatrics*, vol. 76, no. 3, pp. 437–444, 1985.

[8] M. O. Savage, A. Lienhardt, M.-C. Lebrethon et al., "Cushing's disease in childhood: presentation, investigation, treatment and long-term outcome," *Hormone Research*, vol. 55, supplement 1, pp. 24–30, 2001.

[9] G. M. Leong, V. Abad, E. Charmandari et al., "Effects of child- and adolescent-onset endogenous Cushing syndrome on bone mass, body composition, and growth: a 7-year prospective study into young adulthood," *Journal of Bone and Mineral Research*, vol. 22, no. 1, pp. 110–118, 2007.

[10] G. Briassoulis, S. Damjanovic, P. Xekouki, H. Lefebvre, and C. Stratakis, "The glucocorticoid receptor and its expression in the anterior pituitary and the adrenal cortex: a source of variation in hypothalamic-pituitary-adrenal axis function; Implications for pituitary and andrenal tumors," *Endocrine Practice*, vol. 17, no. 6, pp. 941–948, 2011.

[11] G. Briassoulis, A. Horvath, P. Christoforou et al., "Lack of mutations in the gene coding for the hGR (NR3C1) in a pediatric patient with ACTH-secreting pituitary adenoma, absence of stigmata of Cushing's syndrome and unusual histologic features," *Journal of Pediatric Endocrinology and Metabolism*, vol. 25, no. 1-2, pp. 213–219, 2012.

[12] M. A. Magiakou and G. P. Chrousos, "Cushing's syndrome in children and adolescents: current diagnostic and therapeutic strategies," *The Journal of Endocrinological Investigation*, vol. 25, no. 2, pp. 181–194, 2002.

[13] R. I. Gafni, D. A. Papanicolaou, and L. K. Nieman, "Nighttime salivary cortisol measurement as a simple, noninvasive, outpatient screening test for Cushing's syndrome in children and adolescents," *Journal of Pediatrics*, vol. 137, no. 1, pp. 30–35, 2000.

[14] D. L. Batista, J. Riar, M. Keil, and C. A. Stratakis, "Diagnostic tests for children who are referred for the investigation of Cushing syndrome," *Pediatrics*, vol. 120, no. 3, pp. e575–e586, 2007.

[15] A. M. Isidori, G. A. Kaltsas, C. Pozza et al., "Extensive clinical experience—the ectopic adrenocorticotropin syndrome: Clinical features, diagnosis, management, and long-term follow-up," *The Journal of Clinical Endocrinology & Metabolism*, vol. 91, no. 2, pp. 371–377, 2006.

[16] C. A. Stratakis, D. H. Schussheim, S. M. Freedman et al., "Pituitary macroadenoma in a 5-year-old: an early expression of multiple endocrine neoplasia type 1," *Journal of Clinical Endocrinology and Metabolism*, vol. 85, no. 12, pp. 4776–4780, 2000.

[17] D. Batista, N. A. Courkoutsakis, E. H. Oldfield et al., "Detection of adrenocorticotropin-secreting pituitary adenomas by magnetic resonance imaging in children and adolescents with cushing disease," *Journal of Clinical Endocrinology and Metabolism*, vol. 90, no. 9, pp. 5134–5140, 2005.

[18] H. L. Storr, F. Afshar, M. Matson et al., "Factors influencing cure by transsphenoidal selective adenomectomy in paediatric Cushing's disease," *European Journal of Endocrinology*, vol. 152, no. 6, pp. 825–833, 2005.

[19] T. Tamura, R. Tanaka, K. Korii, and H. Okazaki, "Pediatric pituitary adenoma," *Endocrine Journal*, vol. 47, pp. S95–S99, 2000.

[20] D. Batista, M. Gennari, J. Riar et al., "An assessment of petrosal sinus sampling for localization of pituitary microadenomas in children with cushing disease," *Journal of Clinical Endocrinology and Metabolism*, vol. 91, no. 1, pp. 221–224, 2006.

[21] J. L. Doppman, R. Chang, E. H. Oldfield, G. Chrousos, C. A. Stratakis, and L. K. Nieman, "The hypoplastic inferior petrosal sinus: a potential source of false- negative results in petrosal sampling for Cushing's disease," *Journal of Clinical Endocrinology and Metabolism*, vol. 84, no. 2, pp. 533–540, 1999.

[22] A. Lienhardt, A. B. Grossman, J. E. Dacie et al., "Relative contributions of inferior petrosal sinus sampling and pituitary imaging in the investigation of children and adolescents with ACTH-dependent Cushing's syndrome," *The Journal of Clinical Endocrinology & Metabolism*, vol. 86, no. 12, pp. 5711–5714, 2001.

[23] M. A. Magiakou, G. Mastorakos, and G. P. Chrousos, "Final stature in patients with endogenous Cushing's syndrome," *Journal of Clinical Endocrinology and Metabolism*, vol. 79, no. 4, pp. 1082–1085, 1994.

[24] M.-C. Lebrethon, A. B. Grossman, F. Afshar, P. N. Plowman, G. M. Besser, and M. O. Savage, "Linear growth and final height after treatment for Cushing's disease in childhood," *Journal of Clinical Endocrinology and Metabolism*, vol. 85, no. 9, pp. 3262–3265, 2000.

4

SDHB-Associated Paraganglioma in a Pediatric Patient and Literature Review on Hereditary Pheochromocytoma-Paraganglioma Syndromes

Heather Choat,[1] Kerri Derrevere,[1] Lisa Knight,[2] Whitney Brown,[2] and Elizabeth H. Mack[3]

[1] *Department of Pediatrics, University of South Carolina School of Medicine, Columbia, SC 29203, USA*
[2] *Division of Pediatric Endocrinology, Department of Pediatrics, University of South Carolina School of Medicine, 9 Medical Park Drive, Suite 230A, Columbia, SC 29203, USA*
[3] *Division of Pediatric Critical Care, Palmetto Health Children's Hospital, Columbia, SC 29203, USA*

Correspondence should be addressed to Lisa Knight; lisa.knight@uscmed.sc.edu

Academic Editor: Takeshi Usui

Pheochromocytoma and paraganglioma are rare in the pediatric population occurring in approximately 1 in 50,000 children. While some cases are sporadic, they have commonly been associated with syndromes such as von Hippel-Lindau, multiple endocrine neoplasia types IIa and IIb, neurofibromatosis type 1, and hereditary pheochromocytoma-paraganglioma syndromes. In children less than 18 years of age approximately 60% of pheochromocytomas and paragangliomas are associated with a germline mutation. We present an 11-year-old child with an abdominal paraganglioma related to a succinate dehydrogenase subunit B gene mutation whose father had a previously resected abdominal paraganglioma and was found to carry the same mutation. In addition, we review the etiology, genetics, diagnostic approach, and challenges of preoperative management of secretory pheochromocytomas and paragangliomas in children.

1. Introduction

Pheochromocytomas (PCC) and paragangliomas (PGL) are rare tumors in children. PCC are neuroendocrine tumors located within the adrenal gland that arise from chromaffin cells of neural crest origin and commonly produce one or more catecholamines. PGL comprise an extra-adrenal subset of PCC arising from either sympathetic or parasympathetic paraganglia [1–3]. Approximately 10–20% of all PCC/PGL are diagnosed in children with an average age at diagnosis of 11 years [4, 5]. It has been reported that over half of all PCC and PGL in patients <18 years old are associated with a germline mutation and that this percentage seems to increase with decreasing age at diagnosis [6]. They have been commonly associated with heritable conditions such as multiple endocrine neoplasia (MEN) types IIa and IIb, von Hippel-Lindau, and hereditary PCC/PGL syndromes [1–6]. In general, PGL located in the head and neck are more often parasympathetic and nonsecretory whereas PGL within the abdomen are more likely to be sympathetic and are associated with catecholamine secretion [1, 2].

2. Case Report

A previously healthy 11-year-old Caucasian male presented with a chief complaint of periumbilical abdominal pain for one day. He had multiple episodes of nonbloody, nonbilious emesis and decreased oral intake for one day prior to presentation, but no associated fever or diarrhea. Notably he had a two-month history of headaches upon awakening occurring two to three times per week. On presentation, his heart rate was 136 beats per minute and his blood pressure was 160/120 mmHg. An abdominal computed tomography (CT) scan revealed a 3 cm by 2.3 cm retroperitoneal mass between the inferior vena cava and aorta (Figure 1). He was transferred to the pediatric intensive care unit (PICU) for further management of the retroperitoneal mass and hypertensive crisis.

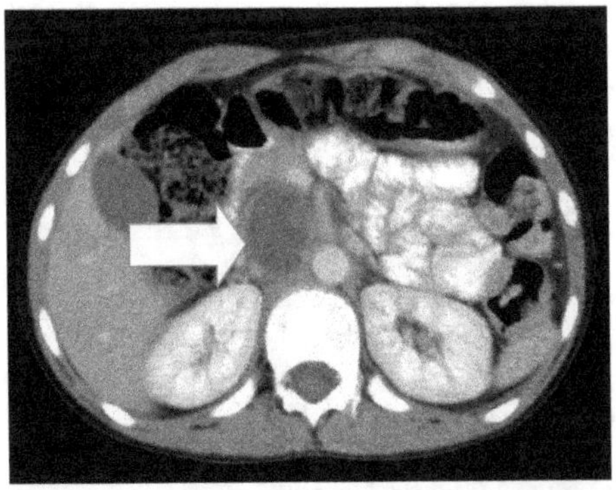

(a)

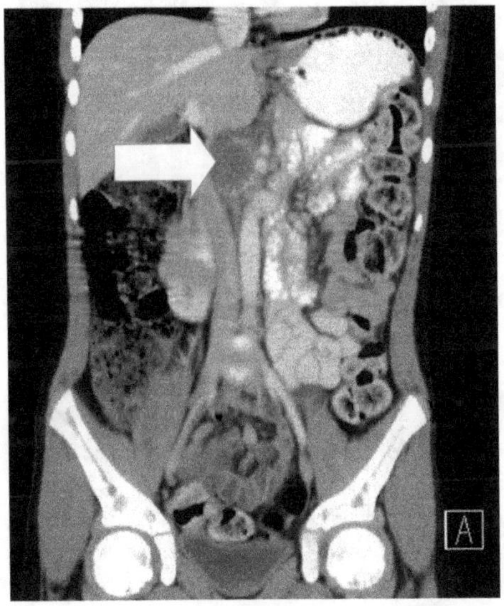

(b)

Figure 1: Axial (a) and coronal (b) images of the 3 × 2.3 cm retroperitoneal mass between aorta and inferior vena cava.

On exam he was nontoxic and no flushing of the skin was present. His abdomen was soft with normal bowel sounds and without palpable masses, guarding, or rebound tenderness. Further questioning revealed that the patient's father underwent resection of abdominal PGL requiring preoperative antihypertensive therapy and postoperative radiation at the age of 24 years. The PGL was found incidentally on imaging performed after a motor vehicle collision. After the patient's diagnosis, further history revealed that the paternal grandfather and a maternal cousin were also diagnosed with PCC. Diagnostic evaluation showed polycythemia with hemoglobin of 17 g/dL, normal echocardiogram, normal electrolytes, and normal renal function.

In the PICU, the patient's hypertension was initially treated with isradipine but was still associated with intermittent tachycardia. Vanillylmandelic acid (VMA) and plasma normetanephrine levels returned elevated, indicating a neuroendocrine secretory tumor. On the third day α-adrenergic blockade was initiated with phenoxybenzamine 0.2 mg/kg/dose orally twice daily. Forty-eight hours later he was started on β-blockade with propranolol 0.15 mg/kg/dose orally twice daily.

Despite gradual increases in α- and β-blockade with phenoxybenzamine, atenolol, and propranolol, he ultimately required an esmolol infusion to maintain the heart rate less than 100 beats per minute. In order to reduce the likelihood of intraoperative and postoperative morbidity, phenoxybenzamine was discontinued 48 hours prior to surgery, and β-blockade was stopped 8 hours prior to surgery. He received α- and β-blockade for 23 days prior to resection.

Laboratory evaluation revealed elevations in the following: plasma normetanephrine 1.72 nmol/L (normal 0–0.89), urine normetanephrine 799 μmol/mol creatinine (normal 0–278), and VMA 15.1 mg/g creatinine (normal < 8.6). Due to the location of the retroperitoneal mass, the patient was not a candidate for laparoscopic approach for its removal. The mass was resected on hospital day 23, and the procedure was uncomplicated (Figure 2). Pathology confirmed the diagnosis of paraganglioma. Following resection, the patient remained normotensive and was discharged home four days postoperatively off all antihypertensive medications. After discharge, a serum genetic panel returned positive for a heterozygous deleterious mutation in the succinate dehydrogenase complex subunit B (SDHB) gene. This gene, located at 1p.36.1-1p.35, was PCR amplified and then sequenced in the forward and reverse directions using automated fluorescent dideoxy sequencing methods. The patient's specific mutation was the splice site-altering change c.541-2A>G located in intron 5 of the gene (Figure 3).

In the pediatric endocrinology clinic two weeks after discharge, the patient was asymptomatic and normotensive. Repeat plasma normetanephrine at that time was decreased but still mildly elevated at 1.15 nmol/L (normal 0–0.89). His family was referred for genetic counseling at this time. The patient's father was found to carry the same genetic mutation, and his younger brother's genetic panel returned normal. Incidentally, a female maternal cousin had previously been found to have a PCC, but she neither did undergo genetic testing nor did the paternal grandfather (Figure 4). One month postoperatively, the patient was seen for follow-up at the National Institutes of Health (NIH) where he had a CT of the neck, chest, abdomen, and pelvis which showed no evidence of residual or metastatic disease. Also, at that time, laboratory assessment showed normal catecholamine levels including urine epinephrine, urine norepinephrine, urine dopamine, urine metanephrines, urine normetanephrines, and total urine metanephrines.

Five months postoperatively, the patient was seen again in the pediatric endocrinology clinic and continued to be asymptomatic and normotensive. Eight months postoperatively at the NIH, magnetic resonance imaging (MRI) of the neck, chest, abdomen, and pelvis showed no evidence of PGL. Laboratory assessment including 24-hour urine epinephrine, norepinephrine, dopamine, metanephrine, normetanephrine, total metanephrines, plasma epinephrine, norepinephrine, and dopamine levels was all within normal range. Thyroid studies at that time were also normal.

Twenty months postoperatively, he was again seen at the NIH and had an unremarkable physical exam and was asymptomatic and normotensive. Repeat MRI of the neck,

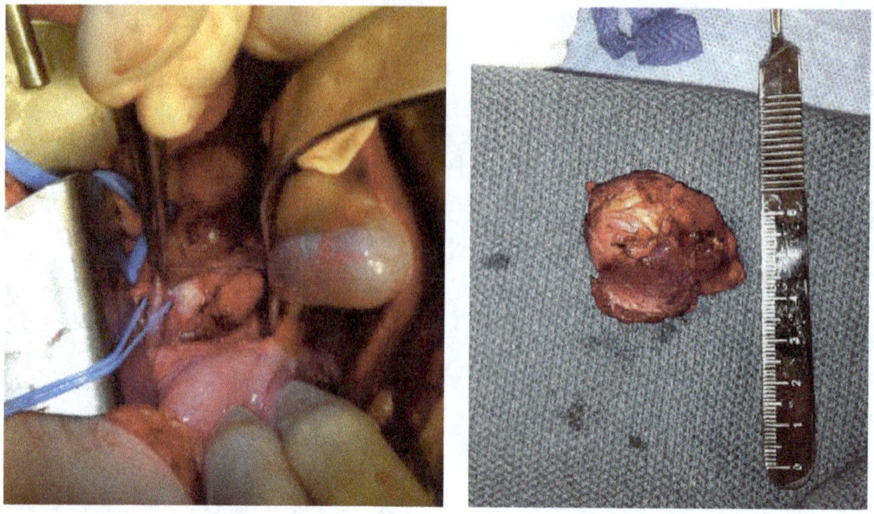

(a) (b)

FIGURE 2: Intraoperative (a) and postoperative (b) views of the retroperitoneal mass.

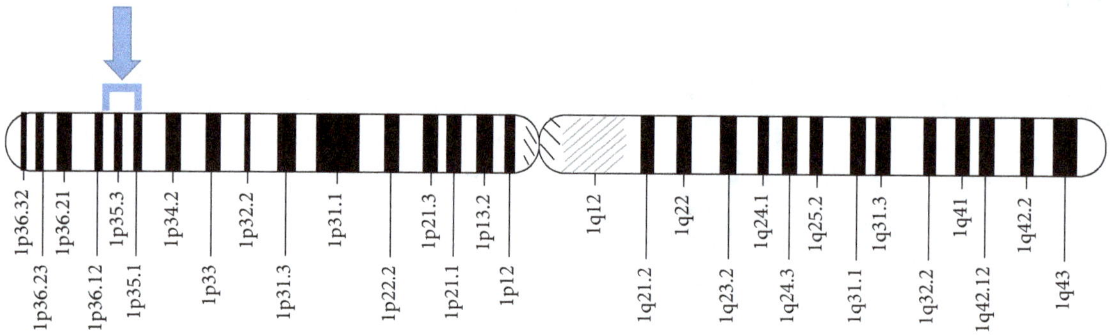

(a) SDH-B cytogenetic location: 1p36.1-p35

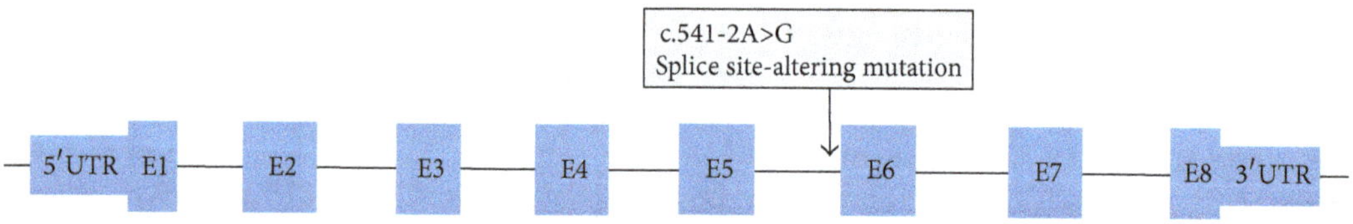

(b) SDH-B germline mutation

FIGURE 3: Chromosomal location of the SDHB gene (a) and site of the patient's specific mutation (b).

chest, abdomen, and pelvis showed no evidence of local or metastatic tumor recurrence. Plasma and urine catecholamines and chromogranin A were again found to be in normal ranges. He is now being followed on an annual basis.

3. Discussion

Our patient presented with many of the typical signs and symptoms of PCC/PGL, most notably with new onset secondary hypertension. With the high incidence of childhood overweight and obesity in the United States (occurring in about 30% of children) the leading cause of pediatric hypertension continues to be essential hypertension, whereas PCC/PGL account for only about 1% of cases [7]. Causes of secondary hypertension in the pediatric population are more commonly associated with certain medications, renal disease, renovascular disease, Cushing syndrome, or hyperthyroidism. However, as our case clearly demonstrates, rare causes including PCC or PGL should always be considered in the setting of secondary hypertension [2, 4, 6].

Diagnostic evaluation for PCC/PGL begins with biochemical evaluation followed by anatomic imaging, with functional imaging if metastatic disease is present, and surgical pathology (Table 1). The tests of choice for biochemical evaluation are plasma free metanephrines and/or fractionated urine metanephrines and normetanephrines, which have a sensitivity approaching 100% for diagnosis of a catecholamine-secreting tumor [1, 8–11]. Chromogranin A

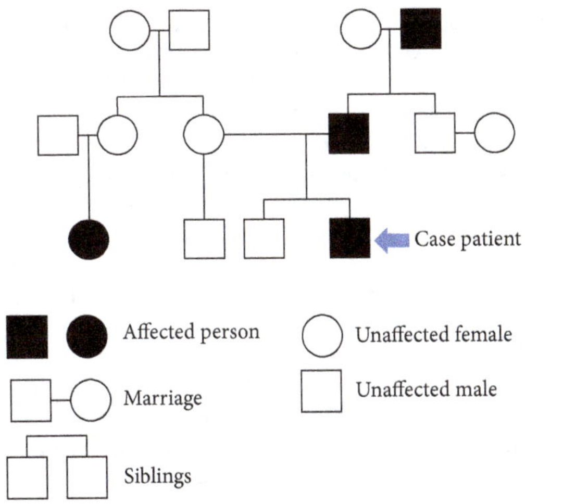

FIGURE 4: Family pedigree of individuals affected with PCC/PGL.

TABLE 1: Work-up of suspected PCC/PGL.

Biochemical testing
Fractionated urine metanephrines
Fractionated plasma free metanephrines
Chromogranin A
Anatomic imaging
Ultrasound (children)
CT
MRI
Functional imaging
^{18}F-Fluorodihydroxyphenylalanine PET
^{18}F-Fluorodopamine PET
^{123}I-MIBG single-positron emission CT

is another biochemical marker that correlates with tumor size, malignant potential, and is a marker for the rare SDHB-related PGL [1, 12]. In addition, patients may have hyperglycemia, increased erythrocyte sedimentation rate, polycythemia, and leukocytosis on preliminary screening. Initial anatomic imaging should include CT of the abdomen and pelvis and then CT of the neck and chest if initial imaging is negative [1, 8]. CT is recommended as the first-choice imaging modality rather than MRI except in cases of known metastatic disease, for detection of skull base and neck PGL, in patients with surgical clips causing image artifact when using CT, in CT contrast-allergic patients, and in patients in whom radiation exposure should be limited such as children, pregnant women, patients with known germline mutations, and those with excessive radiation exposure [13]. For metastatic disease or patients in whom catecholamines are borderline elevated, functional imaging can provide additional diagnostic clarification. Previously, nuclear scintigraphy imaging with ^{123}I-labeled metaiodobenzyl-guanidine (MIBG) was common but has been proven to be less sensitive than newer modalities such as ^{18}F-fluorodihydroxyphenylalanine or ^{18}F-fluorodopamine positron emission tomography (PET) particularly in PGL and metastatic disease [14]. In cases of PCC and PGL, malignancy refers to metastases in locations where paraganglia are not usually found such as bone, lung, and liver.

Definitive treatment of secretory PCC/PGL is surgical resection; however, preoperative medical management of hypertension is equally important to ensure good clinical outcomes. The mainstay of therapy is to first initiate nonselective α-adrenergic blockade with phenoxybenzamine. Once α-blockade has been accomplished, β-blockade is initiated with either a nonselective or a β1-selective blocker such as propranolol or metoprolol, respectively. β-Blockade should not be used initially or as a single agent due to resultant reflex tachycardia and worsening hypertension from unopposed α-adrenergic activation. Treatment should be initiated 1-2 weeks prior to resection to avoid complications from intraoperative catecholamine surges [5, 15, 16]. Also, 1-2 days preoperatively, α-blockade should be stopped and patients may be salt-loaded to avoid postoperative hypotension. Surgical resection is most commonly achieved laparoscopically, but with large tumors or concern for malignancy a laparotomy may be performed [1, 17, 18].

Although some cases of pediatric PCC/PGL are sporadic, it has been reported that 59% of those occurring in children <18 years old and up to 70% of those occurring in children <10 years old are associated with a germline mutation [6]. Syndromes commonly linked to PCC/PGL are von Hippel-Lindau, neurofibromatosis type I, MEN IIa and IIb, and hereditary PCC/PGL syndromes. In the case of our patient and his father, genetic testing revealed the same deleterious mutation in SDHB, reinforcing the diagnosis of a familial paraganglioma syndrome. This particular mutation is not novel, and it is one of over 100 SDH gene mutations which have been reported [19]. The SDH enzyme complex is made up of several subunits (SDHA, SDHB, SDHC, SDHD, and SDH assembly factor 2) and is integral in linking the tricarboxylic acid (TCA) cycle to the process of oxidative phosphorylation within mitochondria. Specifically, SDHB is a known tumor suppressor gene which functions to prevent the accumulation of toxic metabolites during the TCA cycle. While SDH subunit gene mutations have been shown to be associated with neoplasia and cause susceptibility to familial PCC/PGL syndromes, an exact causal mechanism is still unclear [20]. It is widely proposed, however, that the affected subunit determines the phenotype [3].

Hereditary PCC/PGL syndromes have an autosomal dominant mode of inheritance, and approximately 40% of patients with SDHB mutations may go on to develop malignant disease [13, 15, 20]. Overall SDHB mutations are associated with a higher malignancy rate than mutations in the SDHD or SDHC genes and in fact account for 50% or more of malignant PCC and PGL [1]. SDHB mutations usually correlate with disease in the thorax, abdomen, or pelvis while SDHD mutations often manifest as head or neck tumors that are typically benign [6, 12, 17]. A task force selected by the Endocrine Society recently released new practice guidelines recommending that all patients with PCC or PGL be engaged in a shared decision-making process regarding genetic testing [13]. Routine genetic counseling and testing are recommended, however, after the diagnosis of PGL in a child regardless of family history particularly since certain mutations can indicate multisite disease or higher probability of malignancy [17, 21]. Metastatic disease carries a poorer prognosis; 5-year survival probability decreases from 89% in nonmalignant cases to 20–70% in malignant cases depending on location [3]. Therefore, it is important to accurately distinguish between benign and metastatic diseases at the time of diagnosis to ensure sufficient follow-up and treatment. It is currently recommended that mutation-carrying patients who are tumor-free be followed on an annual basis [13]. While a TCA cycle gene mutation database has been created, data are lacking to determine accurate recurrence risk for hereditary PCC and PGL, particularly those diagnosed in children. Research focused in this area is needed to further guide follow-up recommendations and optimize long-term outcomes in the future.

Consent

Written informed consent was obtained from the patient's parent for publication of this case report and any accompanying images. A copy of the consent is available for review by the editor.

References

[1] S. G. Waguespack, T. Rich, E. Grubbs et al., "A current review of the etiology, diagnosis, and treatment of pediatric pheochromocytoma and paraganglioma," *Journal of Clinical Endocrinology and Metabolism*, vol. 95, no. 5, pp. 2023–2037, 2010.

[2] R. A. DeLellis, R. V. Lloyd, P. U. Heitz, and C. Eng, *Pathology and Genetics of Tumours of Endocrine Organs*, IARC Press, Lyon, France, 2004.

[3] A. J. Lowery, S. Walsh, E. W. McDermott, and R. S. Prichard, "Molecular and therapeutic advances in the diagnosis and management of malignant pheochromocytomas and paragangliomas," *Oncologist*, vol. 18, no. 4, pp. 391–407, 2013.

[4] M. Barontini, G. Levin, and G. Sanso, "Characteristics of pheochromocytoma in a 4- to 20-year-old population," *Annals of the New York Academy of Sciences*, vol. 1073, pp. 30–37, 2006.

[5] R. Armstrong, M. Sridhar, K. L. Greenhalgh et al., "Phaeochromocytoma in children," *Archives of Disease in Childhood*, vol. 93, no. 10, pp. 899–904, 2008.

[6] H. P. H. Neumann, B. Bausch, S. R. McWhinney et al., "Germline mutations in nonsyndromic pheochromocytoma," *The New England Journal of Medicine*, vol. 346, no. 19, pp. 1459–1466, 2002.

[7] T. Wyszynska, E. Cichocka, A. Wieteska-Klimczak, K. Jobs, and P. Januszewicz, "A single pediatric center experience with 1025 children with hypertension," *Acta Paediatrica*, vol. 81, no. 3, pp. 244–246, 1992.

[8] I. Ilias and K. Pacak, "Current approaches and recommended algorithm for the diagnostic localization of pheochromocytoma," *Journal of Clinical Endocrinology and Metabolism*, vol. 89, no. 2, pp. 479–491, 2004.

[9] M. Weise, D. P. Merke, K. Pacak, M. M. Walther, and G. Eisenhofer, "Utility of plasma free metanephrines for detecting childhood pheochromocytoma," *Journal of Clinical Endocrinology and Metabolism*, vol. 87, no. 5, pp. 1955–1960, 2002.

[10] J. W. M. Lenders, H. R. Keiser, D. S. Goldstein et al., "Plasma metanephrines in the diagnosis of pheochromocytoma," *Annals of Internal Medicine*, vol. 123, no. 2, pp. 101–109, 1995.

[11] G. Eisenhofer, J. W. M. Lenders, H. Timmers et al., "Measurements of plasma methoxytyramine, normetanephrine, and metanephrine as discriminators of different hereditary forms of pheochromocytoma," *Clinical Chemistry*, vol. 57, no. 3, pp. 411–420, 2011.

[12] A. Szalat, M. Fraenkel, V. Doviner, A. Salmon, and D. J. Gross, "Malignant pheochromocytoma: predictive factors of malignancy and clinical course in 16 patients at a single tertiary medical center," *Endocrine*, vol. 39, no. 2, pp. 160–166, 2011.

[13] J. W. M. Lenders, Q.-Y. Duh, G. Eisenhofer et al., "Pheochromocytoma and paraganglioma : an endocrine society clinical practice guideline," *Journal of Clinical Endocrinology and Metabolism*, vol. 99, no. 6, pp. 1915–1942, 2014.

[14] F. Imani, V. G. Agopian, M. S. Auerbach et al., "^{18}F-FDOPA PET and PET/CT accurately localize pheochromocytomas," *Journal of Nuclear Medicine*, vol. 50, no. 4, pp. 513–519, 2009.

[15] T. H. Pham, C. Moir, G. B. Thompson et al., "Pheochromocytoma and paraganglioma in children: a review of medical and surgical management at a tertiary care center," *Pediatrics*, vol. 118, no. 3, pp. 1109–1117, 2006.

[16] K. Pacak, "Approach to the patient: Preoperative management of the pheochromocytoma patient," *Journal of Clinical Endocrinology and Metabolism*, vol. 92, no. 11, pp. 4069–4079, 2007.

[17] S. D. Peter, P. A. Valusek, S. Hill et al., "Laparoscopic adrenalectomy in children: a multicenter experience," *Journal of Laparoendoscopic & Advanced Surgical Techniques A*, vol. 21, no. 7, pp. 647–649, 2011.

[18] Y. Heloury, M. Muthucumaru, G. Panabokke, W. Cheng, C. Kimber, and M. D. Leclair, "Minimally invasive adrenalectomy in children," *Journal of Pediatric Surgery*, vol. 47, no. 2, pp. 415–421, 2012.

[19] N. Burnichon, V. Rohmer, L. Amar et al., "The succinate dehydrogenase genetic testing in a large prospective series of patients with paragangliomas," *Journal of Clinical Endocrinology and Metabolism*, vol. 94, no. 8, pp. 2817–2827, 2009.

[20] D. Astuti, F. Latif, A. Dallol et al., "Gene mutations in the succinate dehydrogenase subunit SDHB cause susceptibility to familial pheochromocytoma and to familial paraganglioma," *The American Journal of Human Genetics*, vol. 69, no. 1, pp. 49–54, 2001.

[21] M. Iacobone, F. Schiavi, M. Bottussi et al., "Is genetic screening indicated in apparently sporadic pheochromocytomas and paragangliomas?" *Surgery*, vol. 150, no. 6, pp. 1194–1201, 2011.

5

Moyamoya Disease with Coexistent Hypertriglyceridemia in Pediatric Patient

Jacqueline Chan, Fabiola D'Ambrosio Rodriguez, Deepank Sahni, and Claudia Boucher-Berry

Department of Pediatric, Children's Hospital of the University of Illinois, Chicago, IL, USA

Correspondence should be addressed to Jacqueline Chan; jtchan@uic.edu

Academic Editor: Osamu Isozaki

Moyamoya disease is a rare chronic and progressive cerebrovascular disease of the arteries of the circle of Willis that can affect children and adults. It has been associated with multiple diseases, including immunologic, like Graves' disease, diabetes mellitus, and SLE. Hyperlipidemia has been recognized in patients with Moyamoya disease with an incidence of 27–37%. However, no case in pediatric patients has been reported of the coexistence of Moyamoya disease and hyperlipidemia. Here we present a case of a 9-year-old female diagnosed with Moyamoya disease after a stroke with incidental finding of familial hypercholesterolemia. This finding will make our patient a very unique case, since there has not been any reporting of Moyamoya disease and hypercholesterolemia association.

1. Introduction

Moyamoya disease (MMD) is a rare idiopathic chronic and progressive steno-occlusion of bilateral intracranial arteries of the circle of Willis that develop in children and adults. It is characterized by collateral vessels seen on cerebral angiography. An immunologic basis has been suggested for this disease and recent reports have noted an association between Moyamoya and autoimmune diseases including Graves' disease, diabetes mellitus, and Systemic Lupus Erythematosus. Analysis of the comorbidities may be helpful in determining the pathogenesis of Moyamoya [1]. Usual age of onset of MMD in pediatric is after 5 years and progresses more rapidly than in adults [2].

MMD is mainly found in East Asia, especially in Japan and South Korea [3–6]. Because MMD is extremely uncommon in the western countries, no systemic surveys have been conducted in either Europe or North America although there have been some sporadic reports [7, 8].

Familial combined hyperlipidemia (FCHL) is a dominantly inherited hyperlipidemia that occurs in at least 1% of the adult population and is responsible for 10% of premature coronary artery disease. Several metabolic defects apparently are associated with the FCHL phenotype. Most commonly, excess production of very low density lipoprotein apolipoprotein B can be demonstrated [1, 9].

Hyperlipidemia has been recognized in patients with Moyamoya disease with an incidence of 27.7% in a study done in Mayo Clinic Minnesota 1979–2011 and 37.3% in a study done in Japan 2001–2011 [1, 10]. However, no study has been documented in a pediatric patient with abnormal lipid profile with concurrent Moyamoya disease. We report a case of a 9-year-old female with Moyamoya disease and coexistent hyperlipidemia.

2. Case Presentation

Patient is a 9-year-old previously healthy Caucasian female. She was adopted at 3 weeks of age and the family history is unknown. She has a past medical history of gross motor delay, followed closely by Neurology and Physical Therapy and was well by 3 years of age. The patient presented to the Emergency Department with an acute onset of right arm weakness, described as inability to move her arm and write. No history of recent trauma or illness. On arrival to the Emergency Department, vital signs obtained were BP 113/67, pulse 106, and temp. 36.7. Her weight was 26 kg (20% ile), height was 122 cm (3% cile), and BMI was 17 (70% ile).

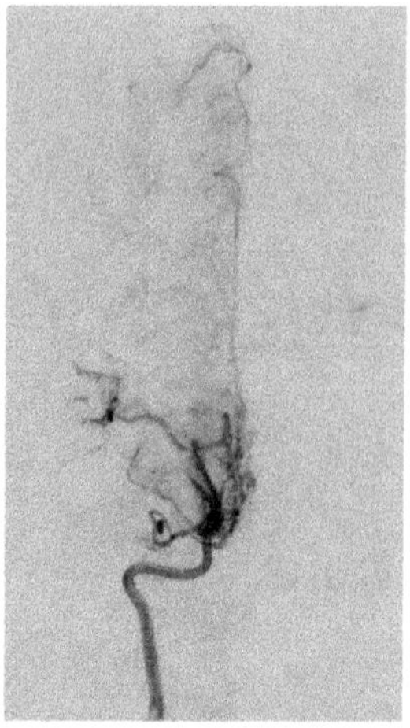

FIGURE 1: Right internal cerebral artery in cerebral angiogram.

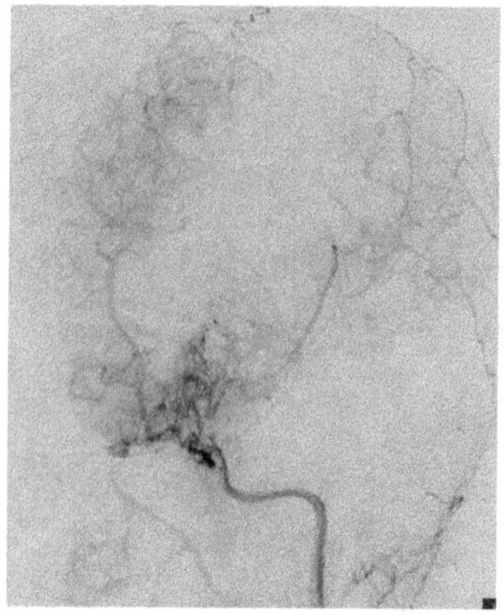

FIGURE 2: Left internal cerebral artery in cerebral angiogram.

Physical exam is only significant for right arm motor weakness 3/5. No sensory deficit was noted. MRI done for stroke protocol revealed small occlusion of the distal internal carotid arteries and numerous small collateral vessels projecting from the circle of Willis region, and MRA was consistent with Moyamoya disease. Six-vessel angiogram confirmed the diagnosis with bilateral internal carotid arteries occlusion as shown in Figures 1 and 2. Baseline fasting lipid profile was abnormal: elevated fasting triglyceride (870 mg/dL, $n <$ 150 mg/dL), elevated total cholesterol (427 mg/dL, $n <$ 200 mg/dL), normal HDL 48 mg/dL, and LDL not measurable due to elevated triglycerides. Apolipoprotein B was elevated at 219 mg/dL (55 mg/dL–125 mg/dL). Thyroid function test was done and revealed slightly elevated TSH of 5.7 mcIU/mL (n 0.35 mcIU/mL–4.0 mcIU/mL) which was not considered clinically significant. She was placed on a pediatric low fat/low cholesterol diet based on nutrition recommendation. She was started on Pravastatin 20 mg daily. Seven days after initial presentation, she developed slurring of speech. MRI demonstrated new acute ischemic infarct involving the left frontal lobe, in the vascular territory of the anterior left middle cerebral artery. Prompt evaluation and revascularization were scheduled. Total cholesterol and triglyceride level decreased to 267 mg/dL and 433 mg/dL, respectively, after fourteen days of Pravastatin therapy, as demonstrated in Figure 3. Patient underwent bilateral superficial temporal artery-middle cerebral artery bypass (STA-MCA) with no complications.

3. Discussion

Moyamoya disease is an uncommon cerebrovascular disease characterized by progressive steno-occlusive changes in the terminal internal carotid arteries (ICA) and their main branches. A bimodal age distribution has been reported for Moyamoya, with a high peak at 5 years and at 40 years [3, 10, 11]. The clinical features of Moyamoya disease differ between children and adults. Moyamoya disease often presents in children initially as a stroke often accompanied by muscular weakness. This is in contrast to adults who typically present with subarachnoid or intraparenchymal hemorrhage [11, 12]. The predominance of ischemic events in childhood, but hemorrhagic strokes in adulthood, has been noted in Taiwanese with MMD [13] Diagnosis is usually possible with a magnetic resonance imaging (MRI) scan to look at the brain and a magnetic resonance angiogram (MRA) to look at the blood vessels of the brain. Although a genetic role has been postulated particularly due to higher incidence of Moyamoya and familial Moyamoya among Asians and Asian-Americans, the pathogenesis underlying this condition among other ethnicities and within North American populations is still unclear. Immunologic basis has been a study of interest due to association of Moyamoya with autoimmune diseases such as Graves' disease and Systemic Lupus Erythematous (SLE). Atherosclerosis and thyroid disease are the most frequent concurrent diseases with MMD especially on the adult population [1, 10].

Long-term prognosis for patients with nonsurgically treated MMD is not fully understood. However, some reports have described its natural clinical course and the results of conservative treatment. Kuroda et al. [14] reported a disease progression rate of approximately 20% over 6 years. Being female was identified as an independent risk factor for disease progression by multivariate analysis. Other investigations on the progression rate of the unaffected side of surgically treated unilateral MMD reported that six of the 41 cases (14.6%) exhibited contralateral progression during the mean follow-up of 34 months [15]. Considering these reports, MMD seems to have a progressive nature. Among many studies examining risk factors for MMD progression, the presence of thyroid disease such as Graves' disease has been a well-known medical condition linked to rapid progression of MMD [16, 17]. Recently, the RNF213 variant was suggested as a possible causative genetic alteration leading to the development as well as progression of MMD [18]. Because surgical revascularization has been recommended for symptomatic patients with impaired hemodynamics, some studies have described the outcomes of conservative treatment among asymptomatic or hemodynamically stable patients with MMD. A multicenter, nationwide survey for conservative treatment results was conducted in 2007 in Japan. The authors reported the annual

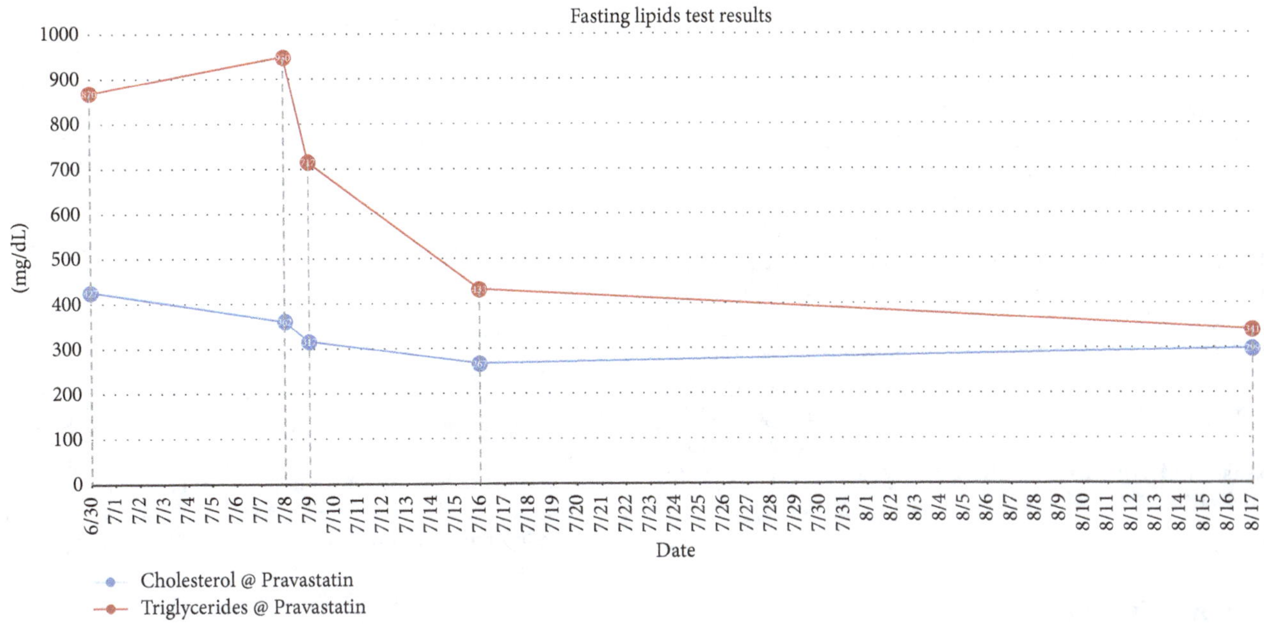

FIGURE 3: Graph showing decrease in cholesterol and triglycerides with Pravastatin treatment.

stroke rate as 3.2% from the observation of 34 asymptomatic patients conservatively followed over 44 months. Hemodynamic disturbance was revealed to be a risk factor for newly developed stroke [19]. In a North American series, the rates of annual ischemic and hemorrhagic stroke rate were reported as 13.3% and 1.7%, respectively. Being female and smoking were risk factors for stroke development [20]. Cho et al. reported an annual stroke rate of 4.5% among 241 hemodynamically stable patients with MMD over 83 months. The annual stroke rate was higher in the hemorrhagic presentation group (5.7%) than the ischemic presentation group (4.2%) or the asymptomatic group (3.4%). They found familial disease and thyroid disease to be risk factors affecting stroke occurrence [21]. As for ischemic presenting MMD, 5.6% of the annual ischemic stroke rate also reported that posterior circulation involvement was a strong risk factor for ischemic stroke [22]. Antiplatelet treatment for preventing stroke in patients with MMD had been utilized by many physicians, especially in non-Asian areas. According to the reports of a worldwide survey, 31% of responders agreed to use long-term acetylsalicylic acid [23]. However, the evidence for antiplatelet treatment is lacking. Recently, the efficacy of antiplatelet therapy for preventing stroke was investigated in a cohort study with a large sample size. According to the authors, antiplatelet therapy could not prevent recurrent cerebral infarction for ischemic presenting patients with MMD. The nature of the ischemic insult in patients with MMD is not an embolic infarction, but instead it is mainly a hemodynamic infarction. The pathologic changes of the MMD vessels near the ICA bifurcation are not a type of endothelial damage, which is prone to platelet adhesion. Therefore, theoretically, antiplatelet drugs will not be effective for preventing ischemic stroke in patients with MMD. Although antiplatelet users are subject to hemorrhagic complications, the therapy was not associated with an increase in cerebral hemorrhage among patients with MMD [24]. Thus, prescribing antiplatelet agents for symptomatic patients with MMD should not yet be considered as an alternative treatment.

Pathologic analysis has demonstrated that affected vessels generally do not exhibit arteriosclerotic or inflammatory changes, even though there may be minimal lipid deposition seen in the intima with fibrous thickening [25, 26]. Rather, vessel occlusion results from a combination of both hyperplasia of smooth muscle cells and luminal thrombosis [10]. The Moyamoya collaterals are dilated perforating arteries believed to be a combination of preexisting and newly developed vessels [26, 27]. A number of growth factors, enzymes, and other peptides have been reported in association with Moyamoya, including basic fibroblast growth factor, transforming growth factor-β1, hepatocyte growth factor, vascular endothelial growth factor, matrix metalloproteinases, intracellular adhesion molecules, and hypoxia-inducing factor-1α, among others [27–34].

In children with primary hyperlipidemia, familial combined hyperlipidemia (FCHL) is expressed three times more commonly than familial hypercholesterolemia and half of the siblings are affected. In our patient, family history is not available. However, FCHL can be defined as elevated fasting cholesterol and triglycerides, with Apo B level of >120 mg/dL, which is consistent with the level seen in our patient. Prognosis includes development of cerebrovascular disease and insulin resistance leading to type 2 diabetes, which itself is a risk factor for atherosclerosis. Long-term prognosis of FCHL in a pediatric patient is not yet well understood as limited pediatric patients with FCHL have been followed through adulthood. Mainstay of treatment of any form of hypertriglyceridemia includes risk-factor control and diet. Children older than 2 years are usually managed with weight control and step-one diet, that is, less than or equal to 30% of total calories being fat [35]. One of the leading comorbidities documented in patients with Moyamoya is hyperlipidemia. However, no study has been reported regarding incidence of Moyamoya coexistent with hypertriglyceridemia on a pediatric patient. Recent case reports and meta-analysis involving patients with Moyamoya and concurrent hyperlipidemia all included patients over 30 years of age. These patients were not diagnosed to have familial hypercholesterolemia (FHC) nor familial combined hyperlipidemia (FCHL). Reasons for elevated cholesterol levels were not clear and were sometimes attributed to other occlusive vascular diseases, as well as untreated hypothyroidism, which is uncommon in the pediatric age group. Our patient by far is the first pediatric patient to have Moyamoya disease and concurrent FCHL, being well managed with Pravastatin.

Acknowledgments

The authors acknowledge the Research Open Access Publishing (ROAAP) Fund of the University of Illinois at Chicago for financial support towards the open access publishing fee for this article.

References

[1] N. E. El Tecle, T. Y. El Ahmadieh, A. M. Bohnen, A. D. Nanney, and B. R. Bendok, "Are hyperlipidemia and autoimmune diseases synergistic in moyamoya disease pathophysiology? Insight from the midwest," *World Neurosurgery*, vol. 82, no. 1-2, p. e398, 2014.

[2] G. M. Burke, A. M. Burke, A. K. Sherma, M. C. Hurley, H. H. Batjer, and B. R. Bendok, "Moyamoya disease: a summary," *Neurosurgical Focus*, vol. 26, no. 4, pp. 1–10, 2009.

[3] W. Miao, P.-L. Zhao, Y.-S. Zhang et al., "Epidemiological and clinical features of Moyamoya disease in Nanjing, China," *Clinical Neurology and Neurosurgery*, vol. 112, no. 3, pp. 199–203, 2010.

[4] R. S. Bower, G. W. Mallory, M. Nwojo, Y. C. Kudva, K. D. Flemming, and F. B. Meyer, "Moyamoya disease in a primarily white, Midwestern us population: increased prevalence of autoimmune disease," *Stroke*, vol. 44, no. 7, pp. 1997–1999, 2013.

[5] L. Berglund, J. D. Brunzell, A. C. Goldberg et al., "Evaluation and treatment of hypertriglyceridemia: an endocrine society clinical practice guideline," *Journal of Clinical Endocrinology and Metabolism*, vol. 97, no. 9, pp. 2969–2989, 2012.

[6] C.-C. Hung, Y.-K. Tu, C.-F. Su, L.-S. Lin, and C.-J. Shih, "Epidemiological study of Moyamoya disease in Taiwan," *Clinical Neurology and Neurosurgery*, vol. 99, no. 2, pp. S23–S25, 1997.

[7] Y. Yonekawa, J. Fandino, M. Hug, M. Wiesli, M. Fujioka, and N. Khan, *Moyamoya Angiopathy in Europe. Moyamoya Disease Update*, Springer, Tokyo, Japan, 2010.

[8] H. Fodstad, M. Bodosi, A. Forssell, and D. Perricone, "Moyamoya disease in patients of Finno-Ugric origin," *British Journal of Neurosurgery*, vol. 10, no. 2, pp. 179–186, 1996.

[9] A. V. Gaddi, A. F. G. Cicero, F. O. Odoo, A. Poli, and R. Paoletti, "Practical recommendations for familial combined hyperlipidemia diagnosis and management: an update," *Vascular Disease Prevention*, vol. 4, no. 3, pp. 229–236, 2007.

[10] Y.-C. Wei, C.-H. Liu, T.-Y. Chang et al., "Coexisting diseases of moyamoya vasculopathy," *Journal of Stroke and Cerebrovascular Diseases*, vol. 23, no. 6, pp. 1344–1350, 2014.

[11] R. M. Scott and E. R. Smith, "Moyamoya disease and moyamoya syndrome," *The New England Journal of Medicine*, vol. 360, no. 12, pp. 1226–1237, 2009.

[12] J.-I. Takanishi, *Moyamoyan Disease in Children, Brain and Development*, Elsevier, 2011.

[13] C.-C. Hung, Y.-K. Tu, C.-F. Su, L.-S. Lin, and C.-J. Shih, "Epidemiological study of moyamoya disease in Taiwan," *Clinical Neurology and Neurosurgery*, vol. 99, supplement 2, pp. S23–S25, 1997.

[14] S. Kuroda, T. Ishikawa, K. Houkin, R. Nanba, M. Hokari, and Y. Iwasaki, "Incidence and clinical features of disease progression in adult moyamoya disease," *Stroke*, vol. 36, no. 10, pp. 2148–2153, 2005.

[15] S. C. Lee, J. S. Jeon, J. E. Kim et al., "Contralateral progression and its risk factor in surgically treated unilateral adult moyamoya disease with a review of pertinent literature," *Acta Neurochirurgica*, vol. 156, no. 1, pp. 103–111, 2014.

[16] S. J. Kim, K. G. Heo, H. Y. Shin et al., "Association of thyroid autoantibodies with moyamoya-type cerebrovascular disease: a prospective study," *Stroke*, vol. 41, no. 1, pp. 173–176, 2010.

[17] S.-H. Im, C. W. Oh, O. K. Kwon, J. E. Kim, and D. H. Han, "Moyamoya disease associated with Graves disease: special considerations regarding clinical significance and management," *Journal of Neurosurgery*, vol. 102, no. 6, pp. 1013–1017, 2005.

[18] Y. Mineharu, Y. Takagi, J. C. Takahashi et al., "Rapid progression of unilateral moyamoya disease in a patient with a family history and an RNF213 risk variant," *Cerebrovascular Diseases*, vol. 36, no. 2, pp. 155–157, 2013.

[19] S. Kuroda, N. Hashimoto, T. Yoshimoto, Y. Iwasaki, and Research Committee on Moyamoya Disease in Japan, "Radiological findings, clinical course, and outcome in asymptomatic moyamoya disease: results of multicenter survey in Japan," *Stroke*, vol. 38, pp. 1430–1435, 2007.

[20] B. A. Gross and R. Du, "The natural history of Moyamoya in a North American adult cohort," *Journal of Clinical Neuroscience*, vol. 20, no. 1, pp. 44–48, 2013.

[21] W.-S. Cho, Y. S. E. Chung, J. E. U. Kim et al., "The natural clinical course of hemodynamically stable adult moyamoya disease," *Journal of Neurosurgery*, vol. 122, no. 1, pp. 82–89, 2015.

[22] H. J. Noh, S. J. Kim, J. S. Kim et al., "Long term outcome and predictors of ischemic stroke recurrence in adult moyamoya disease," *Journal of the Neurological Sciences*, vol. 359, no. 1-2, pp. 381–388, 2015.

[23] M. Kraemer, P. Berlit, F. Diesner, and N. Khan, "What is the expert's option on antiplatelet therapy in moyamoya disease? Results of a worldwide Survey," *European Journal of Neurology*, vol. 19, no. 1, pp. 163–167, 2012.

[24] S. Yamada, K. Oki, Y. Itoh et al., "Effects of surgery and antiplatelet therapy in ten-year follow-up from the registry study of research committee on moyamoya disease in Japan," *Journal of Stroke and Cerebrovascular Diseases*, vol. 25, no. 2, pp. 340–349, 2016.

[25] M. Fukui, S. Kono, K. Sueishi, and K. Ikezaki, "Moyamoya disease," *Neuropathology*, vol. 20, supplement 1, pp. S61–S64, 2000.

[26] A. M. I. Andeejani, M. A. M. Salih, T. Kolawole et al., "Moyamoya syndrome with unusual angiographic findings and protein C deficiency: review of the literature," *Journal of the Neurological Sciences*, vol. 159, no. 1, pp. 11–16, 1998.

[27] P. Cerrato, M. Grasso, A. Lentini et al., "Atherosclerotic adult Moya-Moya disease in a patient with hyperhomocysteinaemia," *Neurological Sciences*, vol. 28, no. 1, pp. 45–47, 2007.

[28] F. Booth, R. Yanofsky, I. B. Ross, P. Lawrence, and K. Oen, "Primary antiphospholipid syndrome with moyamoya-like vascular changes," *Pediatric Neurosurgery*, vol. 31, no. 1, pp. 45–48, 1999.

[29] H. Tsuda, S. Hattori, S. Tanabe et al., "Thrombophilia found in patients with Moyamoya disease," *Clinical Neurology and Neurosurgery*, vol. 99, supplement 2, pp. S229–S233, 1997.

[30] H. C. Jeong, Y. J. Kim, W. Yoon, S. P. Joo, S. S. Lee, and Y. W. Park, "Moyamoya syndrome associated with systemic lupus erythematosus," *Lupus*, vol. 17, no. 7, pp. 679–682, 2008.

[31] T. Czartoski, D. Hallam, J. M. Lacy, M. R. Chun, and K. Becker, "Postinfectious vasculopathy with evolution to moyamoya syndrome," *Journal of Neurology, Neurosurgery and Psychiatry*, vol. 76, no. 2, pp. 256–259, 2005.

[32] N. J. Ullrich, R. Robertson, D. D. Kinnamon et al., "Moyamoya following cranial irradiation for primary brain tumors in children," *Neurology*, vol. 68, no. 12, pp. 932–938, 2007.

[33] S. R. Levine, J. E. Knake, and A. B. Young, "Atypical progressive stroke syndrome associated with oral contraceptives and cigarette use," *Stroke*, vol. 18, no. 2, pp. 519–523, 1987.

[34] J. C. Drees, J. A. Stone, and A. H. B. Wu, "Morbidity involving the hallucinogenic designer amines MDA and 2C-I," *Journal of Forensic Sciences*, vol. 54, no. 6, pp. 1485–1487, 2009.

[35] M. S. Tullu, A. V. Advirkar, R. G. Ghildiyal, and S. Tambe, "Familial hypertriglyceridemia," *Indian Journal of Pediatrics*, vol. 75, no. 12, pp. 1257–1258, 2008.

6

A Case of Acute Psychosis in an Adolescent Male

Ghufran Babar[1] **and Ramin Alemzadeh**[2]

[1] *Section of Pediatric Endocrinology, Children's Mercy Hospitals and Clinics, 3101 Broadway Boulevard, Kansas City, MO 64111, USA*
[2] *Division of Pediatric Endocrinology, University of Illinois College of Medicine at Chicago, 1853 W. Polk Street, Chicago, IL 60612, USA*

Correspondence should be addressed to Ghufran Babar; ghufransaeed@hotmail.com

Academic Editors: C. Capella and A. J. O'Sullivan

Primary hyperparathyroidism (PHPT) is a disorder of calcium homeostasis. We report the case of a 17-year-old adolescent male, who presented with an acute psychosis coinciding with severe hypercalcemia and markedly elevated intact parathyroid hormone (iPTH) level and low vitamin D level. A Sestamibi scan showed a positive signal inferior to the left lobe of the thyroid gland. He had only a partial response to the initial medical and psychiatric management. The enlarged parathyroid gland was resected surgically and postoperatively serum calcium and iPTH levels normalized. The histopathology was compatible with a benign adenoma. Patient's acute psychotic symptoms resolved gradually after surgery; however he remained under psychiatric care for the behavioral issues for about 6 months after surgery. While psychosis is a rare clinical manifestation of hypercalcemia secondary to PHPT in pediatric population, it should be considered as a clinical clue in an otherwise asymptomatic pediatric patient.

1. Introduction

Primary hyperparathyroidism (PHPT) is a disorder of calcium homeostasis. It is rare in pediatric population (age < 18 years) and is usually caused by a single parathyroid adenoma (PA) [1–3]. PA has an incidence of 2–5 per 100,000 children [1]. Elevated levels of intact parathyroid hormone (iPTH) lead to persistent hypercalcemia. PA commonly involves the inferior parathyroid glands, although it can be found in several ectopic sites including thyroid gland, thymus, pericardium, and retroesophageal areas [4]. Hypercalcemia due to PA presents initially as nonspecific symptoms like polyuria, weakness, fatigue, irritability, anorexia, abdominal pain, nausea, emesis, and weight loss. Therefore, the diagnosis of hypercalcemia is often delayed due to subtle clinical symptoms until the complications emerge [1]. These include renal stones, osteopenia and osteoporosis, osteitis fibrosa cystica, peptic ulcer disease, pancreatitis, constipation, hypertension, arrhythmias (shortening of QT interval) [5], and neuropsychiatric diseases [6].

PHPT should be included in the differential diagnosis of all cases of hypercalcemia. Common causes of hypercalcemia include William's syndrome, idiopathic infantile hypercalcemia, malignancy, and toxicity with drugs like thiazides and vitamin A. Rare causes include familial hypocalciuric hypercalcemia, multiple endocrine neoplasia I and II syndromes, subcutaneous fat necrosis, granulomatous disorders, hypervitaminosis D, malignancies, adrenal insufficiency [7], hyperthyroidism, hypothyroidism, and limb fracture with immobilization [2].

The laboratory diagnosis of PHPT is made by demonstrating elevated serum iPTH and calcium levels. A Sestamibi scan of the parathyroid gland can localize the overactive sites. We are presenting a unique patient with hypercalcemia due to a PA. His only symptom at presentation was frank psychosis; however, we were not able to find such a presentation of PHPT in pediatric population by a careful literature review.

2. Case

Our patient is a 17-year-old African American male who was transferred to the Children's Hospital of Wisconsin (CHW) emergency room from a local inpatient psychiatric unit, for further workup of elevated serum calcium and iPTH levels. The patient had been admitted with acute psychosis a week prior to his transfer to CHW, where on a routine laboratory screening he was found to have serum calcium of 16.5 mg/dL

Table 1: Biochemical characteristics of our patient with PHPT.

Laboratory results	BT	AMT	ASMT
Serum iCa (4.5–5.3 mg/dL)	8.0	6.6	4.8
Serum total calcium (8.9–10.7 mg/dL)	18.0	11.8	9.6
Serum iPTH (9–69 pg/mL)	350.0	242.0	<2.5
Serum 25-OH vitamin D (20–100 ng/mL)	18.0	22.0	61.0
Serum phosphate (2.5–4.8 mg/dL)	3.1	3.0	3.5
Serum alkaline phosphatase (50–130 IU/L)	156.0	143.0	122.0
Urine calcium/creatinine ratio (<0.21)	0.6	ND	ND
Urinary calcium excretion rate (<4 mg/kg/day)	12.0	ND	ND
Phosphate/creatinine clearance ratio (0.02–0.22)	0.22	ND	ND
Tubular reabsorption of phosphate (TRP) (78–98)%	78.0	ND	ND

BT: before treatment; AMT: after medical treatment; ASMT: after surgery and medical treatment; ND: not done.

(8.9–10.7). The serum iPTH level was markedly elevated: 315 pg/mL (9–69). During the preceding 2-3 weeks, the patient had intermittent episodes of aggressive, hostile, and angry moods associated with paranoia. He reported hearing of voices, visual hallucinations, and delusional ideation. His mother reported that he had been having difficulty initiating sleep and frequently paced in his bedroom throughout the night. He also had frequent arguments with his father and girlfriend and was reported to have suicidal and homicidal ideations. He subsequently suffered a fracture of the right radius after jumping out of a moving car. Consequently, he was admitted to an inpatient psychiatric unit with diagnosis of acute psychosis.

At the time of presentation, he was in the 12th grade with average school performance. He reported being sexually active and smoked marijuana about 2-3 times per week. He denied history of bone pain, abdominal pain, passage of red colored urine, or stones in the urine. He had a normal birth history and developmental milestones during childhood and no history of head injury. He had a history of behavioral problems since the 2nd grade and was assessed by the school social worker and the psychologist, who attributed them to underlying learning disability, and was placed in special education. He never had any prior psychiatric evaluation nor was he ever placed on psychiatric medications. His past medical and surgical history was unremarkable. There was no family history of hypercalcemia or major medical or mental illnesses.

On physical exam he appeared healthy looking, alert, oriented, and cooperative. He had normal vitals, physical exam, and speech. He appeared to be of average intelligence and moderately agitated. His psychiatric symptoms were unchanged since his first presentation in the local psychiatric hospital. He had no hyperactivity, tics, or stereotypic movements, gait was normal, and recent and remote memories were intact.

He had an elevated serum iPTH 242.0 (9–69 pg/mL) and alkaline phosphatase 156 IU/L (50–130), low serum 25 hydroxy vitamin D 18 ng/mL (20–100), and an elevated 1,25-dihydroxy vitamin D 102 pg/mL (27–71) (Quest Diagnostics, San Juan Capistrano, CA), consistent with PHPT. Thyroid hormone screening, electrolytes, urine drug screen, and vitamin A levels were normal. His 24-hour urinary calcium to creatinine ratio (mg Ca/mg Cr) was 0.60 (<0.21), and urinary calcium excretion rate was 12 mg/kg/day (<4). Phosphate/creatinine clearance ratio was 0.22 (0.02–0.22) and the percentage tubular reabsorption of phosphate (%TRP) was 78 (78–98). Urinary vanillyl mandelic acid was 2.2 mg/24 hours (<3.9) and urinary homovanillic acid was 2.2 mg/24 hours (1.4–7.2). He had a normal electrocardiogram, ultrasound, and MRI of neck and ultrasound of the kidney. A Sestamibi scan showed a positive signal just inferior to the left lobe of the thyroid gland. Multiple endocrine neoplasias type 1 (MEN-1) and MEN-2 gene analysis were negative (Mayo Medical Laboratories, Rochester, MN). Hypercalcemia was treated with intravenous fluids and calcitonin. His calcium levels were moderately decreased by intravenous calcitonin (2–4 U/kg/day); however calcitonin effect was not sustained. The patient underwent surgery for the removal of the parathyroid gland, 5 days after hospitalization (about a month after the acute onset of psychotic symptoms). Intraoperative and postoperative serum iPTH were <2.5 pg/mL, confirming the completeness of the procedure. The calcium levels gradually normalized in 48 hours (9.7 to 10.7 mg/dL), Table 1. The gland weighed 1.3 grams and its histopathology evaluation revealed a hypercellular parathyroid gland containing oxyphil and chief cells with no features of malignancy. Although his paranoid and violent behavior gradually resolved about 2-3 months after surgery, he remained under psychiatric care for behavioral issues for about 6 months after surgery.

3. Discussions

Psychosis may be the earliest manifestation of an endocrine disorder [8]. It has been described in patients with Cushing's syndrome [9], hyperthyroidism [10], and hypothyroidism in pediatric and adult patients [11]. It has not been associated with PHPT in the pediatric age group. Most of the available information on this subject is through the adult literature describing patients with PHPT who have presented with psychosis [12, 13], as well as with other psychiatric symptoms like delirium or dementia, depression, anxiety, lethargy or apathy, stupor, or even coma [13]. The usual symptoms are divided into three categories: (1) confusional state with clouding of consciousness, which ranged from drowsiness to stupor; (2) clear sensorium with depression, psychosis with paranoid delusions and violent or bizarre behavior; and (3) a "pseudoneurotic" form [14].

The pathogenesis of psychosis in PHPT has not been established. However, since calcium appears to play an important role in determining changes in monoamine metabolism of the central nervous system, such as modification of dopaminergic and cholinergic metabolism and release at several neuroregulatory stages, it may affect behavior and mood in some patients [15, 16]. Indeed, calcium channel blockers have been used in treating schizophrenia [16]. Prolonged periods of subclinical hypercalcemia usually precede the development of psychiatric symptoms; however there are conflicting reports regarding the relationship of the severity of the symptoms and the degree of hypercalcemia [17]. An alternate hypothesis is that the psychiatric symptoms may be related to a number of factors like premorbid adjustment and sociocultural influences [18]. In our patient, there is a history of "behavioral problems" with learning disability requiring special education since early elementary school. In adults most cases of PHPT (56%) can be asymptomatic at diagnosis [19] versus the children (16%) [20]. This may be because adults are more likely to have a screening for calcium done, although asymptomatic disease may still be common in pediatric population [21].

Depending upon the severity of hypercalcemia in PHPT, different treatment options can be utilized including hydration and by using loop diuretics like furosemide to cause calciuresis. Bisphosphonates and calcitonin have also been effective in lowering serum calcium concentrations in hypercalcemic children [5]. The other treatment options include using oral phosphate, glucocorticoids [22], and peritoneal dialysis [23]. The definitive treatment is surgery, which should be carried out as soon as possible [24]. It is effective in lowering serum calcium but may not reverse end-organ damage that has already occurred [24].

In PHPT, decreased percent tubular reabsorption of phosphate (TRP) usually results in low serum phosphate [25]; however, in some instances serum phosphate levels may fall in the low normal range as observed in our patient.Our patient's serum iPTH and calcium levels normalized after the parathyroidectomy. In addition, his serum 25-OH vitamin D levels normalized after replacement therapy.

Fujikawa et al. observed that neurobehavioral symptoms in mild primary hyperparathyroidism related to hypercalcemia might not improve after the parathyroidectomy [26]. The recovery from the psychosis secondary to the PHPT after the surgery is not related to the duration of disease, severity of changes, or the age of the patient [27].

In conclusion, we present a case of PHPT due to a parathyroid adenoma presenting with psychosis. Physicians should know that PHPT might be responsible for a wide spectrum of symptoms. Although psychotic symptoms are uncommon, as compared to affective or cognitive symptoms, they may occur as a sole manifestation of this disorder and may lead to dangerous behaviors. A screening serum calcium level should be checked in a patient presenting with psychiatric symptoms, since a delayed diagnosis can result in more severe complications. The disease is usually due to a single PA, and surgery is an extremely safe and effective method of preventing the complications of this disease and perhaps the reversal of psychiatric symptoms.

References

[1] J. Kollars, A. E. Zarroug, J. van Heerden et al., "Primary hyperparathyroidism in pediatric patients," *Pediatrics*, vol. 115, no. 4, pp. 974–980, 2005.

[2] J. M. Ruda, C. S. Hollenbeak, and B. C. Stack Jr., "A systematic review of the diagnosis and treatment of primary hyperparathyroidism from 1995 to 2003," *Otolaryngology: Head and Neck Surgery*, vol. 132, no. 3, pp. 359–372, 2005.

[3] D. Melliere, D. Berrahal, L. Perlemuter, E. Hindie, and D. Simon, "Primary hyperparathyroidism. Symptoms related to age, sex, calcaemia, anatomic lesions and weight of the glands," *Presse Medicale*, vol. 24, no. 39, pp. 1889–1893, 1995.

[4] T. R. S. Prasad and V. Bhatnagar, "Giant solitary parathyroid adenoma presenting with bone disease," *Indian Pediatrics*, vol. 39, no. 11, pp. 1044–1047, 2002.

[5] M. F. Carroll and D. S. Schade, "A practical approach to hypercalcemia," *American Family Physician*, vol. 67, no. 9, pp. 1959–1966, 2003.

[6] M. A. Levine, "Primary hyperparathyroidism: 7,000 years of progress," *Cleveland Clinic Journal of Medicine*, vol. 72, no. 12, pp. 1084–1098, 2005.

[7] A. Montoli, G. Colussi, and L. Minetti, "Hypercalcaemia in Addison's disease: calciotropic hormone profile and bone histology," *Journal of Internal Medicine*, vol. 232, no. 6, pp. 535–540, 1992.

[8] V. I. Reus, "Behavioral disturbances associated with endocrine disorders," *Annual Review of Medicine*, vol. 37, pp. 205–214, 1986.

[9] D. Hirsch, G. Orr, V. Kantarovich, H. Hermesh, E. Stern, and L. Blum, "Gushing's syndrome presenting as a schizophrenia-like psychotic state," *Israel Journal of Psychiatry and Related Sciences*, vol. 37, no. 1, pp. 46–50, 2000.

[10] C.-L. Lu, Y.-C. Lee, S.-J. Tsai, P.-G. Hu, and C.-B. Sim, "Psychiatric disturbances associated with hyperthyroidism: an analysis report of 30 cases," *Zhonghua Yi Xue Za Zhi (Taipei)*, vol. 56, no. 6, pp. 393–398, 1995.

[11] V. Bhatara, M. G. Alshari, P. Warhol, J. M. McMillin, and A. Bhatara, "Coexistent hypothyroidism, psychosis, and severe obsessions in an adolescent: a 10-year follow-up," *Journal of Child and Adolescent Psychopharmacology*, vol. 14, no. 2, pp. 315–323, 2004.

[12] B. Spivak, M. Radvan, R. Ohring, and A. Weizman, "Primary hyperparathyroidism, psychiatric manifestations, diagnosis and management," *Psychotherapy and Psychosomatics*, vol. 51, no. 1, pp. 38–44, 1989.

[13] G. R. Geffken, H. E. Ward, J. P. Staab, S. L. K. Carmichael, and D. L. Evans, "Psychiatric morbidity in endocrine disorders," *Psychiatric Clinics of North America*, vol. 21, no. 2, pp. 473–489, 1998.

[14] P. J. Velasco, M. Manshadi, K. Breen, and S. Lippmann, "Psychiatric aspects of parathyroid disease," *Psychosomatics*, vol. 40, no. 6, pp. 486–490, 1999.

[15] G. Athanassenas, E. Papadopoulos, A. Kourkoubas et al., "Serum calcium and magnesium levels in chronic schizophren-

ics," *Journal of Clinical Psychopharmacology*, vol. 3, no. 4, pp. 212–216, 1983.

[16] S. H. Snyder, "Molecular mechanism of psychotropic drug action," in *Proceedings of the 136th American Psychiatric Association Annual Meeting*, New York, NY, USA, 1983.

[17] C. Joborn, J. Hetta, H. Johansson et al., "Psychiatric morbidity in primary hyperparathyroidism," *World Journal of Surgery*, vol. 12, no. 4, pp. 476–481, 1988.

[18] R. D. Alarcon and J. A. Franceschini, "Hyperparathyroidism and paranoid psychosis: case report and review of the literature," *British Journal of Psychiatry*, vol. 145, pp. 477–486, 1984.

[19] J. A. van Heerden and C. S. Grant, "Surgical treatment of primary hyperparathyroidism: an institutional perspective," *World Journal of Surgery*, vol. 15, no. 6, pp. 688–692, 1991.

[20] C. R. Harman, J. A. van Heerden, D. R. Farley, C. S. Grant, G. B. Thompson, and K. Curlee, "Sporadic primary hyperparathyroidism in young patients: a separate disease entity?" *Archives of Surgery*, vol. 134, no. 6, pp. 651–656, 1999.

[21] C. B. Huang, S. C. Huang, F. F. Chou, and W. J. Chen, "Primary hyperparathyroidism in children: report of a case and a brief review of the literature," *Journal of the Formosan Medical Association*, vol. 92, no. 12, pp. 1095–1098, 1993.

[22] D. H. Fulmer, A. B. Dimich, E. O. Rothschild, and W. P. Myers, "Treatment of hypercalcemia. Comparison of intravenously administered phosphate, sulfate, and hydrocortisone," *Archives of Internal Medicine*, vol. 129, no. 6, pp. 923–930, 1972.

[23] U. Querfeld, I. B. Salusky, and R. N. Fine, "Treatment of severe hypercalcemia with peritoneal dialysis in an infant with end-stage renal disease," *Pediatric Nephrology*, vol. 2, no. 3, pp. 323–325, 1988.

[24] H. Lauschke, M. Kaminski, H. Stratmann, and A. Hirner, "The parathyrotoxic crisis—a surgical emergency," *Chirurg*, vol. 71, no. 1, pp. 58–62, 2000.

[25] Y. Ohata, T. Yamamoto, Y. Kitai et al., "A case of primary hyperparathyroidism in childhood found by a chance hematuria," *Clinical Pediatric Endocrinology*, vol. 16, no. 1, pp. 11–16, 2007.

[26] Y. Fujikawa, M. Koga, H. Sugao et al., "Neurobehavioral symptoms in mild primary hyperparathyroidism: related to hypercalcemia but not improved by parathyroidectomy," *Henry Ford Hospital Medical Journal*, vol. 35, no. 4, pp. 211–215, 1987.

[27] C. K. Smith, J. Barish, J. Correa, and R. H. Williams, "Psychiatric disturbance in endocrinologic disease," *Psychosomatic Medicine*, vol. 34, no. 1, pp. 69–86, 1972.

7

Acanthosis Nigricans Associated with an Adrenocortical Tumor in a Pediatric Patient

Elizabeth Isaacoff,[1] Filippina Filia Dimitriadi,[2] Frank Barrows,[3] Bruce Pawel,[4] Peter Mattei,[5] and Sogol Mostoufi-Moab[1]

[1] *Department of Pediatrics, The Children's Hospital of Philadelphia, 34th Street and Civic Center Boulevard, 3535 Market Street, Room 1562, Philadelphia, PA 19104, USA*
[2] *Division of Pediatric Endocrinology, St. Christopher's Hospital for Children, 3601 A. Street, Philadelphia, PA 19134, USA*
[3] *Division of Pediatric Endocrinology, Monmouth Medical Children's Hospital, 180 Avenue at the Commons, Suite 7B, Shrewsbury, NJ 07702, USA*
[4] *Department of Pathology, The Children's Hospital of Philadelphia, 34th Street and Civic Center Boulevard, Philadelphia, PA 19104, USA*
[5] *Department of General Surgery, The Children's Hospital of Philadelphia, 34th Street and Civic Center Boulevard, Philadelphia, PA 19104, USA*

Correspondence should be addressed to Elizabeth Isaacoff; isaacoffe@email.chop.edu

Academic Editors: C. Capella, M. Demura, N. Islam, and M. P. Kane

Malignant acanthosis nigricans (AN) is a rare paraneoplastic syndrome seen primarily in adults with an underlying diagnosis of gastrointestinal adenocarcinoma. Malignant AN is characterized by hyperpigmentation and velvety hyperplasia of the epidermis. This condition is generally not associated with tumors in pediatric populations or in the adrenal gland. We present a case of malignant AN in a pediatric patient with a nonmalignant, functional adrenocortical tumor.

1. Introduction

Childhood adrenocortical tumors (ACTs) generally present during the first 5 years of life, with a second, smaller peak noted during adolescence [1–4]. Majority of these tumors come to medical attention subsequent to overproduction of adrenal cortical hormones. Virilization is the most common presenting sign (84.3%), either alone (55.1%) or in combination with overproduction of other adrenal hormones including aldosterone or glucocorticoids (29.2%), followed by 5.5% with isolated Cushing's syndrome, and 10.2% with nonfunctional tumors [4].

The diagnosis of ACTs in pediatric patients is generally made within 5–8 months of the first presenting signs and symptoms [2, 4, 5]; however, one-third of pediatric patients have either unresectable or metastatic disease at the time of diagnosis. The remaining two-thirds have disease confined to the adrenals [4]. An elevated blood or urine concentration of adrenocortical hormones and a suprarenal mass generally suggest a preoperative diagnosis of ACT. Imaging studies are necessary for sufficient staging and surgery planning [6]. Surgery is the best treatment plan for those with ACTs, and cisplatin-based chemotherapy with mitotane is indicated for metastatic disease or when complete resection is not possible at presentation [6]. In children with localized ACTs, tumor weight ≤200 g, virilization alone, stage I disease, absence of spillage during surgery, and age ≤3 years are considered important favorable prognostic indicators [4].

Malignant acanthosis nigricans (AN) is a rare paraneoplastic syndrome seen mainly in adults with adenocarcinomas, primarily of gastric origin [7, 8]. Malignant AN appears concurrently at the time of tumor diagnosis in 61.3%, but may also appear before (17.6%) or after (21.1%) cancer diagnosis [9]. Malignant AN is usually not a recognized paraneoplastic

Table 1: Pre- and postoperative endocrine laboratory values.

Hormone	Preoperative hormone level	Postoperative hormone level				Normal range
	4/19/2010	5/11/2010	6/30/2010	4/20/2011	9/26/2012	
Glucose (mg/dL)	88	71	127	83	78	74–127
Nonfasting insulin (uU/mL)	43.7	—	30.7	—	—	—
Hemoglobin A1C (%)	4.9	—	—	4.7	4.7	3.8–5.9
Testosterone (ng/dL)	150	<3.0	<3.0	<2.5	<2.5	Tanner 1 range <3–10 Tanner 2 range 18–150
Androstenedione (ng/dL)	72	<10	—	<10	<10	Tanner 1 range <10–17 Tanner 2 range 31–65
Dehydroepiandrosterone sulfate (ug/dL)	73	<10	—	—	—	Range for 1–5 years of age <5–57 Tanner 2 range 42–109
IGF-1/Somatomedin-C serum (ng/mL)	325	—	143	101	111	Range for 3-4 years of age 54–178
FSH (mIU/mL)	0.143	—	—	—	—	Tanner 1 range 0.1–3.0
Luteinizing hormone (mIU/mL)	0.010	—	—	—	—	Tanner 1 range 0.01–0.3

finding associated with pediatric tumors. Here, we report the first case of malignant AN in a pediatric patient with a non-malignant, functional ACT at the time of tumor diagnosis.

2. Case Presentation

A previously healthy 33-month-old Caucasian male presented with a three-month history of rapid virilization and a neck rash. Height and weight remained unchanged over the preceding months at the 50th percentile. Blood pressure at the time of diagnosis was 123/65 mmHg and heart rate 112 bpm. Physical examination was notable for coarse facial features, facial acne, anterior and posterior cervical acanthosis nigricans, Tanner 2 pubic hair, and pubertal phallus (8 cm in length and 2 cm in diameter), but prepubertal testes at 3 mL volume bilaterally. Laboratory evaluation revealed an elevated nonfasting insulin level with normal values for glucose, random cortisol 19.6 mcg/dL (normal range 9–22 mcg/dL), ACTH 8.35 pg/mL (normal range 5–46 pg/mL), and hemoglobin A1C 4.7% (normal range 3.8–5.9%). Abnormal laboratory findings for age included elevated testosterone, androstenedione, dehydroepiandrosterone sulfate (DHEAS), all within Tanner 2-3 range. IGF-I level was increased for age. Gonadotropins were Tanner stage 1, confirming a peripheral source for androgen production. Serum electrolytes, beta-HCG, and alpha-fetoprotein levels were all within normal limits. Table 1 is a summary of pertinent laboratory results.

MRI of the abdomen revealed a 2.3 × 3 cm mass within the right adrenal cortex, absent retroperitoneal lymphadenopathy, and lack of tumor thrombus within the IVC. The patient underwent a successful right adrenalectomy and retroperitoneal lymph node dissection without any complications. Postoperative screening morning cortisol was undetectable (<1.0 mcg/dL), indicating suppression of contralateral unaffected adrenal gland. He was treated with stress-dose hydrocortisone and subsequently transitioned to and slowly weaned off of physiologic replacement postoperatively. Follow-up random cortisol level one year postoperatively was normal at 7.1 mcg/dL (normal range 1.5–9.0 mcg/dL). Pathology review revealed a 12.5-gram encapsulated tumor without hemorrhage, necrosis, or capsular invasion (Figure 1). Tumor cells exhibited rare mitotic figures, favoring the diagnosis of a non-malignant adrenal cortical tumor. He demonstrated marked clinical improvement of all symptoms, including normalization of all laboratory values three weeks after surgery and complete resolution of the acanthosis nigricans three months postoperatively.

3. Discussion

ACT peaks during the first and fourth decades of life [10]. The incidence of ACT varies internationally, with particularly high rates noted in southern Brazil, where the incidence is approximately 10–15 times that observed in the USA [6]. Predisposing genetic factors may be responsible for this increased incidence [6]. ACT in children is exceptionally rare, composing only 0.2% of pediatric cancers [11]. Only 25 new cases are expected to occur annually in the USA, for an estimated annual incidence of 0.2–0.3 cases per million [11].

Acanthosis nigricans (AN), a common cutaneous finding, is characterized by hyperpigmentation and velvety hyperplasia of the epidermis [12]. In general, it affects flexural areas including the neck, antecubital, and, the popliteal fossa [12]. Benign AN usually presents between birth and puberty and can have a possible genetic component [8]. Benign AN often occurs in individuals exhibiting insulin resistance, such as patients with a diagnosis of diabetes mellitus, obesity, and polycystic ovarian syndrome [12]. Although benign forms of AN are relatively common, malignant AN can occur as a rare paraneoplastic syndrome with approximately 1,000 reported worldwide cases [13]. It is most often seen in adults with an underlying diagnosis of gastrointestinal adenocarcinoma [7, 8]. Malignant AN tends to worsen with progression of the neoplasm, lessen with treatment, and return with tumor

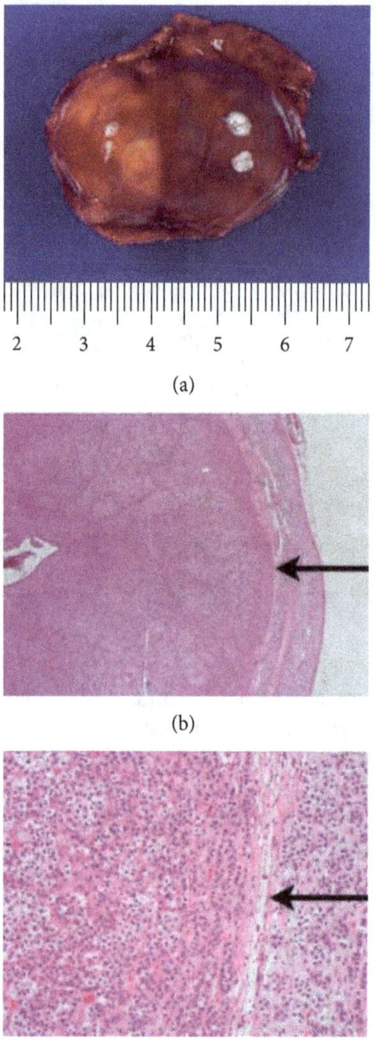

(a)

(b)

(c)

FIGURE 1: (a) Gross photograph of resected adrenal mass. (b) Low power photomicrograph of adrenocortical tumor. The tumor is encapsulated (arrow) and has a pushing border, with compressed normal adrenal cortex on the right. (H&E, 20x). (c) High power photomicrograph of adrenocortical tumor. Arrow is pointing to a thin fibrous capsule. The tumor has similar cytologic features to the normal adrenal seen on the right. Features that have been associated with malignancy (capsular invasion, necrosis, and increased mitotic activity) are not present (H&E, 200x).

recurrence and/or metastases [8]. Malignant AN is extremely uncommon in pediatric tumors [14, 15] with only one reported pediatric case of malignant AN associated with a malignant adrenal tumor [16].

The pathophysiology of malignant AN is not well understood. Elevated levels of growth factors released from tumors, such as transforming growth factor alpha (TGF-alpha), can bind to epidermal growth factor receptors (EGFR) in the epidermis and stimulate keratinocyte growth [7, 12, 17]. Malignant AN can be associated with the sign of Leser-Trélat (LT), a rare and sudden onset of multiple benign skin growths originating in keratinocytes (seborrheic keratoses) and associated with an internal malignancy [7, 12]. Biopsy specimens of seborrheic keratoses in a patient with LT, malignant AN, and melanoma revealed elevated levels of urinary TGF-alpha and increased epidermal staining of EGFRs, with decreased levels of both after treatment of the melanoma [17]. Hereditary diseases associated with AN demonstrate activating germ line mutations in the fibroblast growth factor receptor 3 (FGFR3) gene, which increase keratinocyte growth [18–21]. A positive association of FGFR3 expression has been reported in two cases of malignant AN, with expression throughout the acanthotic lesions [22].

Our patient's AN likely resulted from excess glucocorticoid production by the adrenal tumor, albeit not captured in preoperative laboratory studies. His elevated IGF-1 driven by increased adrenal androgens may have also played a role. Contralateral adrenal cortical suppression with undetectable cortisol and suppressed ACTH after surgery points to excess glucocorticoid hormone secretion by the adrenal mass in addition to the noted elevated adrenal androgens. The excess glucocorticoid production likely contributed to glucocorticoid-induced insulin resistance, resulting in AN. This case represents the first reported association of malignant AN with a nonmalignant, functional cortical adrenal mass in a pediatric patient and an important clue to a possible underlying cortical adrenal tumor as a contributing cause for this unusual phenomenon.

References

[1] P. C. Ribeiro, R. S. Neto, M. J. Schell, L. Lacerda, G. A. Sambaio, and I. Cat, "Adrenocortical carcinoma in children: a study of 40 cases," *Journal of Clinical Oncology*, vol. 8, no. 1, pp. 67–74, 1990.

[2] J. A. Wieneke, L. D. R. Thompson, and C. S. Heffess, "Adrenal cortical neoplasms in the pediatric population: a clinicopathologic and immunophenotypic analysis of 83 patients," *The American Journal of Surgical Pathology*, vol. 27, no. 7, pp. 867–881, 2003.

[3] R. Sandrini, R. C. Ribeiro, and L. DeLacerda, "Extensive personal experience: childhood adrenocortical tumors," *Journal of Clinical Endocrinology and Metabolism*, vol. 82, no. 7, pp. 2027–2031, 1997.

[4] E. Michalkiewicz, R. Sandrini, B. Figueiredo et al., "Clinical and outcome characteristics of children with adrenocortical tumors: a report from the international pediatric adrenocortical tumor registry," *Journal of Clinical Oncology*, vol. 22, no. 5, pp. 838–845, 2004.

[5] A. O. Ciftci, M. E. Şenocak, F. C. Tanyel, and N. Büyükpamukçu, "Adrenocortical tumors in children," *Journal of Pediatric Surgery*, vol. 36, no. 4, pp. 549–554, 2001.

[6] C. Rodriguez-Galindo, B. C. Figueiredo, G. P. Zambetti, and R. C. Ribeiro, "Biology, clinical characteristics, and management of adrenocortical tumors in children," *Pediatric Blood and Cancer*, vol. 45, no. 3, pp. 265–273, 2005.

[7] R. L. Moore and T. S. Devere, "Epidermal manifestations of internal malignancy," *Dermatologic Clinics*, vol. 26, no. 1, pp. 17–29, 2008.

[8] H. Curth, "Cancer associated with acanthosis nigricans: review of literature and report of a case of acanthosis nigricans with

cancer of the breast," *Archives of Surgery*, vol. 47, no. 6, pp. 517–552, 1943.

[9] M. Ramos-e-Silva, J. C. Carvalho, and S. C. Carneiro, "Cutaneous paraneoplasia," *Clinics in Dermatology*, vol. 29, no. 5, pp. 541–547, 2011.

[10] M. D. Wooten and D. K. King, "Adrenal cortical carcinoma. Epidemiology and treatment with mitotane and a review of the literature," *Cancer*, vol. 72, no. 11, pp. 3145–3155, 1993.

[11] L. Bernstein and J. G. Gurney, "Carcinomas and other malignant epithelial neoplasms," in *Cancer Incidence and Survival Among Children and Adolescents: United States SEER Program 1975–1995*, pp. 139–148, National Cancer Institute, Bethesda, Md, USA, 1999.

[12] S. Boyce and J. Harper, "Paraneoplastic dermatoses," *Dermatologic Clinics*, vol. 20, no. 3, pp. 523–532, 2002.

[13] H. O. Sedano and R. J. Gorlin, "Acanthosis nigricans," *Oral Surgery Oral Medicine and Oral Pathology*, vol. 63, no. 4, pp. 642–467, 1987.

[14] P. Bhargava, S. Bhargava, D. Mathur, U. S. Agarwal, and R. Bhargava, "Malignant acanthosis nigricans in a 2 year old child with Wilm's tumour," *Indian Journal of Dermatology, Venereology and Leprology*, vol. 64, no. 1, pp. 29–30, 1998.

[15] T. C. Garrott, "Malignant acanthosis nigricans associated with osteogenic sarcoma," *Archives of Dermatology*, vol. 106, no. 3, pp. 384–385, 1972.

[16] M. Hiranandani, I. Kaur, S. C. Singhi, and U. Bhoria, "Malignant acanthosis nigricans in adrenal carcinoma," *Indian pediatrics*, vol. 32, no. 8, pp. 920–923, 1995.

[17] D. L. Ellis, S. P. Kafka, J. C. Chow et al., "Melanoma, growth factors, acanthosis nigricans, the sign of leser-trelat, and multiple acrochordons. A possible role for alpha-transforming growth factor in cutaneous paraneoplastic syndromes," *The New England Journal of Medicine*, vol. 317, no. 25, pp. 1582–1587, 1987.

[18] G. A. Meyers, S. J. Orlow, I. R. Munro, K. A. Przylepa, and E. W. Jabs, "Fibroblast growth factor receptor 3 (FGFR3) transmembrane mutation in Crouzon syndrome with acanthosis nigricans," *Nature Genetics*, vol. 11, no. 4, pp. 462–464, 1995.

[19] P. L. Tavormina, G. A. Bellus, M. K. Webster et al., "A novel skeletal dysplasia with developmental delay and acanthosis nigricans is caused by a Lys650Met mutation in the fibroblast growth factor receptor 3 gene," *The American Journal of Human Genetics*, vol. 64, no. 3, pp. 722–731, 1999.

[20] L. Castro-Feijóo, L. Loidi, A. Vidal et al., "Hypochondroplasia and acanthosis nigricans: a new syndrome due to the p.Lys650Thr mutation in the fibroblast growth factor receptor 3 gene?" *European Journal of Endocrinology*, vol. 159, no. 3, pp. 243–249, 2008.

[21] D. R. Berk, E. B. Spector, and S. J. Bayliss, "Familial acanthosis nigricans due to K650T FGFR3 mutation," *Archives of Dermatology*, vol. 143, no. 9, pp. 1153–1156, 2007.

[22] Y. Hida, Y. Kubo, Y. Nishio et al., "Malignant acanthosis nigricans with enhanced expression of fibroblast growth factor receptor 3," *Acta Dermato-Venereologica*, vol. 89, no. 4, pp. 435–437, 2009.

8

A Rare and Potentially Fatal Etiology of Hypercalcemia in an Infant

Ambreen Sonawalla,[1] Vildan Tas,[2] Manish Raisingani,[3] and Emir Tas[3]

[1] *Pediatric Residency Program, University of Arkansas for Medical Sciences, Little Rock, AR, USA*
[2] *Department of Pediatrics, University of Arkansas for Medical Sciences, Little Rock, AR, USA*
[3] *Department of Pediatrics, Division of Endocrinology and Diabetes, University of Arkansas for Medical Sciences, Little Rock, AR, USA*

Correspondence should be addressed to Emir Tas; etas@uams.edu

Academic Editor: Lucy Mastrandrea

Hypercalcemia is an uncommon finding in children. Hypercalcemia has various etiologies including parathyroid dependent and independent mechanisms. Increased activity of the 1-alpha-hydroxylase enzyme in granulomatous diseases is a well-defined but an extremely rare cause of hypercalcemia in pediatric patients, particularly in infants. We describe the case of an infant who presented with failure to thrive, hepatosplenomegaly, and hypercalcemia who was initially treated with steroids but was later diagnosed with disseminated histoplasmosis in the absence of an underlying immunodeficiency. Extra caution should be used before considering steroids for the treatment of hypercalcemia and, whenever possible, steroids should not be initiated until a definite etiology is identified.

1. Introduction

Serum calcium level is tightly regulated as calcium is important for numerous cellular functions including cell membrane integrity, muscle contraction, and neuronal excitability [1]. Calcium regulation involves a very-well orchestrated interplay between parathyroid hormone, 1,25-dihydroxy vitamin D, phosphorus, and multiple organ systems including the gut, kidneys, skin, and liver.

Hypercalcemia is an infrequently encountered biochemical abnormality in the pediatric age group [2]. The most common causes, unlike in adults, are parathyroid hormone independent processes. Among them, granulomatous diseases, such as fungal infections, are an uncommon but recognized cause of hypercalcemia [3]. Granulomatous diseases lead to increased activity of the 1alpha-hydroxylase enzyme which converts 25-hydroxy vitamin D to 1,25-dihydroxy vitamin D, the biologically active form.

Hypercalcemia of any cause is initially treated symptomatically, with the ultimate treatment decided by the underlying cause. Steroids have typically been used in the treatment of hypercalcemia when it is secondary to excess vitamin D ingestion or increased 1alpha-hydroxylase activity such as in granulomatous disorders [4].

2. Case Presentation

A 7-month-old ex-30-week preterm female infant presented to the emergency department of our hospital with a two-month history of worsening intermittent vomiting and failure to thrive despite nutritional optimization and trial of different infant formulas. Past medical history was notable for prolonged NICU stay mainly due to delays in oral feeding. She had no pulmonary, cardiac, or intestinal complications of prematurity. She did not require any surgical procedure or hospital admission following NICU discharge at around 6 weeks of age. History is also negative for recent fevers or recurrent infections.

On presentation, she was in no acute distress and had normal vital signs. Weight and height were both below the first percentile. Physical examination was significant for the presence of hepatosplenomegaly. Laboratory workup was notable for elevated transaminases and significant hypercalcemia (4.47 mmol/L; Normal Range: 2.12-2.74mmol/L).

TABLE 1: Calcium metabolism markers at each of the hospital admissions.

	Initial presentation (Baseline)	Second admission (+7 weeks)	Third admission (+15 weeks)
Total calcium (RR: 2.12-2.74 mmol/L)	4.47	3.37	2.47
Ionized calcium (RR: 1.1-1.3 mmol/L)	2.43	1.83	1.35
25 hydroxy vit D (RR: 20-200 nmol/L)	153		50.2
1,25 dihydroxy vit D (RR: 49.7-197.9 pmol/L)	364		92.9
Parathyroid hormone (RR: 12-65 ng/L)	5.3		
Phosphorus (RR: 1.39-2.39 mmol/L)	1.55		1.1
Albumin (RR: 3.5 – 4.5 g/L)	4.4	4.1	2.4
Urine Ca:Cr ratio	1.85		

Baseline phosphorus level was normal and the parathyroid hormone level was appropriately suppressed as seen in Table 1. She was admitted to hospital for management and further workup.

Aggressive intravascular fluid resuscitation with normal saline only partially improved serum calcium levels. Furosemide and calcitonin were used in succession, but they also failed to have a noticeable impact on serum calcium levels. Two doses of pamidronate, 0.5 mg/kg each two days apart, were eventually successful in restoring normal calcium levels. She also switched to low calcium infant formula, Calcilo- XD.

An extensive workup for viral and fungal etiologies was negative, as was the evaluation for metabolic, genetic, and oncologic causes of hypercalcemia. The skeletal survey did not show any lytic lesions; CT scan of the chest, abdomen, and pelvis was negative for the presence of lymphadenopathy or pulmonary lesions. Hepatosplenomegaly was confirmed with a CT scan; however, the underlying pathology was not revealed until a liver biopsy was performed for persistently elevated liver enzymes and massive hepatomegaly. Liver biopsy showed lobular histiocytic infiltrate with well-formed granulomas, hemophagocytosis, and increased portal/periportal and pericellular fibrosis with bridging indicating chronicity, with no further evidence to indicate an underlying etiology of the granulomas.

She was discharged home after 3 weeks of hospitalization once adequate weight gain and normal and stable calcium levels were achieved. Liver enzymes were improved but remained elevated. She had required readmission after one month for the recurrence of vomiting and poor weight. She had no fevers. Workup on this admission showed leukopenia and return of hypercalcemia (Table 1). Chronic granulomatous disease, immunodeficiency, tuberculosis, and hemophagocytic lymphohistiocytosis (HLH) were considered in the differential; however, screening was negative. HLH genotyping showed only a single allele mutation on UNC13 gene, but this variant did not explain her findings. Despite the lack of a standard definition of infantile sarcoidosis, this disease was considered due to elevated levels of angiotensin-converting enzyme (ACE) at 108 U/L (18-90). In the light of negative results for a possible underlying immunodeficiency and malignancy, she was placed on prednisolone 1 mg/kg/day for hypercalcemia. She remained afebrile and was discharged home in stable condition with prednisolone.

After 5 weeks of prednisolone treatment, she presented with daily emesis and low-grade fevers. Complete blood count showed pancytopenia, peripheral smear showed fungal elements. She was admitted to the intensive care unit for disseminated fungal infection. Urine Histoplasma antigen was found to be positive. Systemic antifungal treatment was started. Of note, serum calcium and liver enzyme levels were normal during the third admission (Table 1). Because of disseminated fungal infection, prednisolone was discontinued and a hydrocortisone taper was initiated. She had an excellent response to antifungal treatment. Hepatosplenomegaly resolved and all other serum markers have improved. She remained on systemic antifungal treatment for 9 months. She made full-recovery and caught up with growth and development.

3. Discussion

Hypercalcemia results when there is increased bone resorption, excessive intestinal absorption, or decreased renal excretion of calcium, or a combination of these processes. It may be asymptomatic or present with hypotonia, poor feeding, vomiting, failure to thrive (FTT), constipation, polyuria, dehydration, seizures, or, even psychiatric symptoms depending on the age of the patient [5]. Establishing the etiology requires concomitant evaluation of serum total and ionized calcium, phosphorus, magnesium, intact parathyroid hormone, 25-hydroxy vitamin D ($25(OH)D_3$), and 1,25-dihydroxy vitamin D ($1,25(OH)_2D_3$) concentrations, as well as renal function and urinary calcium excretion [4]. Unlike in adults, hypercalcemia in children is most commonly secondary to parathyroid hormone independent processes. These include hypervitaminosis D and A, medications, malignancies, granulomatous disorders, endocrinopathies, renal tubular disorders, chronic inflammatory disorders, and infections [5].

Hypervitaminosis D may be from elevated levels of $25(OH)D_3$ concentrations, which is usually due to excess ingestion of vitamin D, or from elevated levels of $1,25(OH)_2D_3$ which may be from malignancy, granulomatous diseases, subcutaneous fat necrosis of the newborn, or idiopathic infantile hypercalcemia [5].

Granulomatous diseases, including fungal infections, are a rare but well-established cause of hypercalcemia [6]. The mechanism is extra-renal production of $1,25(OH)_2D_3$ by 1alpha-hydroxylase in activated macrophages within the granulomas, best described in sarcoidosis [7]. The elevated level of the active vitamin D metabolite causes hypercalcemia by a combination of increased intestinal absorption and reduced bone resorption of calcium, as well as increased renal tubular reabsorption. These macrophages are not responsive to negative feedback from elevated levels of $1,25(OH)_2D_3$ but respond to steroids.

Initial management of hypercalcemia depends on the presence of symptoms and degree of elevation of serum calcium, but ultimate treatment depends on the underlying cause. Symptomatic patients are treated with hydration and furosemide. If hypercalcemia persists, calcitonin and bisphosphonates may be used. The latter is effective especially when the primary cause of the hypercalcemia is increased mobilization of bone calcium. Our patient's severe, symptomatic hypercalcemia (Table 1) did not respond to any of the first line treatments. She had a temporary response to IV bisphosphonates but returned with hypercalcemia after only 4 weeks of the infusion therapy as the bisphosphonate did not target the underlying etiology. The role of steroids in the treatment of hypercalcemia in granulomatous diseases is well-established [3, 5]. Steroids exert their action by suppressing the excess 1alpha-hydroxylase activity and decreasing extra-renal production of $1,25(OH)_2D_3$ [8]. Prednisone or prednisolone at a dose of 1 mg/kg/day divided into two doses is the recommended treatment regimen [4]. Our patient's calcium level remained normal and stable following initiation of the steroid treatment.

Histoplasmosis, a granulomatous fungal infection, is the most common endemic fungus in the United States. Most patients remain asymptomatic and have a self-limited illness [9]. Fever, respiratory symptoms, lymphadenopathy, splenomegaly, and poor weight gain are among the most common signs and symptoms, but hypercalcemia is a rare manifestation. None of the 40 infants described by Odio et al. had hypercalcemia as a finding of disseminated histoplasmosis [10]. Surprisingly, our patient had an atypical presentation for fungal infection and did not present with any of the classic symptoms.

The literature is scarce on hypercalcemia in children and adults with histoplasmosis. Steele et al. [11] described a 10-month-old infant with disseminated histoplasmosis who presented with FTT, vomiting, hepatosplenomegaly, and hypercalcemia. Hypercalcemia in this infant was successfully managed with dietary calcium restriction alone; however, it is not clear whether the timing of antifungal treatment in the course of the fungal infection had prevented worsening hypercalcemia. Surprisingly, the infant had to be maintained on a low calcium diet even at 3-year follow up. This is in contrast to our patient who, though was initially placed on a low calcium and vitamin D formula, did not continue to require it when the underlying cause of the hypercalcemia, the fungal infection, had been controlled. Two adult cases with histoplasmosis related hypercalcemia were initially diagnosed with sarcoidosis based on the presenting clinical and laboratory data. One of the patients was found to have histoplasmosis soon after steroid treatment was begun for presumed sarcoidosis [12]. Hypercalcemia in this case resolved with the treatment of the fungal infection. The patient described by Walker et al. [13], however, presented with prolonged malaise, fever, nausea, vomiting, and weight loss. He was readmitted to the hospital after initiation of steroids, with recurrent fever and died from widespread organ disease and cardiac arrest. A postmortem examination found evidence of disseminated histoplasmosis.

Our patient was also initially placed on steroid treatment due to presumed sarcoidosis. Although there are no well-established diagnostic criteria for infantile sarcoidosis, the constellation of her signs and symptoms along with laboratory data including elevated angiotensin-converting enzyme activity in the absence of other explanation for hypercalcemia was the reason of this decision. The correct diagnosis was reached when she presented with pancytopenia, a few weeks into prednisone treatment.

4. Conclusion

Hypercalcemia is an uncommon biochemical abnormality in the pediatric age group. Disseminated fungal infections such as histoplasmosis are also uncommon in an otherwise healthy infant, and hypercalcemia is a rare presenting symptom in such patients. However, even in the absence of classic signs of fungal infections, as was the case in our patient, it is important to consider fungal causes in hypercalcemia with granulomas and evidence of hypervitaminosis D.

Steroids are a well-established treatment for hypercalcemia in granulomatous diseases. Although steroids may resolve several of the overlapping symptoms, they can also unmask the fungal infection and have potentially lethal consequences. It is therefore important to exclude infectious granulomatous etiologies prior to initiating steroid therapy for hypercalcemia.

Disclosure

The abstract of this case was presented as a poster at the 101st Annual Meeting of the Endocrine Society, 2019, New Orleans, LA; and abstract was published in the supplemental issue of the *Journal of the Endocrine Society* (JES).

References

[1] D. Goltzman, *Pediatric Endocrinology 5th edition*, Fima Lifshitz, Ed., vol. 2, Disorders of Calcium and Mineral Metabolism, 2016, Section IV , Chapter 23, page 539.

[2] J. D. McNeilly, R. Boal, M. G. Shaikh, and S. F. Ahmed, "Frequency and aetiology of hypercalcaemia," *Archives of Disease in Childhood*, vol. 101, no. 4, pp. 344–347, 2016.

[3] P. J. Tebben, R. J. Singh, and R. Kumar, "Vitamin D-mediated hypercalcemia: mechanisms, diagnosis, and treatment," *Endocrine Reviews*, vol. 37, no. 5, pp. 521–547, 2016.

[4] F. Lifshitz, "Pediatric endocrinology: growth, adrenal, sexual, thyroid, calcium, and fluid balance disorders," 2019, https://www.barnesandnoble.com/p/pediatric-endocrinology-fifth-edition-volume-2-fima-lifshitz/1112253732/2678657265790?st=PLA&sid=BNB_New+Marketplace+Shopping+Books&sourceId=PLAGoNA&dpid=tdtve346c&2sid=Google_c&gclid=EAIaIQobChMIia-Ynbzu4AIVmrrACh1XzgFvEAYYAiABEgInS_D_BwE.

[5] V. J. Stokes, M. F. Nielsen, F. M. Hannan, and R. V. Thakker, "Hypercalcemic disorders in children," *Journal of Bone and Mineral Research*, vol. 32, no. 11, pp. 2157–2170, 2017.

[6] T. P. Jacobs and J. P. Bilezikian, "Clinical review: rare causes of hypercalcemia," *The Journal of Clinical Endocrinology & Metabolism*, vol. 90, no. 11, pp. 6316–6322, 2005.

[7] R. S. Mason, T. Frankel, Y. L. Chan, D. Lissner, and S. Posen, "Vitamin D conversion by sarcoid lymph node homogenate," *Annals of Internal Medicine*, vol. 100, no. 1, pp. 59–61, 1984.

[8] L. M. Sandler, C. G. Winearls, L. J. Fraher, T. L. Clemens, R. Smith, and J. L. O'Riordan, "Studies of the hypercalcaemia of sarcoidosis: effect of steroids and exogenous vitamin D3 on the circulating concentrations of 1, 25-dihydroxy vitamin D3," *The Quarterly Journal of Medicine*, vol. 53, no. 210, pp. 165–180, 1984.

[9] L. J. Wheat, M. M. Azar, N. C. Bahr, A. Spec, R. F. Relich, and C. Hage, "Histoplasmosis," *Infectious Disease Clinics of North America*, vol. 30, no. 1, pp. 207–227, 2016.

[10] C. M. Odio, M. Navarrete, J. M. Carrillo, L. Mora, and A. Carranza, "Disseminated histoplasmosis in infants," *The Pediatric Infectious Disease Journal*, vol. 18, no. 12, pp. 1065–1068, 1999.

[11] C. J. Steele and M. B. Kleiman, "Disseminated histoplasmosis, hypercalcemia and failure to thrive," *The Pediatric Infectious Disease Journal*, vol. 13, no. 5, pp. 421-422, 1994.

[12] K. V. Liang, J. H. Ryu, and E. L. Matteson, "Histoplasmosis with tenosynovitis of the hand and hypercalcemia mimicking sarcoidosis," *JCR: Journal of Clinical Rheumatology*, vol. 10, no. 3, pp. 138–142, 2004.

[13] J. V. Walker, D. Baran, N. Yakub, and R. B. Freeman, "Histoplasmosis with hypercalcemia, renal failure, and papillary necrosis. Confusion with sarcoidosis," *Journal of the American Medical Association*, vol. 237, no. 13, pp. 1350–1352, 1977.

9

"Primary Hyperparathyroidism (PHPT) in Children: Two Case Reports and Review of the Literature"

Gerdi Tuli,[1,2] Jessica Munarin,[1,2] Daniele Tessaris,[1,2] Raffaele Buganza,[1,2] Patrizia Matarazzo,[1,2] and Luisa De Sanctis[1,2]

[1]*Department of Pediatric Endocrinology, Regina Margherita Children's Hospital of Turin, Turin, Italy*
[2]*Department of Sciences of Public Health and Pediatrics, University of Turin, Turin, Italy*

Correspondence should be addressed to Gerdi Tuli; gerdi.tuli@unito.it

Academic Editor: Lucy Mastrandrea

Primary hyperparathyroidism (PHPT) is a rare disorder in children and adolescents. Typical biochemical features are hypercalcemia and hypophosphatemia, but the clinical features can be heterogeneous, and in some cases, symptoms are vague and nonspecific, leading to misdiagnosis or late diagnosis. Herein, we report two cases of PHPT in pediatric age with different presenting symptoms, pain in the foot, and progressive alteration of the gait in the first case and recurrent abdominal pain with emotional lability in the second. Biochemical and radiological assessment confirmed PHPT. Both cases were treated surgically as definitive treatment, but in the second case, previous medical treatment with cinacalcet, a calcimimetic agent, was required to reduce serum PTH and calcium levels. After surgery, despite conventional treatment with calcium and calcitriol, case 1 developed a hungry bone syndrome. The analysis of the MEN-1 (Multiple Endocrine Neoplasia) gene was negative in both cases. A diagnosis of PHPT should be considered when children or adolescents present bone pain with radiological imaging of osteolytic lesion and biochemical feature of hypercalcemia associated with hypophosphatemia. In PHPT, the gold standard treatment is represented by surgery followed by strict postoperative endocrine monitoring to maintain adequate homeostasis of calcium and bone metabolism.

1. Introduction

Primary hyperparathyroidism (PHPT), a rare disorder in pediatric age, with an estimated incidence of 2–5 cases in 100,000 live births, is characterized by excessive secretion of parathyroid hormone (PTH), responsible for hypercalcemia and hypophosphatemia [1–3]. Most cases of PHPT are not hereditary, and the familial PHPT accounts for 10–20% of cases [4–7].

The main clinical features involve the skeleton and the kidney. Bone pain, skeleton deformities, and the increased fracture risk at any skeleton sites are the most important symptoms. Rarely, the first manifestation of PHPT can be rickets or osteomalacia, associated with short stature [1,7]. Nephrocalcinosis and nephrolithiasis are the main complications of PHPT, and hypercalciuria is the most common risk factor for renal stone development.

Other clinical features related to PHPT include neurological symptoms (attention-deficit disorders, irritable behaviours, depression, weakness, seizures, proximal myopathy, and lethargy), gastrointestinal symptoms (vomiting, nausea, diarrhea, and acute pancreatitis), and cardiovascular complications, including prolonged QT interval (7–10).

Radiological assessment includes parathyroid and thyroid ultrasound and 99mTC-sestamibi scintigraphy, total body bone scintiscan, jaw X-ray, and X-ray evaluation of the skeletal site with bone pain.

The gold standard treatment in children is surgery [8, 9]. In the presence of severe hypercalcemia, parenteral isotonic solutions or calciomimetic agents such as cinacalcet, which lower serum calcium and PTH, but do not improve bone mass density (BMD), are required [10]. An alternative presurgical therapeutic option includes the use of bisphosphonates that improve BMD and lower biochemical markers of bone turnover in patients with PHPT, but have less effect on lowering calcium and PTH [7].

Similarly to adults, solitary parathyroid adenoma is the most common finding in children with sporadic PHPT [2, 11], but unlike in adult patients, PHPT symptoms are frequently present at diagnosis in pediatric age. However, in the absence of a family history of PHPT, since PHPT symptoms can be vague and nonspecific, the disease may be misdiagnosed or delayed in the diagnosis [8, 9, 11], especially in pubertal age, when rapid bone growth may unmask certain skeletal manifestations of PHPT [1, 2].

We report the clinical history of two female adolescents with PHPT who differed in clinical presentation at diagnosis, both referred to the pediatric endocrinologist 12 months after the onset of symptoms. In the first case, skeletal manifestations of osteolytic lesion at the right calcaneus were present, whereas in the second case, the main symptoms were abdominal pain and irritability.

2. Case Reports

2.1. Case 1. A 16-year-old girl of Philippine origin was referred to our department as she complained of right foot pain and progressive gait abnormalities in the last 12 months. Auxological parameters showed short stature (141.1 cm, <3° Tanner percentile), within a familial short stature context, and normal weight (48 kg, 10° Tanner percentile) and BMI (24.1 kg/m^2).

Radiographic evaluation of the lower limb demonstrated an osteolytic lesion to the right heel and a concomitant lesion of unclear interpretation to the left cuboid bone, both then confirmed at CT scan and MRI.

Biochemical investigations revealed elevated serum PTH levels (598 pg/ml; normal range 15–57), elevated serum calcium concentration (3.02 mmol/L; normal range 2.2–2.7), and low serum phosphate levels (0.56 mmol/L; normal range 1–1.8), as shown in Table 1. The urinary calcium to creatinine ratio was 0.25 mg/mg, and renal ultrasound and ECG were normal.

Total body bone scintiscan with 99Tc-oxidronate revealed increased absorption at the right heel, consistent with a brown tumor finding.

Parathyroid ultrasound did not show any significant pathological signs, but the Tc99/sestaMIBI parathyroid scan revealed an abnormal and persistent focal retention of the tracer in the right inferior thyroid pole, consistent with the hyperactivity of the right inferior parathyroid.

Therefore, the biochemical and radiological features indicated a PHPT condition; to rule out MEN-1, pituitary function was analyzed and showed normal hormonal profile. Fasting glucose, insulin, and calcitonin levels were normal; no lipoma, angiofibroma, or jaw tumors were present; both parents and siblings had normal serum PTH levels. Genetic analysis of the MEN-1 gene was negative for mutations.

The girl underwent right inferior parathyroidectomy through a minimally invasive approach, after intraoperative evaluation of the parathyroid hormone. Histological examination confirmed the presence of an adenoma (dimension 3.3 × 1.7 × 0.5 cm, weight 3 gr). To control the hypocalcemia caused by the transient hypoparathyroidism of the remaining parathyroid glands previously inhibited by the adenoma, conventional treatment with oral administration of calcitriol (0.75 mcg/day) and calcium carbonate was started; the latter was initially given at 2 g/day and then increased up to 3 g/day for numbness; finger paraesthesia and positive Chvostek and Trousseau signs were associated with low serum calcium despite high parathyroid hormone levels (Ca 1.85 mmol/L, PTH 113 ng/ml). Subsequently, the patient no longer presented signs or symptoms of hypocalcemia; laboratory analyses showed adequate calcium-phosphate metabolism and normal serum PTH levels (31 pg/ml).

Three months after surgery, biochemical evaluation again showed an increase in the PTH value (146 pg/ml), with sightly low serum calcium levels (2.02 mmol/L), configuring a hungry bone syndrome (HBS) condition, characterized by an elevated uptake of calcium by the bones after a prolonged period of hypercalcemia due to hyperparathyroidism. The oral calcium carbonate dose was, therefore, increased to 4 g/day, with normalization of serum calcium level (2.4 mmol/L) and partial response of PTH levels (67 pg/ml).

2.2. Case 2. A 14-year-old girl was referred to our department, having complained of recurrent abdominal pain and emotional lability for the last 12 months. Auxological parameters showed normal height (153.7 cm, 10–25° Tanner percentile), weight (47 kg, 10–25° Tanner percentile), and BMI (19.9 kg/m^2). Biochemical investigations revealed high serum calcium concentration (3.36 mmol/L, normal range 2.2–2.7), low phosphate level (0.6 mmol/L; normal range 1–1.8), and elevated PTH levels (320 pg/ml; normal range 15–57), as shown in Table 1.

The parathyroid ultrasound evaluation showed the presence of a hypoechoic nodule in the right inferior thyroid pole (22 × 12 mm), confirmed by the Tc99/sestaMIBI scan which revealed an abnormal and persistent retention of the tracer in the same area, therefore compatible with hyperactivity of the right inferior parathyroid.

To rule out the presence of multiple endocrine neoplasia, pituitary function was investigated and showed normal hormone secretion. Fasting glucose, insulin, and calcitonin levels were normal, and no lipoma, angiofibroma, or jaw tumors were present; parents and siblings had normal serum PTH levels. Genetic analysis for MEN-1 mutations was negative.

The urinary calcium/creatinine ratio was 0.35 mg/mg, and abdominal ultrasound displayed the presence of a small hyperechoic image (5 mm) in the upper pole of the right kidney, consistent with nephrolithiasis, although asymptomatic. Spinal X-ray showed generalized bone rarefaction, evident in all vertebral bodies, and the whole-body bone scan revealed regular ^{99}Tc-oxidronate uptake.

Biochemical and radiological investigations confirmed the diagnosis of PHPT. Prior to surgery, as high serum calcium levels represented a high intraoperative risk, treatment with a calcimimetic agent (cinacalcet) was started,

TABLE 1: Laboratory data of cases reported at diagnosis, after surgery, and at the last evaluation.

		Case 1	Case 2
	Diagnosis	3.02	3.36
Serum calcium (mmol/l)	After surgery	1.85	2.35
	Last evaluation	2.3	2.3
	Diagnosis	0.56	0.6
Phosphate (mmol/l)	After surgery	0.84	1.04
	Last evaluation	0.84	1.13
	Diagnosis	598	320
PTH (pg/ml)	After surgery	113	131
	Last evaluation	67	46
	Diagnosis	6.8*	16.2*
25-hydroxyvitamin D (ng/ml)	After surgery	—	61.9*
	Last evaluation	—	43*
	Diagnosis	0.25	0.35
CaU/CrU	After surgery	0.06	0.1
	Last evaluation	0.01	0.05
Adenoma weight (gr)		3	2.5

at 60 mg/day dose for three months, with an improvement in calcium and phosphate metabolism (Ca 2.97 mmol/L, P 0.6 mmol/L), with still elevated PTH levels (457.9 pg/mL). Since cinacalcet is an off-label drug in pediatric age, permission of the local Ethics Committee and informed consent from the parents were obtained prior to its administration.

The girl, therefore, underwent right inferior parathyroidectomy through a mini-invasive approach, with intraoperative monitoring of the PTH; histological examination confirmed the presence of adenomatous tissue (dimension 2,5 × 1.4 × 0.5 cm, weight 2.5 gr). Biochemical investigations after surgery showed a rapid decrease in calcium level (2.35 mmol/L), with lowering of PTH levels (131 pg/ml); subsequently, as the girl had lip and finger tremors with mild hypocalcemia (Ca 2.01 mmol/L), conventional treatment with oral administration of calcium carbonate (1 g/day) and oral calcitriol (62.5 mcg/day) was started, with no further signs or symptoms of hypocalcemia and normalization of calcium-phosphate homeostasis and normal level of PTH (46 pg/ml) on biochemical monitoring. Calcium treatment was stopped after one month, while calcitriol after two years; currently, after 6 years from the onset of primary hyperparathyroidism, there is no recurrence of the disease and calcium-phosphate metabolism is adequate.

3. Discussion

PHPT is a very rare condition among children and adolescents; Table 2 indicates the data emerging from the literature describing pediatric cohorts with at least 5 subjects [1–25, 27].

The two cases of PHPT reported here showed a different clinical onset at diagnosis, with bone pain in the first case and vague symptoms such as abdominal pain and behavioural problems in the second. Both patients were referred to the pediatric endocrinologist 12 months after the onset of symptoms.

The first presented case highlights that, in case of laboratory data suggestive for PHPT, even in the presence of US of the neck negative for pathological findings, a Tc^{99}/sestaMIBI parathyroid scan has to be performed [9]. Once PHPT is confirmed, if bone pain is present, an X-ray of the syntomatic skeletal site and of the jaw and whole-body scintiscan should be performed, as well as an ECG evaluation.

Parathyroid adenoma represents the most frequent PHPT etiology in pediatric age, with higher aggressive behaviour than adults and higher serum and urinary calcium levels.

It is noteworthy that, in the presence of significant hypercalcemia, especially if associated with cardiac arrhythmia, the intraoperative risk is high; therefore, in such cases, the utilization of a calcimimetic agent, i.e., cinacalcet (Mimpara) or bisphosphonates, for short periods could allow to lower calcium levels, despite high levels of PTH, and to act in a safer surgical context, although few data on their use as calcium-lowering agents in pediatric age are present in the literature so far.

After successful removal of one or more hyperfunctioning parathyroid glands, patients with PHPT show a rapid transient decrease in serum calcium levels due to functional inhibition of healthy parathyroid glands. This hypocalcemia is generally mild, lasts a maximum of 2–4 days after surgery, and is independent of the size of the hyperactive glands [26, 28]. Conventional treatment with oral calcium and calcitriol is the gold standard for this condition. However, in case of long-standing PHPT, hungry bone syndrome (HBS) can occur, as shown in the first case presented. This term has been coined to represent the deep (Ca < 2.1 mmol/l) and prolonged (longer than four days after operation) hypocalcemia, following parathyroidectomy in severe hyperparathyroidism [29].

At the time of presentation, nearly 80% of children are symptomatic and have end-organ damage, mostly involving the bone and kidney [2]. The condition can manifest with various signs and symptoms related to hypercalcemia, involving the gastrointestinal, musculoskeletal, renal, and neurological systems; such nonspecific clinical presentation may, therefore, be responsible for misdiagnosis or delayed diagnosis. In the presence of such symptoms, pediatricians should be aware of monitoring bone metabolism, evaluating serum calcium and phosphate levels, as well as PTH, when bone pain or nephrocalcinosis is also present.

Once PHPT is diagnosed in pediatric age, genetic analysis for Multiple Endocrine Neoplasia (MEN) syndromes and PTH assessment, as well as X-ray of jaw and urinary calcium to creatinine ratio, in parents and siblings should be carried out to search for genetic or familial conditions [30].

In conclusion, PHPT is a rare disease in pediatric age that can be misdiagnosed; the presence of PHPT should be considered if children or adolescents present with bone pain or nephrocalcinosis, radiological imaging of osteolytic lesions, or vague gastrointestinal or neurological not otherwise explained.

TABLE 2: Main papers reporting patients with PHPT in the pediatric age.

Author	Year	No. of pediatric patients	Main results
Allo et al. [12]	1982	53	Adenoma in 64.2% of studied patients; hyperplasia in 30.2%, overall in <18 y.o. (38%) vs. >18 y.o. (18.5%) patients
Lawson et al. [13]	1996	11	All sporadic PHPT. Delayed diagnosis in children; at diagnosis, 91% patients were symptomatic (renal stones 45%, abdominal pain 18%, learning difficulties 18%, musculoskeletal abnormalities 9%, and fatigue 9%). Mean serum Ca^{++}: 3.39 mmol/l at diagnosis
Cronin et al. [14]	1996	8	Pediatric cohort with PHPT due to parathyroid adenoma, presenting mostly with hypercalcemic crisis (50%). Mean serum Ca^{++}: 3.5 mmol/l at diagnosis
Loh et al. [15]	1998	22	Pediatric cohort with PHPT due to parathyroid adenoma, presenting mostly with fatigue (77%) or weakness (64%). Mean serum Ca^{++}: 3.07 mmol/l; mean serum PTH 131 pg/ml at diagnosis
Harman et al. [16]	1999	33	Pediatric cohort with PHPT due to parathyroid adenoma, symptomatic in 94% of cases, mostly renal stones (7/33) and bone disease (9/33). Mean serum Ca^{++}: 3.02 mmol/l at diagnosis; mean adenoma weight 0.96 gr
Hsu and Levine [17]	2002	16	Single adenomas in 11 patients; multiple-gland disease in 2 patients, including 1 with MEN2
Kollars et al. [2]	2005	52	Symptomatic in 79% of cases; end-organ damage (nephrocalcinosis or lithiasis, acute pancreatitis, or bone involvement) in 44%. Mean serum Ca^{++}: 3.1 mmol/l; mean serum P 1.8 mmol/l; mean serum PTH 76.3 pg/ml at diagnosis
Bhadada et al. [18]	2008	14	Single parathyroid adenoma in 85.7%, 1 patient with four-gland hyperplasia and 1 MEN-1. Main reported symptoms were bone disease, recurrent nephrolithiasis, and pancreatitis. Mean serum Ca^{++}: 2.77 mmol/l; mean P 0.9 mmol/l; mean serum PTH 781 pg/ml at diagnosis
Libansky et al. [19]	2008	10	Pediatric cohort with parathyroid adenoma and 1 ectopic adenoma. Mean serum Ca^{++}: 3.21 mmol/l; mean serum PTH 217.6 pg/ml at diagnosis
Mallet E [4]	2008	55	31 adenomas and 11 hyperplasias underwent surgery. Medical management (i.v. diphosphonates) in 11 neonates. Mean serum Ca^{++}: 3.64 mmol/l; mean serum P 1.3 mmol/l; mean serum PTH 536 pg/ml at diagnosis
Al-shanafey et al. [20]	2010	5	Surgical management in neonates with severe hyperparathyroidism, all symptomatic with lethargy, poor feeding, and irritability. In all patients, surgical treatment was curative. Mean serum Ca^{++}: 3.84 mmol/l; mean serum PTH 3607 pg/ml at diagnosis
George et al. [5]	2010	15	Single parathyroid adenoma in 100% of patients. Main reported symptoms were bone pain, fractures, proximal myopathy, and renal calculi; 33.3% had postoperative HBS. Mean serum Ca^{++}: 3.35 mmol/l; mean serum P 0.98 mmol/l; mean serum PTH 801 pg/ml at diagnosis; mean adenoma weight 3.84 gr
Shah et al. [21]	2012	19	Pediatric cohort with adenoma, presenting mostly bone pain (68%), weakness (68%), or fractures (52.6%)
Li et al. [22]	2012	12	Parathyroid adenoma in 100% (4/12 ectopic adenoma), presenting mostly urinary and bone tissue impairment. Mean serum Ca^{++}: 3.82 mmol/l; mean serum P 1.18 mmol/l; mean serum PTH 1016 pg/ml at diagnosis
Belcher et al. [8]	2013	230	Literature review of studies regarding PHPT in the youth and adolescents. Single adenomas in 80% of patients, multiple-gland hyperplasia in 16.5% (MGH), double adenomas in 0.9%, and normal parathyroid gland in 2.6%. Of MGH, 50% were MEN I, MEN II, or familial non-MEN. Tc(99m)-sestamibi and ultrasound were 86% (37/43) and 74.5% (70/94) sensitive
Burke et al. [27	2013	19	Study aiming to enhance the radioguided parathyroidectomy. Adenoma in 74% and hyperplasia in 26%. No complications were noted in the pediatric patients after surgery. Mean serum Ca^{++}: 3.05 mmol/; mean serum PTH 177 pg/ml at diagnosis. Mean serum Ca^{++}: 2.35 mmol/; mean serum PTH 33 pg/ml after the surgery. Mean adenoma weight 0.44 gr
Alagaratnam S and Kurzawinski [9]	2014	29	Pediatric cohort with adenoma presenting mostly gastrointestinal symptoms (41%) and skeletal manifestations (20.7%)
Roizen and Levine [6]	2014	268	A meta-analysis comparing biochemical profiles in the youth and adults: greater hypercalcemia and hypercalciuria in youths at similar concentrations of serum intact PTH. Mean serum Ca^{++}: 3.2 mmol/; mean serum P 0.9 mmol/l; mean serum PTH 331 pg/ml; mean ALP 995 UI/l at diagnosis. Mean gland weight 2 gr
Mancilla et al. [23]	2017	16	Pediatric cohort with parathyroid and thymic (2/16) adenoma, mostly symptomatic (75%). Mean serum Ca^{++}: 3.02 mmol/; mean serum PTH 177.3 pg/ml at diagnosis

Table 2: Continued.

Author	Year	No. of pediatric patients	Main results
Lou et al. [11]	2017	40	Pediatric cohort with different patterns at diagnosis; increasing rate of diagnosis in asymptomatic subjects, higher postoperative complications, and disease recurrence in patients with positive familial history. Mean serum Ca^{++}: 2.91 mmol/; mean serum PTH 152.5 pg/ml at diagnosis
Vannucci et al. [24]	2018	22	Pediatric cohort with MEN-1 mutation presenting PHPT in 50% of cases, mostly asymptomatic (10/11)
Saponaro et al. [25]	2018	31	Young and adult population with PHPT: significantly lower PTH, higher serum in the younger group. Nephrolithiasis, fragility, fracture, and densitometric parameter rates did not differ between groups. Mean serum Ca^{++}: 2.73 mmol/; mean serum P 0.77 mmol/l; mean serum 25-hydroxyvitamin D 19.6 ng/ml, mean serum PTH 111 pg/ml; mean ALP 232 UI/l at diagnosis
Wang et al. [7]	2018	59	Pediatric cohort reporting bone pain as the most common manifestation, high rate of rickets (45.8%) compared to adults (23.7%), and an important correlation to short stature. Hypercalciuria, more frequent in pediatrics, hypophosphatemia, and urolithiasis among adults. Mean serum Ca^{++}: 3.01 mmol/; mean serum PTH 177 pg/ml; mean serum ALP 374 UI/l; mean serum 25-hydroxyvitamin D 12.9 ng/ml at diagnosis
Rampp et al. [26]	2020	86	Pediatric cohort with parathyroid and thymic (22/86) adenoma presenting systemic and neurocognitive symptoms in 64% and nephrolithiasis in 20%. Mean serum Ca^{++}: 2.93 mmol/; mean serum PTH 110 pg/ml at diagnosis. Mean gland weight 0.3 gr. Mean serum Ca^{++}: 2.42 mmol/l after the surgery
Jovanovic et al. [3]	2020	14	Adults and youth comparison; bone disease in the youth (42.9%) and asymptomatic disease in adults (39.3%). Preoperative serum calcium and PTH significantly higher in the youth than in adults. Mean serum Ca^{++}: 3.47 mmol/; mean serum P 0.8 mmol/l; mean serum PTH 572.6 pg/ml at diagnosis. Mean serum Ca^{++}: 2.42 mmol/; mean serum P 0.92 mmol/l; mean serum PTH 22.8 pg/ml; 25-hydroxyvitamin D 39.5 ng/ml after the surgery

References

[1] A. A. Khan, D. A. Hanley, R. Rizzoli et al., "Primary hyperparathyroidism: review and recommendations on evaluation, diagnosis, and management. A Canadian and international consensus," *Osteoporosis International*, vol. 28, no. 1, pp. 1–19, 2017.

[2] J. Thakker, A. E. Zarroug, J. Van Heerden et al., "Primary hyperparathyroidism in pediatric patients," *Pediatrics*, vol. 115, no. 4, pp. 974–980, 2005.

[3] M. Moir, I. Paunovic, V. Zdravkovic et al., "Case-control study of primary hyperparathyroidism in juvenile vs. adult patients," *International Journal of Pediatric Otorhinolaryngology*, vol. 131, Article ID 109895, 2020.

[4] E. Slijepcevic, "Primary hyperparathyroidism in neonates and childhood," *Hormone Research in Paediatrics*, vol. 69, no. 3, pp. 180–188, 2008.

[5] J. George, S. V. Acharya, T. R. Bandgar, P. S. Menon, and N. S. Shah, "Primary hyperparathyroidism in children and adolescents," *The Indian Journal of Pediatrics*, vol. 77, no. 2, pp. 175–17810, 2010.

[6] J. Roizen and M. A. Levine, "A meta-analysis comparing the biochemistry of primary hyperparathyroidism in youths to the biochemistry of primary hyperparathyroidism in adults," *The Journal of Clinical Endocrinology & Metabolism*, vol. 99, no. 12, pp. 4555–4564, 2014.

[7] W. Wang, J. Kong, M. Nie et al., "Primary hyperparathyroidism in Chinese children and adolescents: a single-centre experience at peking union medical college hospital," *Clinical Endocrinology*, vol. 87, no. 6, pp. 865–873, 2017.

[8] R. Meng, A. M. Metrailer, D. L. Bodenner, and B. C. Stack, "Characterization of hyperparathyroidism in youth and adolescents: a literature review," *International Journal of Pediatric Otorhinolaryngology*, vol. 77, no. 3, pp. 318–322, 2013.

[9] S. Alagaratnam and T. R. Kurzawinski, "Aetiology, diagnosis and surgical treatment of primary hyperparathyroidism in children: new trends," *Hormone Research in Paediatrics*, vol. 83, no. 6, pp. 365–37510, 2015.

[10] P. Schwarz, J. J. Body, J. Cáp et al., "The PRIMARA study: a prospective, descriptive, observational study to review cinacalcet use in patients with primary hyperparathyroidism in clinical practice," *European Journal of Endocrinology*, vol. 171, no. 6, pp. 727–73510, 2014.

[11] I. Lou, D. F. Schneider, R. S. Sippel, H. Chen, and D. M. Elfenbein, "The changing pattern of diagnosing primary hyperparathyroidism in young patients," *The American Journal of Surgery*, vol. 213, no. 1, pp. 146–15010, 2017.

[12] M. Kuhn, N. W. Thompson, J. K. Harness, and R. H. Nishiyama, "Primary hyperparathyroidism in children, adolescents, and young adults," *World Journal of Surgery*, vol. 6, no. 6, pp. 771–77510, 1982.

[13] M. L. Lawson, S. F. Miller, G. Ellis, R. M. Filler, and S. W. Kooh, "Primary hyperparathyroidism in a paediatric hospital," *QJM: An International Journal of Medicine*, vol. 89, no. 12, pp. 921–932, 1996.

[14] C. Cronin, T. Reeve, B. Robinson, P. Clifton-Bligh, A. Guinea, and L. Delbridge, "Primary hyperparathyroidism in childhood and adolescence," *Journal of Paediatrics and Child Health*, vol. 32, no. 5, pp. 397–39910, 1996.

[15] K.-C. Loh, Q.-Y. Duh, D. Shoback, L. Gee, A. Siperstein, and O. H. Clark, "Clinical profile of primary hyperparathyroidism

in adolescents and young adults," *Clinical Endocrinology*, vol. 48, no. 4, pp. 435–443, 1998.

[16] C. R. Harman, J. A. van Heerden, D. R. Farley, C. S. Grant, G. B. Thompson, and K. Curlee, "Sporadic primary hyperparathyroidism in young patients," *Archives of Surgery*, vol. 134, no. 6, pp. 651–655, 1999.

[17] S. C. Hsu and M. A. Levine, "Primary hyperparathyroidism in children and adolescents: the Johns Hopkins Children's Center experience," *Journal of Bone and Mineral Research*, vol. 17, no. 2, pp. N44–N50, 2002.

[18] S. K. Bhadada, A. Bhansali, P. Dutta, A. Behera, G. V. Chanukya, and B. R. Mittal, "Characteristics of primary hyperparathyroidism in adolescents," *Journal of Pediatric Endocrinology and Metabolism*, vol. 21, no. 12, pp. 1147–1153, 2008.

[19] P. Libánský, J. Astl, S. Adámek et al., "Surgical treatment of primary hyperparathyroidism in children: report of 10 cases," *International Journal of Pediatric Otorhinolaryngology*, vol. 72, no. 8, pp. 1177–1182, 2008.

[20] S. Foltán, R. Al-Hosaini, A. Al-Ashwal, and A. Al-Rabeeah, "Surgical management of severe neonatal hyperparathyroidism: one center's experience," *Journal of Pediatric Surgery*, vol. 45, no. 4, pp. 714–717, 2010.

[21] V. N. Shah, S. K. Bhadada, A. Bhansali, A. Behera, B. R. Mittal, and V. Bhavin, "Influence of age and gender on presentation of symptomatic primary hyperparathyroidism," *Journal of Postgraduate Medicine*, vol. 58, no. 2, pp. 107–111, 2012.

[22] C.-C. Li, C. Yang, S. Wang, J. Zhang, X.-R. Kong, and J. Ouyang, "A 10-year retrospective study of primary hyperparathyroidism in children," *Experimental and Clinical Endocrinology & Diabetes*, vol. 120, no. 04, pp. 229–233, 2012.

[23] E. E. Mancilla, M. A. Levine, and N. S. Adzick, "Outcomes of minimally invasive parathyroidectomy in pediatric patients with primary hyperparathyroidism owing to parathyroid adenoma: a single institution experience," *Journal of Pediatric Surgery*, vol. 52, no. 1, pp. 188–191, 2017.

[24] L. Vannucci, F. Marini, F. Giusti, S. Ciuffi, F. Tonelli, and M. L. Brandi, "MEN1 in children and adolescents: data from patients of a regional referral center for hereditary endocrine tumors," *Endocrine*, vol. 59, no. 2, pp. 438–448, 2018.

[25] F. Saponaro, C. Marcocci, F. Cacciatore et al., "Clinical profile of juvenile primary hyperparathyroidism: a prospective study," *Endocrine*, vol. 59, no. 2, pp. 344–352, 2018.

[26] R. D. Materazzi, E. E. Mancilla, N. S. Adzick et al., "Single gland, ectopic location: adenomas are common causes of primary hyperparathyroidism in children and adolescents," *World Journal of Surgery*, vol. 44, no. 5, pp. 1518–1525, 2020.

[27] J. F. Burke, K. Jacobson, A. Gosain, R. S. Sippel, and H. Chen, "Radioguided parathyroidectomy effective in pediatric patients," *Journal of Surgical Research*, vol. 184, no. 1, pp. 312–317, 2013.

[28] J. E. Iyer, S. Van Thiel, J. A. Romijn, and N. A. T. Hamdy, "Therapy OF endocrine disease: hungry bone syndrome: still a challenge in the post-operative management of primary hyperparathyroidism: a systematic review of the literature," *European Journal of Endocrinology*, vol. 168, no. 3, pp. R45–R5310, 2013.

[29] J. Westerdahl, P. Lindblom, S. Valdemarsson, S. Tibblin, and A. Bergenfelz, "Risk factors for postoperative hypocalcemia after surgery for primary hyperparathyroidism," *Archives of Surgery*, vol. 135, no. 2, pp. 142–147, 2000.

[30] C. D. C. Kamilaris and C. A. Stratakis, "Multiple endocrine neoplasia type 1 (MEN1): an update and the significance of early genetic and clinical diagnosis," *Front Endocrinol (Lausanne)*, vol. 11, 2019.

10

New-Onset Diabetes in Children during COVID-19: Clinical Case Report

M. Aabdi,[1] **A. Aarab**,[2] **O. Es-Saad,[1] K. Malki,[1] H. Bkiyar,[1] and B. Housni[1]**

[1]*Anesthesiology and Intensive Care Unit Department, MOHAMMED VI University Hospital Center, Oujda, Morocco*
[2]*Laboratory Unit Department, MOHAMMED VI University Hospital Center, Oujda, Morocco*

Correspondence should be addressed to M. Aabdi; med.aabdi@gmail.com

Academic Editor: Suat Simsek

Introduction. Data of COVID-19 in newborns and children are limited, and clinical manifestations are nonspecific and might delay the diagnosis, which might lead to severe complications. In this clinical case, we will describe new-onset diabetes with consciousness impairment as an atypical revealing way of COVID-19. *Case.* A 3-year-old child presented to the Emergency Department with loss of consciousness (without fever), lethargy, and stupor. Clinical assessment on admission found an unconscious child with a pediatric Glasgow Coma Scale of 10/15 with no localizing signs or meningeal syndrome, polypneic of 35 breaths/min, pulse oximetry of 90%, with signs of overall dehydration: skin folds, sunken eyes, tachycardia of 160 beats/minute, and recoloring time superior at 3 seconds. Laboratory findings showed hyperleukocytosis of 16000/mm^3, lymphopenia of 450/mm^3, glycemia of 5 g/L with a correct ionogram : corrected natremia of 139 mmol/L, serum potassium of 4.5 mmol/L, glycosuria of 3+, ketonuria of 2+, and HbA1c of 10%, and COVID-19 RT-PCR came back positive. *Conclusion.* COVID-19 might be revealed with atypical symptoms including new-onset diabetes and diabetic ketoacidosis; therefore, clinicians must suspect it in children with blood glucose and HbA1c at the time of admission. This will help to manage patients with hyperglycemia early.

1. Introduction

From March 2020, Anesthesiology and Intensive Care Unit Department, Mohammed VI University Hospital Center, Oujda, Morocco, has been facing an unprecedented outbreak of coronavirus disease and spread of 2019 novel coronavirus or severe acute respiratory syndrome coronavirus 2 (SARS-CoV-2), which has now become a global pandemic [1, 2]. The disease caused by SARS-CoV-2 was termed "COVID-19," and the World Health Organization declared the COVID-19 outbreak a public health emergency of international concern and officially was declared a pandemic on March 11, 2020 [2].

Data from the early months of 2020 suggest that there is a bidirectional relationship between COVID-19 and diabetes [3]. Diabetes is associated and is continuously suggested as a risk factor that contributes to the severity and mortality of COVID-19 [1]. Multiple forms of diabetes might be observed in patients with COVID-19 including new-onset diabetes and metabolic complications such as diabetic ketoacidosis and hyperosmolarity [4]. Nonetheless, data on new-onset type 1 diabetes during the COVID-19 pandemic, particularly in children, are limited [5]. In this article, we describe a clinical case of a 3-year-old child who presented to the Emergency Department (ED) in a ketoacidosis decompensation state, a recent diagnosis with COVID-19 infection, and who was retrospectively diagnosed with new-onset diabetes.

2. Clinical Case

A 3-year-old child presented to the ED with loss of consciousness (without fever), lethargy, and stupor. Clinical assessment on admission found an unconscious child with a pediatric Glasgow Coma Scale (GCS) of 10/15 with no localizing signs or meningeal syndrome, polypneic of 35 breaths/min, pulse oximetry of 90%, with signs of overall dehydration (skin folds), sunken eyes, tachycardia of 160 beats/minute, and recoloring time superior at 3 seconds.

Laboratory findings showed hyperleukocytosis of 16000 mm^3, lymphopenia of 450 mm^3, glycemia of 5 g/L with a correct ionogram : corrected natremia of 139 mmol/L, serum potassium of 4.5 mmol/L, glycosuria of 3+, ketonuria of 2+, and HbA1c of 10%.

Brain computed tomography (CT) came back normal; the search for a primary infection site led us to carry out a chest X-ray showing an alveolar-interstitial syndrome (Figure 1), supplemented by a thoracic CT revealing a bilateral ground-glass opacification consistent with viral pneumopathy, with moderate impairment with a level of suspicion scored CO-RADS 4 (Figure 2). Given the epidemiological context, a COVID-19 RT-PCR came back positive.

Diabetic ketoacidosis (DKA) is the most common hyperglycemic emergency and is associated with increased morbidity and mortality. In children and adolescents with type 1 diabetes, DKA accounts for the most common cause of death. DKA is characterized by hyperglycemia, ketosis, and metabolic acidosis [6].

Management of DKA consisted of rehydration with Ringer's lactate 20 ml/kg initially and physiological serum as well as insulin therapy with a dose of 0.05 IU/kg/h along with monitoring of blood sugar levels and any complications. The prognosis was favorable with neurological, respiratory, and metabolic improvement; the child was transferred to the pediatric endocrinology department for further assessment.

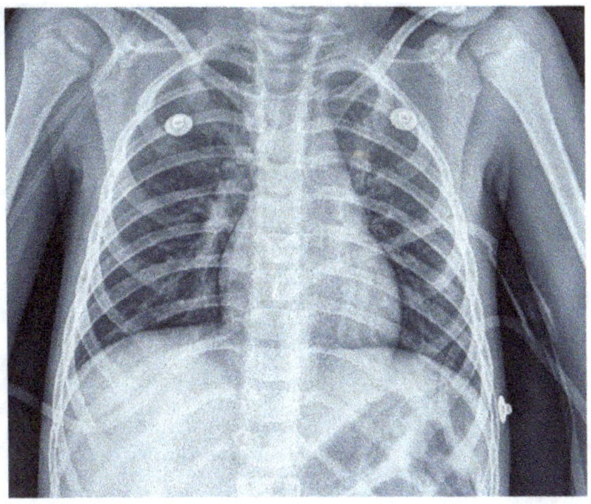

FIGURE 1: Chest X-ray showing an alveolar-interstitial syndrome.

3. Discussion

Coronaviruses are positive-strand ribonucleic, large viruses. Only two genera of the viruses can infect humans: a and b types, and they are called human coronaviruses (HCoVs) [7].

HCoVs are used to be mild phenotypes in humans because of their inconsequential pathogenic effect. However, two epidemics emerging in the early 21st century (severe acute respiratory syndrome (SARS) and Middle East respiratory syndrome (MERS)) with a high rate of morbidity and mortality changed the knowledge about this [8].

COVID-19 is generally more frequent among adults more than 15 years old with less confirmed cases among children [9]. However, the number of children infected has increased due to the pathogen detection campaigns and the lack of protective measures [10].

A report of a multicenter regional data from North West London of new-onset type 1 diabetes and DKA in children has estimated an increase of 80% of new type 1 diabetes cases during the COVID-19 pandemic and postulates that COVID-19 exposure contributed to the observed increase in cases by precipitating or accelerating type 1 diabetes onset [5]. A previous paper reported that children accounted for 5% of confirmed COVID-19 cases and presented with a milder disease symptom, and they have a better prognosis compared with adults, with very low mortality rate [7, 9]. But children with newly diagnosed diabetes, either it is new--onset or previously undiagnosed, tend to have increased levels of inflammatory markers and indicators of multiorgan injury leading to severe or critical illness of COVID-19 [11]. They also present severe hyperglycemic complications such as DKA and hyperosmolar hyperglycemic syndrome requiring high doses of insulin [12]. COVID-19 patients with newly diagnosed diabetes have higher mortality rate than those with known diabetes [11].

The pathophysiological mechanisms implicated with the increased frequency and severity of COVID-19 in people with diabetes are not yet elucidated, and several hypotheses have been elaborated to explain the link between COVID-19 and high rate and worst outcomes in diabetic people [2].

Diabetes is associated with an increased risk of infections, including viral ones due to defects in the innate immunity affecting phagocytosis, neutrophil chemotaxis, and cell-mediated immunity [1, 13]. Besides, diabetes and insulin resistance are associated with endothelial dysfunction and increased platelet aggregation and activation leading to the hypercoagulable prothrombotic state [13]. The latter associated with the low-grade chronic inflammation might promote the cytokine storm, a severe complication of COVID-19 characterized by excessive production of inflammatory cytokines [14]. Furthermore, COVID-19 spike protein gains entry to its target cells by using the angiotensin-converting enzyme 2 (ACE2) as the receptor, which has protective effects primarily regarding inflammation [1]. COVID-19 infection reduces ACE2 expression inducing cellular damage, hyperinflammation, and respiratory failure and can lead to a direct effect on β-cell function, which not only explains that diabetes might be a risk factor for a severe form of COVID-19 disease but also explains that infection could induce new-onset diabetes [1, 9, 15–18].

New-onset diabetes must be detected in all nondiabetic patients especially those at high risk for metabolic disease who have contracted the viral infection. Besides, most patients present multiple stresses with COVID-19 including respiratory failure and sepsis requiring intravenous infusion of insulin and fluid balance to control the glycemia levels [19]. In addition, potassium balance must be carefully considered in the context of insulin treatment, as hypokalemia is a common feature of COVID-19 and may be exacerbated after the introduction of insulin [19].

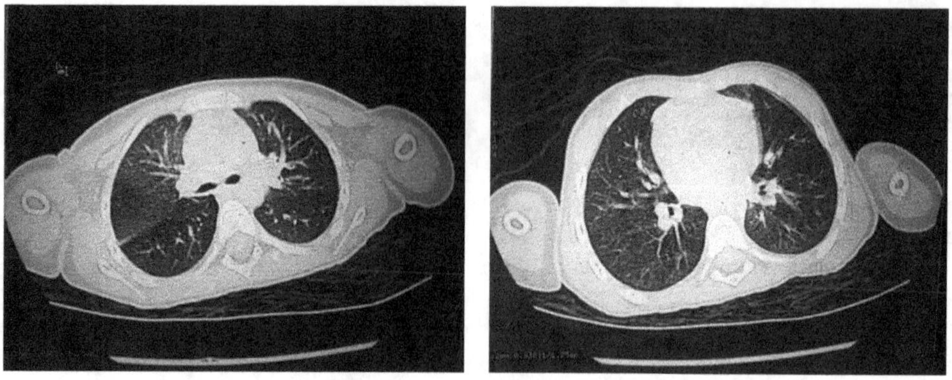

(a) (b)

FIGURE 2: Chest CT scan showing images in favor of pneumopathy COVID-19 CO-RADS 4.

4. Conclusion

This clinical case supports the strong link between COVID-19 infection and diabetes. Therefore, physicians should consider this in all nondiabetic children and screen them at their admission with blood glucose and HbA1C for appropriate and early management.

Consent

Written informed consent was obtained from the child holder for publication of this case report and accompanying images.

Authors' Contributions

Dr. Aabdi Mohammed contributed to conceptualization, methodology, validation, formal analysis, and visualization and wrote the original draft. Dr. Aarab Adnane contributed to formal analysis and visualization and reviewed and edited the manuscript. Dr. Es-Saad Ounci provided resources and developed software and was responsible for data curation. Dr. Malki Khalil, Pr. Housni Brahim, and Pr. Houssam Bkiyar were responsible for visualization. Pr. Houssam Bkiyar reviewed and edited the manuscript. Pr. Housni Brahim was responsible for project administration; provided resources; contributed to conceptualization, methodology, and validation; and reviewed and edited the manuscript. Dr. Aarab Adnane, Dr. Es-Saad Ounci, Dr. Malki Khalil, Pr. Housni Brahim, and Pr. Houssam Bkiyar approved the final version of the manuscript.

Acknowledgments

The authors acknowledge the frontline medical staff working day and night in Morocco to rescue critical cases and protect the public health. The authors know that these great efforts are now and will be in the future crucial in overcoming COVID-19.

References

[1] S. R. Bornstein, F. Rubino, K. Khunti et al., "Practical recommendations for the management of diabetes in patients with COVID-19," *The Lancet Diabetes & Endocrinology*, vol. 8, no. 6, pp. 546–550, 2020.

[2] E. Papadokostaki, N. Tentolouris, and E. Liberopoulos, "COVID-19 and diabetes: what does the clinician need to know?" *Primary Care Diabetes*, vol. 14, no. 5, pp. 558–563, 2020.

[3] Y. Chen, X. Gong, L. Wang, and J. Guo, "Effects of hypertension, diabetes and coronary heart disease on COVID-19 diseases severity: a systematic review and meta-analysis MedRxiv," p. 280, 2020.

[4] M. Paul Zimmet, M. D. George Alberti, M. D. Stefan Bornstein et al., "New-onset diabetes in COVID-19," *The New England Journal of Medicine*, vol. 383, no. 8, pp. 787–789, 2020.

[5] R. Unsworth, S. Wallace, N. S. Oliver et al., "New-onset type 1 diabetes in children during COVID-19: multicenter regional findings in the UK," *Diabetes Care*, vol. 43, no. 11, pp. e170–e171, 2020.

[6] M. Fayfman, F. J. Pasquel, and G. E. Umpierrez, "Management of hyperglycemic crises," *Medical Clinics of North America*, vol. 101, no. 3, pp. 587–606, 2017.

[7] Y. Dong, Y. Dong, X. Mo, Y. Hu, X. Qi, and F. Jiang, "Epidemiology of COVID-19 among children in China," *Pediatrics*, vol. 145, no. 6, 2020.

[8] A. H. De Wilde, J. Eric, M. K. Snijder, and M. J. Van, "Host factors in coronavirus replication," in *Assessment & Evaluation in Higher Education*, p. 435, Springer International Publishing, New York, NY, USA, 2012, Available from: http://books.google.com/books?id=_DDwCqx6wpcC&printsec=frontcover&dq=unwritten+rules+of+phd+research&hl=&cd=1&source=gbs_api%255Cnpapers2://publication/uuid/48967E01-55F9-4397-B941-310D9C5405FA%255Cnhttp://medcontent.metapress.com/index/A65RM03P4874243N.p.

[9] J. She, L. Liu, and W. Liu, "COVID-19 epidemic: disease characteristics in children," *Journal of Medical Virology*, vol. 92, no. 7, pp. 747–754, 2020.

[10] C. Jiehao, X. Jin, L. Daojiong et al., "A case series of children with 2019 novel coronavirus infection: clinical and epidemiological features," *Clinical Infectious Diseases*, vol. 71, no. 6, pp. 1547–1551, 2020.

[11] T. Sathish, Y. Cao, and N. Kapoor, "Newly diagnosed diabetes in COVID-19 patients," *Primary Care Diabetes*, vol. 15, no. 1, p. 194, 2020.
[12] Y. Jie, S. Jia, H. Ng, and E. Yeoh, "Diabetic ketoacidosis precipitated by COVID-19 in a patient with newly diagnosed diabetes mellitus," *Diabetes Research and Clinical Practice*, vol. 164, Article ID 108166, 2020.
[13] W. Abu-ashour, L. Twells, J. Valcour et al., "The association between diabetes mellitus and incident infections : a systematic review and meta-analysis of observational studies," *BMJ Open Diabetes Research and Care*, vol. 5, no. 1, 2017.
[14] W. Guo, M. Li, Y. Dong et al., "Diabetes is a risk factor for the progression and prognosis of COVID-19," *Diabetes Metabolism Research and Reviews*, vol. 36, no. 6, Article ID e3319, 2020.
[15] S. M. Bindom and E. Lazartigues, "The sweeter side of ACE2: physiological evidence for a role in diabetes," *Molecular and Cellular Endocrinology*, vol. 302, no. 2, pp. 193–202, 2020.
[16] M. Apicella, M. C. Campopiano, M. Mantuano, L. Mazoni, A. Coppelli, and S. Del Prato, "COVID-19 in people with diabetes: understanding the reasons for worse outcomes," *The Lancet Diabetes & Endocrinology*, vol. 8, no. 9, pp. 782–792, 2020.
[17] J.-K. Guo, S.-S. Lin, X.-J. Ji, and L.-M. Guo, "Binding of SARS coronavirus to its receptor damages islets and causes acute diabetes," *Acta Diabetologica*, vol. 47, no. 3, pp. 193–199, 2010.
[18] L. Fang, G. Karakiulakis, and M. Roth, "Are patients with hypertension and diabetes mellitus at increased risk for COVID-19 infection?" *The Lancet Respiratory Medicine*, vol. 8, no. 4, p. e21, 2020.
[19] R. P. Dellinger, M. M. Levy, A. Rhodes et al., "Surviving sepsis campaign : international guidelines for management of severe sepsis and septic shock ," *Critical Care Medicine*, vol. 41, no. 2, pp. 580–637, 2013.

11

Endogenous Cushing's Syndrome with Precocious Puberty in an 8-Year-Old Boy due to a Large Unilateral Adrenal Adenoma

Muhammad Rajib Hossain,[1] Md. Mashiul Alam,[2] Junaid Nabi,[3] and Mahzabin Kibria[1]

[1] *Department of Medicine, Shaheed Suhrawardy Medical College Hospital, Sher-e-Bangla Nagar, Dhaka 1207, Bangladesh*
[2] *Department of Pediatrics, Dhaka Medical College Hospital, 100 Ramna, Dhaka 1000, Bangladesh*
[3] *Department of Surgery, Shaheed Suhrawardy Medical College Hospital, Sher-e-Bangla Nagar, Dhaka 1207, Bangladesh*

Correspondence should be addressed to Muhammad Rajib Hossain; rajibssmc@gmail.com

Academic Editors: M. T. Garcia-Buitrago, H. Hattori, H. Kang, and N. Sakane

Adrenocortical tumors (ACTs) causing Cushing's syndrome are extremely rare in children and adolescents. Bilateral macronodular adrenocortical disease which is a component of the McCune-Albright syndrome is the most common cause of endogenous Cushing's syndrome. We report the case of a boy with Cushing's syndrome who presented with obesity and growth retardation. The child was hypertensive. The biochemical evaluation revealed that his serum cortisol levels were 25.80 μg/dL, with a concomitant plasma ACTH level of 10.0 pg/mL and nonsuppressed serum cortisol on high-dose dexamethasone suppression test (HDDST) to be 20.38 μg/dL. Computed tomography of the abdomen demonstrated a $8 \times 6 \times 5$ cm left adrenal mass with internal calcifications. Following preoperative stabilization, laparotomy was carried out which revealed a lobulated left adrenal mass with intact capsule weighing 120 grams. Histopathological examination revealed a benign cortical neoplastic lesion, suggestive of adrenal adenoma; composed of large polygonal cells with centrally placed nuclei and prominent nucleoli without capsular and vascular invasion. On the seventh postoperative day, cortisol levels were within normal range indicating biochemical remission of Cushing's syndrome. On followup after three months, the patient showed significant clinical improvement and had lost moderate amount of weight and adrenal imaging was found to be normal.

1. Introduction

Adrenocortical tumors (ACTs) are quite rare in children and adolescents. Iatrogenic hypercortisolism is the most common cause of Cushing's syndrome (CS) in infancy and childhood [1]. In infants and children less than 7 years of age, adrenal tumors and predominantly malignant adrenal carcinoma constitute the most common causes of Cushing's syndrome [2] and that of those older than 7 years is ACTH secreting pituitary adenoma. ACTH-independent CS in children has been reported to be due to bilateral macronodular adrenocortical disease encountered in cases of McCune-Albright syndrome (MAS) [3]. The prevalence of the syndrome is reported to be between 1/100,000 and 1/1,000,000 and has been observed more commonly in females [4], with a tendency of severe presentation.

We report the case of an 8-year-old boy who was diagnosed with Cushing's syndrome due to a left sided adrenal adenoma who had presented with generalized obesity and growth retardation with features of precocious puberty. Subsequently, a left adrenal adrenalectomy was performed and clinical stabilization resulted in weight loss and biochemical resolution of Cushing's syndrome.

2. Case Report

An 8-year-old Bangladeshi boy presented to our out patient department (OPD) with complaints of gaining weight for the last 9 months. The parents were also concerned that the boy was not attaining the height according to his age. The child was born to nonconsanguineous parents at term, by

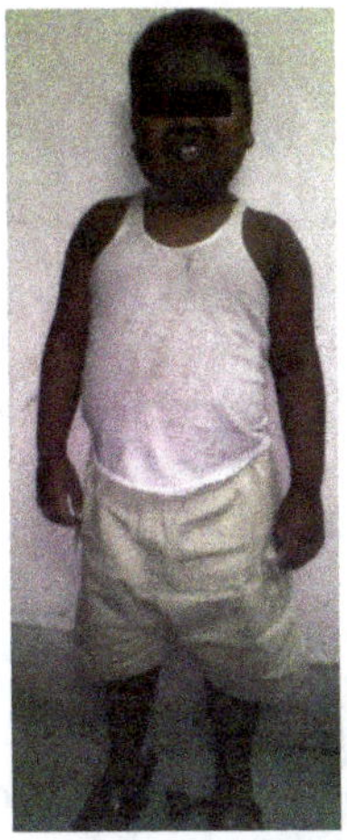

FIGURE 1: Typical appearance of Cushings syndrome (note moon face and abdominal distension).

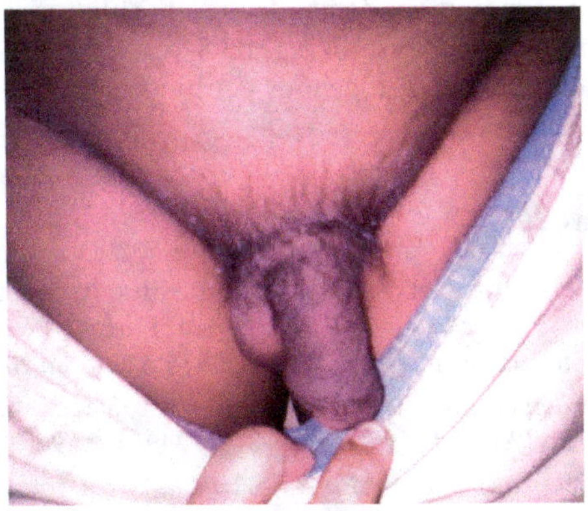

FIGURE 2: The unexpected finding of enlarged phallus more than normal for age and growth of child and coarse pubic hair.

normal vaginal delivery. Birth weight was 2.6 kg. Physical examination revealed a chubby boy with moon face and protruding abdomen (Figure 1). Increased body hair, striae, and other stigmata of MAS such as café-au-lait spots were absent. An unexpected finding was an abnormally large phallus with coarse pubic hair (Figure 2). On enquiry, the parents gave no history of steroid intake. His IQ scores were appropriate for his age and there was no history of voice change, and his sibling was in good health. The patient's body length was 92 cm (<3rd percentile; standard deviation score (SDS) −6.5) and his weight was 29 kg (80th percentile; SDS +1.6).

Blood pressure was 220/140 mmHg. Biochemical evaluation revealed a cortisol level of 25.80 μg/dL with a concurrent plasma ACTH level of 10.0 pg/mL (within normal limits). His serum cortisol following high-dose dexamethasone suppression test (HDDST) (0.25 mg of dexamethasone every 6 hours for 48 hours (20 μg/kg/dose)) was 20.38 μg/dL and fasting blood sugar was 110 mg/dL (Table 1).

Ultrasonography revealed a left suprarenal mass with parenchymal disease of kidneys. Patient underwent a contrast-enhanced abdominal computed tomography

TABLE 1: Biochemical evaluation of the patient.

Parameter	Value
An 8 am cortisol (μg/dL) (4.4–22.6)	25.80
ACTH (pg/mL) (4–20)	10.0
HDDST Cortisol (μg/dL) (41)	20.38
Fasting blood glucose (mg/dL) (119)	110
Sodium (mmol/L) (135–145)	138
Potassium (mmol/L) (3.0–5.5)	3.9
Creatinine (mg/dL) (0.4–1.2)	0.8
Hemoglobin (g/dL) (>11)	12.4

ACTH: adrenocorticotrophic hormone, HDDST: high-dose dexamethasone suppression test.

(CECT) scan which divulged a large, well-circumscribed mildly enhancing adrenal mass (8 × 6 × 5 cm approx.) having few internal calcifications at left suprarenal region, which had displaced left kidney slightly downwards (Figures 3 and 4).

The patient underwent left adrenal adrenalectomy following laparotomy, which revealed a 8.2 × 6.3 × 5.2 cm lobulated mass with capsule being intact and weighing 130 gm. There were no adhesions to adjacent organs, no lymphadenopathy, and the inferior vena was spared. Histopathological evaluation revealed a benign cortical neoplastic lesion, suggestive of adrenal adenoma, composed of large polygonal cells with centrally placed nuclei and abundant pale eosinophilic cytoplasm. Some of the cells showed endocrine atypia albeit capsular and vascular invasion being absent.

In the postoperative management, the patient was given hydrocortisone (I/M) which was tapered off slowly. After one week, cortisol levels were within normal limits demonstrating biochemical remission of Cushing's syndrome. There was also moderate decline in the weight of the patient. The patient was discharge on post-operative day 10. Followup was done after three months and patient had lost more weight and adrenal imaging was normal.

3. Discussion

The most common cause of hypercortisolism with clinical manifestations of Cushing's syndrome is administrationof synthetic glucocorticoids [5]. Pediatric adrenocortical tumors (ACTs) are rare in infancy and occur primarily in children between one and five years of age (60%), with a peak in incidence below 4 years of age (0.4 cases per million). Nearly half of these ACTs are adrenocortical carcinoma [6]. Adrenal cortical tumors (ACTs) constitute less than 0.2% of all pediatric neoplasms and account for 6% of all adrenal tumors in children with an estimated incidence of 0.3 million population [7]. There seems to be a bimodal incidence of these tumors, with one peak at under 5 years of age and the second one in the fourth or fifth decades of life. Increased androgen production in infancy and early childhood ACTs is attributed to the structure of the adrenal gland at the time of birth when the inner fetal zone constitutes 85%–90% of the gland; the primary steroid product of the inner fetal zone is dehydroepiandrosterone sulphate [8].

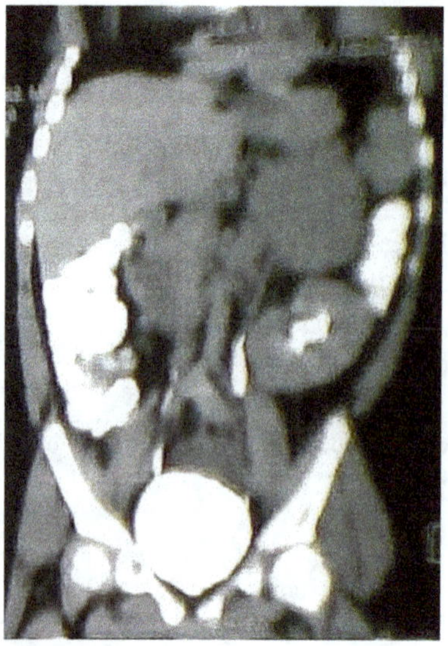

Figure 3: Contrast-enhanced abdominal computed tomography (CECT) scan in axial view revealed a large, well-circumscribed mildly enhancing adrenal mass (8 × 6 × 5 cm approx.) having few internal calcifications at left suprarenal region, which had displaced left kidney slightly downwards (arrow-mass; triangle-left kidney).

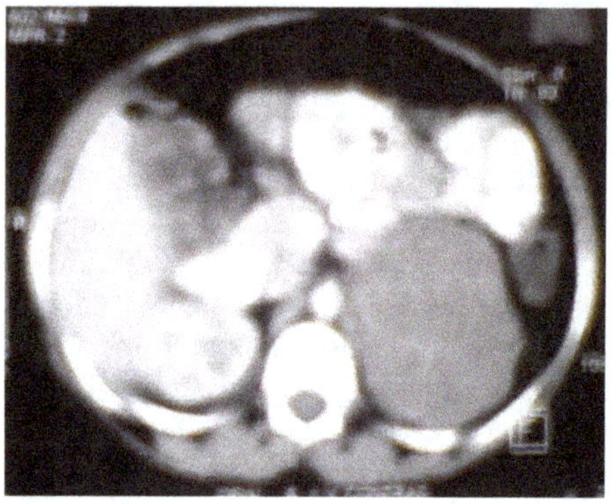

Figure 4: Enlarged view of CT scan image in cross section, showing a large well-circumscribed mildly enhancing mass having few calcification at left suprarenal region.

The physical changes that occur in Cushing's syndrome such as the moon face, hirsutism, and acne as well as the bulging of the cervicodorsal region (buffalo hump) are a result of the intense action of the glucocorticoids which favor the accumulation of fat in the abdomen, chest, and face (central obesity). Growth hormone and β-adrenergic receptor antagonists also induce lipolysis which facilitates increase in triglycerides and free fatty acids. Hypertension is a consequence of increased renin substrate and sodium retention, facilitating the expansion of extracellular volume. In our case, the patient presented with precocious puberty which is in line with the observations made by Michalkiewicz et al. [9] who found in a registry of 254 pediatric patients with ACTs that 55% with virilization alone. Twenty-nine percent presented with mixed overproduction of adrenal hormones. Only 5.5% percent of this group presented with isolated Cushings syndrome, and this tended to occur in older children (median age 12.6 years).

Several laboratory investigations are helpful in establishing the diagnosis and differentiating between suprarenal or hypophyseal origin. These include serum cortisol levels, plasma ACTH, and high-dose dexamethasone suppression test (HDDST) which has better sensitivity [10]. Radiological evaluation includes ultrasonography, computed tomography (CT) scan of abdomen, and MRI of the brain. CT scan has been shown to be more sensitive in identification and localization of tumor mass [11]. The recommended procedure is surgical removal of the tumor (adrenalectomy) [12], which resulted in rapid weight loss in our patient. Postoperative hydrocortisone supplementation following surgery for adrenal adenoma causing CS is necessary as the contralateral adrenal gland is usually hypoplastic secondary to prolonged suppressed ACTH secretion from the pituitary due to CS.

Pediatric adrenocortical tumors (ACTs) are most commonly encountered in females and in children less than four years. But our case being an 8-year-old boy forms a rare presentation of endogenous Cushing's syndrome due to adrenal adenoma.

References

[1] C. J. Migeon and R. Lanes, "Adrenal cortex: hypo and hyperfunction," in *Pediatric Endocrinology*, F. Lifshitz, Ed., vol. 8, p. 214, Informa Healthcare, London, UK, 5th edition, 2007.

[2] L. Loridan and B. Senior, "Cushing's syndrome in infancy," *The Journal of Pediatrics*, vol. 75, no. 3, pp. 349–359, 1969.

[3] J. M. W. Kirk, C. E. Brain, D. J. Carson, J. C. Hyde, and D. B. Grant, "Cushing's syndrome caused by nodular adrenal hyperplasia in children with McCune-Albright syndrome," *Journal of Pediatrics*, vol. 134, no. 6, pp. 789–792, 1999.

[4] C. E. Dumitrescu and M. T. Collins, "McCune-Albright syndrome," *Orphanet Journal of Rare Diseases*, vol. 3, no. 1, article 12, 2008.

[5] D. N. Orth, "Cushing's syndrome," *The New England Journal of Medicine*, vol. 332, pp. 791–803, 1995.

[6] W. L. Miller, J. J. Townsend, M. M. Grumbach, and S. L. Kaplan, "An infant with Cushing's disease due to an adrenocorticotropin-producing pituitary adenoma," *Journal of Clinical Endocrinology and Metabolism*, vol. 48, no. 6, pp. 1017–1025, 1979.

[7] K. S. Budhwani, K. Ghritlaharey, and M. Debbarma, "Adrenal cortex tumor in a six year girl—a report and review of literature," *Indian Journal of Medical and Pediartric Oncology*, vol. 25, no. 3, pp. 71–75, 2004.

[8] C. L. Coulter, "Fetal adrenal development: insight gained from adrenal tumors," *Trends in Endocrinology and Metabolism*, vol. 16, no. 5, pp. 235–242, 2005.

[9] E. Michalkiewicz, R. Sandrini, B. Figueiredo et al., "Clinical and outcome characteristics of children with adrenocortical tumors: a report from the international pediatric adrenocortical tumor registry," *Journal of Clinical Oncology*, vol. 22, no. 5, pp. 838–845, 2004.

[10] L. Forga, E. Anda, and J. P. Martinez de Esteban, "Sindromes paraneoplasicos," *Anales del Sistema Sanitario de Navarra*, vol. 28, pp. 213–226, 2005.

[11] S. K. Mayer, L. L. Oligny, C. Deal, S. Yazbeck, I. N. Gagné, and H. Blanchard, "Childhood adrenocortical tumors: case series and reevaluation of prognosis—a 24-year experience," *Journal of Pediatric Surgery*, vol. 32, no. 6, pp. 911–915, 1997.

[12] S. Agarwala, D. K. Mitra, V. Bhatnagar, P. S. N. Menon, and A. K. Gupta, "Aldosteronoma in childhood: a review of clinical features and management," *Journal of Pediatric Surgery*, vol. 29, no. 10, pp. 1388–1391, 1994.

12

Premature Menarche Associated with Primary Hypothyroidism in a 5.5-Year-Old Girl

Dhrubajyoti Sharma,[1] Devi Dayal,[1] Anju Gupta,[1] and Akshay Saxena[2]

[1] *Departments of Pediatrics, Advanced Pediatrics Center, Postgraduate Institute of Medical Education and Research, Chandigarh-160012, India*

[2] *Departments of Radiodiagnosis, Advanced Pediatrics Center, Postgraduate Institute of Medical Education and Research, Chandigarh-160012, India*

Correspondence should be addressed to Devi Dayal, drdevidayal@indiatimes.com

Academic Editors: Y. Moriwaki and S. Simsek

Children with hypothyroidism generally have delayed pubertal development. Rare association with precocious puberty may occur especially in long standing untreated patients. The cardinal features of hypothyroidism induced pseudo precocious pubertal development include thelarche, galactorrhea and menarche. Other characteristics features are an absence of sexual hair and retardation of linear growth. Its manifestation as isolated menarche has been rarely reported. Recently, a five and half year old girl presented to us with history of one episode of vaginal bleeding. A pelvic ultrasonogram revealed multiple cysts in both ovaries and subsequent investigations led to a diagnosis of autoimmune hypothyroidism.

1. Case Report

A five- and half-year-old girl presented with history of one episode of vaginal bleeding seven days prior to admission. The amount of bleeding was small, noticed by mother as blood spots on undergarments. There was no history of local trauma or discharge, foreign body insertion, bleeding from any other site, and difficulty in micturition. There was no history to suggest prior central nervous system insult, raised intracranial pressure, polyuria, polydipsia, or ingestion of hormonal preparations. She was the second child born at term to a low socioeconomic status family. Her physical and mental development was said to be normal by the parents. There was no family history of a thyroid disorder or precocious puberty.

On examination, child appeared pale. There was no edema, goiter, or lymphadenopathy. Her weight and height were 17.2 kilograms and 96.5 centimeters, respectively, (both below 3rd percentiles according to CDC growth charts). Head circumference was 51 centimeters. Heart rate was 90 per minute and blood pressure 90/70 mm Hg. Breast and pubic hair development was Tanner stage 1. Abdomen was protuberant without organomegaly or palpable mass. Neurological and ophthalmologic examinations were normal. A thorough gynaecological examination revealed normal genitalia for age and ruled out local trauma or foreign body. Menstrual bleeding (menarche) was considered after excluding local causes. In view of short stature, an initial impression of isosexual precocity caused by acquired hypothyroidism was made.

Investigations revealed hemoglobin of 8.8 g/dL, total leukocyte count 6800/mm^3, platelet count 1,50,000/mm^3, and macrocytic hypochromic anemia on peripheral smear examination. Thyroid function tests showed gross hypothyroidism with total triiodothyronine (T_3) 0.45 pg/mL (normal, 0.7–2 pg/mL), total thyroxine (T_4) 32 ng/mL (normal, 55–135 ng/mL), and thyroid-stimulating hormone (TSH) 133.4 mIU/mL (normal, 0.17–4 mIU/mL). Follicle stimulating hormone (FSH) was 10 mIU/mL (normal, 1.0–4.2 mIU/mL), Luteinizing hormone (LH) 0.5 mIU/mL (normal, 0.02–0.18 mIU/mL), estradiol (E_2) 127.58 pg/mL (normal, 6–27 pg/mL), and prolactin (PRL) 26.30 ng/mL (normal, 3–24 ng/mL). Antithyroid microsomal antibodies (anti-TMA) determined by semiquantitative microtiter particle

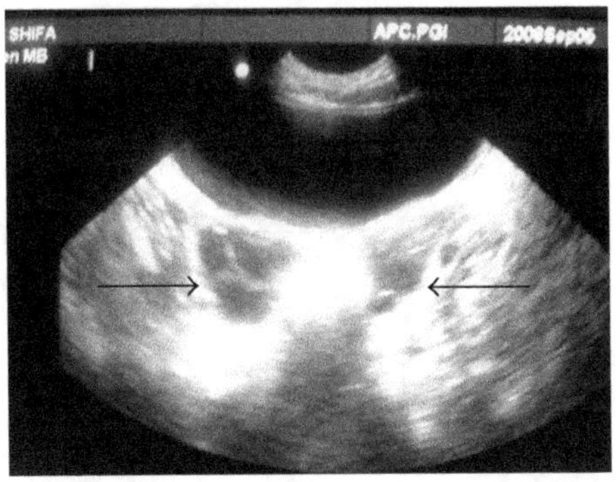

FIGURE 1: Ultrasonogram showing multicystic ovaries (Rt > Lt).

agglutination method were strongly positive (3+). Her bone age corresponded to 3 years. A pertechnetate thyroid scan revealed normal sized lobes with adequate tracer uptake. Thyroid ultrasound showed mild reduction in echogenicity and normal volume for age. Pelvic ultrasonography revealed normal sized uterus and enlarged ovaries (right ovary 5.6 cc and left 5.5 cc). Both ovaries had multiple cysts with largest measuring 1.2 cms diameter on right side and 1.2 × 1 cms on left side (Figure 1).

Levothyroxine (5 μg/kg/d) therapy was initiated. There was no recurrence of vaginal bleeding till the first follow-up visit one and half months after hospital discharge. Repeat hormonal estimations were normal (T_3 2.05 ng/mL, T_4 131.9 ng/mL, TSH 2.42 mIU/mL, FSH 1.27 mIU/mL, LH 0.352 mIU/mL, E_2 16.4 pg/mL, and PRL 18 ng/mL). However, ultrasonogram done after 3 months of thyroxine therapy still showed multiple cysts in the right ovary and single cyst in left one (right ovary 3 cc and left ovary 2 cc). Repeat sonography a month later demonstrated absence of cysts. She has remained symptoms-free and showed a catch-up height increase of 9 centimeters over 1 year followup.

2. Discussion

Delayed pubertal development is a common manifestation of long standing untreated hypothyroidism. Precocious puberty may occur rarely as the presenting feature [1]. The onset is with thelarche with or without galactorrhea followed by menarche with absence of hair development as a characteristic feature. Another clinical clue to hypothyroidism in these cases is the decreased linear growth, quite opposite of what is seen in patients with true precocious puberty [1]. Isolated menarche, as seen in our patient, is an extremely rare presentation of hypothyroidism-related precocity [2]. Only a few cases have been reported so far. The typical clinical clues of short stature and delayed bone age were present in our case, so diagnosis of hypothyroidism could be easily entertained after excluding local causes of bleeding. In addition, important manifestations that were reported previously and detected in our case as well were bilateral ovarian enlargement with multiple cysts, hyperprolactinemia, and increased levels of gonadotropins, mainly FSH and E_2 [2–4]. This association of precocious pubertal development and hypothyroidism, although seemingly unphysiologic, may occur in almost 50% of children with severe hypothyroidism of long duration [1]. The cause of hypothyroidism in these patients is often undiagnosed lymphocytic thyroiditis although it may be seen in association with congenital hypothyroidism also [5]. In our patient, the bone age delay and skeletal retardation indicated that the pathology began at about 3 years of age. Since autoimmune thyroiditis is uncommon before 6 years of age, we performed a thyroid scan that excluded dysgenesis or ectopia, the usual congenital causes of thyroid decompensation during growing years. Presence of anti-TMA favoured a diagnosis of autoimmune thyroiditis.

The underlying hormonal mechanisms in hypothyroidism-associated precocity remain obscure. Wyk and Grumbach tried to explain precocious puberty by an overlap in negative feedback regulation with overproduction of gonadotropins as well as thyrotropin (both share common α subunit) in response to thyroid deficiency [6]. But although gonadotropins are elevated in these patients, these have been observed to be GnRH unresponsive or bioinactive in earlier studies [7]. Also advancement of skeletal maturation characteristically associated with elevated gonadotropin states is not seen. So, gonadotropin excess does not appear to cause sexual precocity associated with hypothyroidism. The FSH and E_2 levels were elevated in our patient although the clinical presentation with short stature, delayed BA and loss of consonance of pubertal development along with laboratory evidence of severe primary hypothyroidism indicated hypothyroidism-induced pseudoprecocity. We however could not do GnRH test to definitely exclude gonadotropin-dependent precocious puberty.

Another theory is that extreme TSH elevation seen in profound hypothyroidism induces FSH like-effects on the gonads resulting in multicystic ovaries, uterine bleeding, and breast enlargement. Hence, precocious puberty secondary to hypothyroidism behaves like an incomplete form of gonadotropin-dependant precocious puberty [8]. According to prolactin theory, hyperprolactinemia as a result of chronic stimulation of TRH enhances the sensitivity of ovaries to even trace amounts of circulating gonadotropins prepubertally [8]. Although PRL increase in the index patient was only mild, the increased sensitivity of ovaries to gonadotropins along with extremely elevated TSH having FSH-like effects could have caused multicystic ovaries.

References

[1] L. Garibaldi, "Disorders of Pubertal development," in *Nelson Text Book of Pediatrics*, R. M. Kliegman, R. E. Behrman, H. B. Jenson, and B. F. Stanton, Eds., vol. 2, pp. 2309–2316, Elsevier, New Delhi, India, 18th edition, 2007.

[2] V. K. Piziak and H. B. Hahn Jr., "Isolated menarche in juvenile hypothyroidism," *Clinical Pediatrics*, vol. 23, no. 3, pp. 177–179, 1984.

[3] K. V. Kumar, J. Muthukrishnan, R. Sinha, and K. D. Modi, "Two cases describing the effects of hypothyroidism on puberty and growth," *International Journal of Gynecology and Obstetrics*, vol. 103, no. 2, pp. 183–184, 2008.

[4] C. K. Indumathi, G. Bantwal, and M. Patil, "Primary hypothyroidism with precocious puberty and bilateral cystic ovaries," *Indian Journal of Pediatrics*, vol. 74, no. 8, pp. 781–783, 2007.

[5] T. Asami, T. Kikuchi, T. Kamimura, S. Kinoshita, and M. Uchiyama, "Precocious puberty in a girl with congenital hypothyroidism receiving continuous L-thyroxine-replacement therapy," *Pediatrics International*, vol. 43, no. 1, pp. 87–90, 2001.

[6] J. J. V. Wyk and M. M. Grumbach, "Syndrome of precocious menstruation and galactorrhea in juvenile hypothyroidism: an example of hormonal overlap in pituitary feedback," *The Journal of Pediatrics*, vol. 57, no. 3, pp. 416–435, 1960.

[7] I. Z. Beitins and H. H. Bode, "Hypothyroidism with elevated gonadotropin secretion," *Pediatric Research*, vol. 14, no. 4, pp. 475–476, 1980.

[8] M. P. Desai, "The thyroid gland," in *Pediatric Endocrine Disorders*, M. P. Desai, V. Bhatia, and P. S. N. Menon, Eds., pp. 183–202, Orient Longman Limited, 2001.

13

Short-Term PTH(1-34) Therapy in Children to Correct Severe Hypocalcemia and Hyperphosphatemia due to Hypoparathyroidism: Two Case Studies

Pooja E. Mishra,[1] Betsy L. Schwartz,[2] Kyriakie Sarafoglou,[3] Kristen Hook,[4] Youngki Kim,[5] and Anna Petryk[3]

[1]*St John's Medical College, Bangalore, India*
[2]*Pediatric Endocrinology, Park Nicollet, Minneapolis, MN, USA*
[3]*Pediatric Endocrinology, University of Minnesota, Minneapolis, MN, USA*
[4]*Pediatric Dermatology, University of Minnesota, Minneapolis, MN, USA*
[5]*Pediatric Nephrology, University of Minnesota, Minneapolis, MN, USA*

Correspondence should be addressed to Anna Petryk; petry005@umn.edu

Academic Editor: Osamu Isozaki

The standard treatment of hypoparathyroidism is to control hypocalcemia using calcitriol and calcium supplementation. However, in severe cases this approach is insufficient, and the risks of intravenous (i.v.) calcium administration and prolonged hospitalization must be considered. While the use of recombinant human parathyroid hormone 1-34 [rhPTH(1-34)] for long-term control of hypocalcemia has been established, the benefits of short-term rhPTH(1-34) treatment in children have not been explored. We report two patients with hypoparathyroidism treated with rhPTH(1-34). Patient 1 is a 10-year-old female with polyglandular autoimmune syndrome type 1. Patient 2 is a 12-year-old female with hypoparathyroidism after total thyroidectomy. Both patients showed poor response to i.v. and oral calcium and calcitriol, and patient 1 did not respond to phosphate binders. Patient 1 had rapid increase in serum calcium with a decrease in serum phosphate after a 3-day course of subcutaneous rhPTH(1-34). Patient 2 had normalization of calcium and phosphate levels after a 7-day course of rhPTH(1-34). These cases support a role for rhPTH(1-34) in the acute management of hypoparathyroidism in hospitalized patients to more rapidly correct hypocalcemia and hyperphosphatemia, shorten hospitalization, and reduce the need for frequent i.v. calcium boluses.

1. Introduction

Hypoparathyroidism may be due to a number of causes, including autoimmune destruction of parathyroid glands, accidental removal of or damage to the parathyroid glands following thyroid surgery, or genetic disorders such as 22q11.2 deletion. Hypoparathyroidism manifests as hypocalcemia and hyperphosphatemia with a low serum parathyroid hormone (PTH) level. Acute hypocalcemia is typically controlled with calcium and calcitriol supplementation. However, in some children these standard measures are insufficient, requiring prolonged hospitalization and even transfer to the pediatric intensive care unit (PICU) for intravenous (i.v.) calcium administration. Alternate therapeutic options for these children should be considered.

Use of recombinant human (rh) PTH(1-34) (teriparatide) has been documented in adults, with successful control of serum calcium and phosphate levels [1]. However, due to occurrence of osteosarcoma in rat toxicology studies of rhPTH(1-34) there is concern about its long-term use in a pediatric population [2].

Recent studies have demonstrated the advantage of using rhPTH(1-34) to control hypocalcemia in children for periods up to 3 years [3–5]. The two cases presented here suggest a role for rhPTH(1-34) in the acute management of hypocalcemia and hyperphosphatemia. This treatment can accelerate

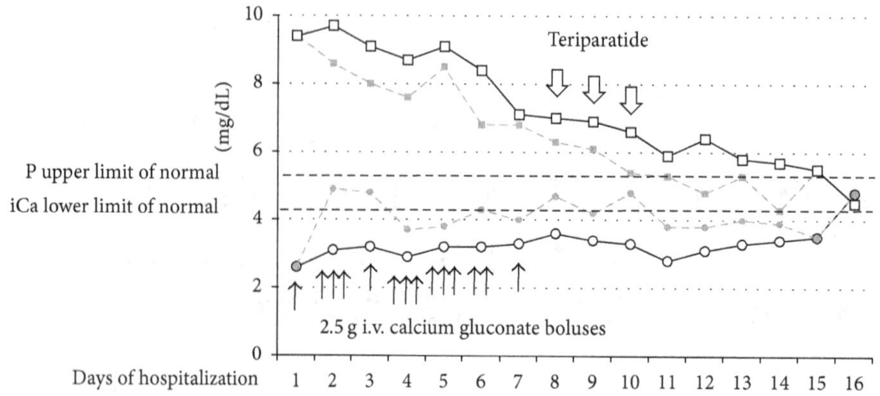

Days of hospitalization	1	2	3	4	5	6	7	8	9	10	11	12	13	14	15	16
Total ECa (g/day)	0.2	3.9	3.4	3.9	2.0	1.8	1.5	1.3	1.3	1.3	1.3	1.3	3.0	3.6	3.6	3.6
Total ECa (mg/kg/day)	8.5	147	130	147	75	66	58	49	49	49	49	49	114	136	136	136
Oral ECa (g/day)	3.2	3.2	3.2	3.2	1.3	1.3	1.3	1.3	1.3	1.3	1.3	1.3	3.0	3.6	3.6	3.6
Oral ECa (mg/kg/day)	121	121	121	121	49	49	49	49	49	49	49	49	114	136	136	136
Calcitriol (mcg/day)	0.25	0.5	1.0	1.0	1.0	0.5	0.5	0.5	0.5	0.5	0.5	0.5	0.5	0.5	0.5	0.5

FIGURE 1: Trends in serum ionized calcium and phosphorus levels in a 10-year-old girl with hypoparathyroidism over the course of hospitalization. Minimum and maximum daily levels of iCa (circles and solid and dashed lines, resp.) and P (squares and dashed and solid lines, resp.) are shown. Black arrows indicate individual calcium gluconate boluses (2.5 g each). Open arrows point to once daily subcutaneous administration of teriparatide. Oral supplementation consisted of calcium carbonate except for Days 5–12 when calcium glubionate was given. ECa, elemental calcium.

normalization of serum calcium and phosphate, reduce the need for i.v. calcium, and shorten the period of hospitalization.

2. Case Presentations

2.1. Patient 1. A 10-year-old female presented to dermatology clinic with a 4-year history of alopecia universalis and nail dystrophy, hypocalcemic seizures at 4 years of age (seizure-free on calcium and vitamin D supplements), and frequent thrush during infancy. A clinical diagnosis of autoimmune polyglandular syndrome type 1 was made and confirmed with a pathogenic mutation in the autoimmune regulator (*AIRE*) gene. She had a normal ACTH level and adequate peak cortisol level of 17.8 μg/dL after 250 μg of cosyntropin i.v.

A week later, she presented to the Emergency Department with tetany and a 3-day history of cramping in the hands and legs. Her serum iCa level was 2.3 mg/dL (reference range 4.4–5.2 mg/dL) and phosphate level was 9.2 mg/dL (reference range 2.9–5.4 mg/dL). She was given an i.v. bolus of 2.5 g calcium gluconate and 0.25 μg of calcitriol before being transferred to PICU. Repeat testing showed persistent hypocalcemia and hyperphosphatemia and low PTH level (<3 pg/mL, reference range 12–72 pg/mL). She required multiple calcium gluconate boluses. Figure 1 shows trends in iCa and P levels along with calcium and calcitriol doses. She received ergocalciferol 50,000 IU daily by mouth on days 2–4. On Day 5, her 25-hydroxyvitamin D level was normal (43 μg/L, reference range 20–75 μg/L) and ergocalciferol was discontinued.

On Day 3, due to persistently high serum phosphate, she was started on phosphate binder aluminum hydroxide (600 mg three times daily), and then Renagel (up to 9.6 g per day). Despite high dose calcium supplementation (up to 8 g of calcium carbonate per day) and renal protective measures, she continued to have hypocalcemia and hyperphosphatemia. On Day 8, she was started on rhPTH(1-34) (20 μg once a day subcutaneously) and i.v. calcium boluses were discontinued. Within 48 hours, there was a significant rise in iCa and a drop in serum phosphate levels. rhPTH(1-34) was discontinued after 3 days of treatment. Hydrochlorothiazide (12.5 mg twice daily) was added on Day 13 to reduce renal calcium excretion because of nephrocalcinosis found on renal ultrasound. She was discharged on Day 15 with normal iCa (4.8 mg/dL) and P (4.5 mg/dL) levels a day later.

2.2. Patient 2. Patient 2 is a 12-year-old girl diagnosed with Graves' disease five weeks prior to admission, treated with methimazole. Two weeks later she was found to have a thyroid nodule and was diagnosed with papillary thyroid cancer. She underwent total thyroidectomy with central neck dissection without removal of the parathyroid glands. Following surgery she was started on 112 mcg of L-thyroxine daily, calcium carbonate 1000 mg four times a day, and calcitriol 0.25 μg daily. She presented to the Emergency Department five days later with muscle spasms, irritability, and difficulty in swallowing. Laboratory evaluation revealed severe hypocalcemia (iCa 2.8 mg/dL, Figure 2) and hyperphosphatemia (8.6 mg/dL). PTH level was <0.3 pg/mL. Free T4 level was normal (0.99 ng/dL, reference range 0.76–1.46 ng/dL), but TSH was still suppressed at <0.01 mU/L (reference range 0.4–4.0 mU/L).

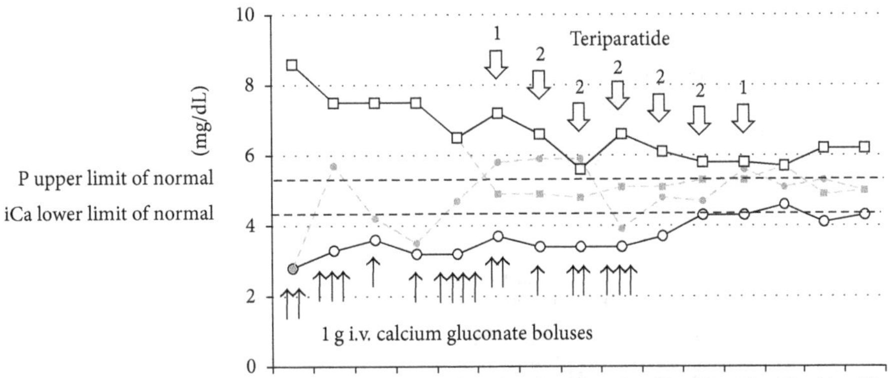

Days of hospitalization	1	2	3	4	5	6	7	8	9	10	11	12	13	14	15
Total ECa dose (g/day)	1.8	2.7	3.9	3.7	5.2	5.0	4.9	5.0	5.1	4.8	4.8	3.2	3.2	2.8	2.4
Total ECa (mg/kg/day)	31	47	69	65	91	88	86	88	89	85	85	56	56	49	42
Oral ECa (g/day)	1.6	2.4	3.8	3.6	4.8	4.8	4.8	4.8	4.8	4.8	4.8	3.2	3.2	2.8	2.4
Oral ECa (mg/kg/day)	28	42	67	63	85	85	85	85	85	85	85	56	56	49	42
Calcitriol (mcg/day)	0.25	0.25	0.5	0.5	1.0	1.0	1.0	2.0	2.0	2.0	2.0	2.0	1.0	0.5	0.5

FIGURE 2: Trends in serum ionized calcium and phosphorus levels in a 12-year-old girl with hypoparathyroidism over the course of hospitalization. Minimum and maximum daily levels of iCa (circles and solid and dashed lines, resp.) and P (squares and dashed and solid lines, resp.) are shown. Black arrows indicate individual calcium gluconate boluses (1 g each). Open arrows point to days of subcutaneous administration of teriparatide with the numbers above the arrows indicating once daily (1) or twice daily (2) injections. Oral supplementation consisted of calcium carbonate except for Days 2-3 when calcium citrate was also given. ECa, elemental calcium.

She was given two i.v. boluses of 1 g calcium gluconate and was transferred to PICU for further management. She required repeated i.v. calcium boluses in addition to oral supplementation with increasing doses of calcium carbonate (up to 12 g per day). The dose of calcitriol was gradually increased to 2 μg per day. Her 25-hydroxy-vitamin D level was 27 μg/L. She received 50,000 IU of ergocalciferol on Days 4 and 11, cholecalciferol 1,000 IU daily on Days 3–7, and then 4,000 IU daily starting on Day 8. Due to persistent signs and symptoms of hypocalcemia (prominent Chvostek sign, paresthesias, and QTc prolongation), rhPTH(1-34) treatment was started on Day 6 at a dose of 20 μg once a day subcutaneously. The same day, serum phosphate level decreased rapidly from 7.2 to 4.9 mg/dL, and serum iCa increased from 3.7 to 5.8 mg/dL. The dose of rhPTH(1-34) was temporarily increased to 20 μg twice daily on Days 7–11 because the effect diminished before the next scheduled dose. After 4 days of rhPTH(1-34) treatment, the patient no longer required i.v. calcium boluses. With near normalization of serum calcium and phosphate levels, rhPTH(1-34) was discontinued on Day 12. On discharge (Day 15), her iCa level was 4.8 mg/dL and phosphate level was 5.6 mg/dL.

3. Discussion

Standard therapeutic approaches in patients with hypoparathyroidism include calcium and vitamin D supplementation. Persistent severe hypocalcemia requires i.v. calcium gluconate administration in the form of i.v. boluses or as a continuous infusion. The latter may have to be continued for a week to ensure enterocyte recovery and adequate intestinal absorption of oral calcium and carries significant risks (cardiac arrhythmia, extravasation, and thrombophlebitis). Moreover, traditional therapy is not causative because it does not replace the deficient hormone.

While there is accumulating evidence for the benefits of rhPTH(1-34) replacement in children on a long-term basis [3], these two cases illustrate that a short-term treatment may also benefit children with refractory hypoparathyroidism by allowing faster normalization of calcium and phosphorus levels and shortening hospitalization, particularly when continuous i.v. calcium infusion is neither feasible nor effective. Similar benefits of short-term rhPTH(1-34) therapy have been demonstrated in adults with postsurgical hypoparathyroidism [6]. Certain patient populations are at a particularly high risk for severe hypocalcemia, for example, after thyroidectomy for thyroid cancer or Graves' disease, partly due to "hungry bone syndrome" in the latter [7], as illustrated by Patient 2.

Twice daily dosing of rhPTH was required in Patient 2 due to significant excursions in serum calcium levels, consistent with previous data showing less variation on a twice daily regimen compared to a once daily injections [8]. It remains to be determined if a longer acting rhPTH(1-84) molecule with favorable long-term safety and efficacy in adults [9] would benefit children as well.

Competing Interests

The authors declare that they have no competing interests.

References

[1] K. K. Winer, C. W. Ko, J. C. Reynolds et al., "Long-term treatment of hypoparathyroidism: a randomized controlled study comparing parathyroid hormone-(1-34) versus calcitriol and calcium," *Journal of Clinical Endocrinology and Metabolism*, vol. 88, no. 9, pp. 4214–4220, 2003.

[2] J. L. Vahle, M. Sato, G. G. Long et al., "Skeletal changes in rats given daily subcutaneous injections of recombinant human parathyroid hormone (1-34) for 2 years and relevance to human safety," *Toxicologic Pathology*, vol. 30, no. 3, pp. 312–321, 2002.

[3] K. K. Winer, N. Sinaii, J. Reynolds, D. Peterson, K. Dowdy, and G. B. Cutler Jr., "Long-term treatment of 12 children with chronic hypoparathyroidism: a randomized trial comparing synthetic human parathyroid hormone 1-34 versus calcitriol and calcium," *Journal of Clinical Endocrinology and Metabolism*, vol. 95, no. 6, pp. 2680–2688, 2010.

[4] P. Matarazzo, G. Tuli, L. Fiore et al., "Teriparatide (rhPTH) treatment in children with syndromic hypoparathyroidism," *Journal of Pediatric Endocrinology and Metabolism*, vol. 27, no. 1-2, pp. 53–59, 2014.

[5] R. I. Gafni, J. S. Brahim, P. Andreopoulou et al., "Daily parathyroid hormone 1–34 replacement therapy for hypoparathyroidism induces marked changes in bone turnover and structure," *Journal of Bone and Mineral Research*, vol. 27, no. 8, pp. 1811–1820, 2012.

[6] M. Shah, I. Bancos, G. B. Thompson et al., "Teriparatide therapy and reduced postoperative hospitalization for postsurgical hypoparathyroidism," *JAMA Otolaryngology—Head and Neck Surgery*, vol. 141, no. 9, pp. 822–827, 2015.

[7] C. E. Pesce, Z. Shiue, H.-L. Tsai et al., "Postoperative hypocalcemia after thyroidectomy for Graves' disease," *Thyroid*, vol. 20, no. 11, pp. 1279–1283, 2010.

[8] K. K. Winer, N. Sinaii, D. Peterson, B. Sainz Jr., and G. B. Cutler Jr., "Effects of once versus twice-daily parathyroid hormone 1–34 therapy in children with hypoparathyroidism," *Journal of Clinical Endocrinology and Metabolism*, vol. 93, no. 9, pp. 3389–3395, 2008.

[9] M. R. Rubin, N. E. Cusano, W. Fan et al., "Therapy of hypoparathyroidism with PTH(1–84): a prospective six year investigation of efficacy and safety," *The Journal of Clinical Endocrinology & Metabolism*, vol. 101, no. 7, pp. 2742–2750, 2016.

14

Effect of Prolonged Discontinuation of L-Thyroxine Replacement in a Child with Congenital Hypothyroidism

Rita Ann Kubicky,[1,2] Evan Weiner,[2,3] Bronwyn Carlson,[2] and Francesco De Luca[1,2]

[1] *Section of Endocrinology and Diabetes, St. Christopher's Hospital for Children, Drexel University College of Medicine, Philadelphia, PA 19134, USA*
[2] *Department of Pediatrics, Drexel University College of Medicine, Philadelphia, PA 19102, USA*
[3] *Department of Emergency Medicine, St. Christopher's Hospital for Children, Drexel University College of Medicine, Philadelphia, PA 19134, USA*

Correspondence should be addressed to Rita Ann Kubicky, ritaann.kubicky@tenethealth.com

Academic Editors: T. Kita and R. Murray

When diagnosed through neonatal screening and treated promptly and adequately, infants with congenital hypothyroidism (CH) experience normal physical growth and neurological development. Here we present a 3-year-old boy diagnosed with CH as a newborn, who was subsequently left untreated and experienced significant growth failure and developmental delay. This case emphasizes the importance of a consistent adherence to treatment in preventing such complications, especially in infancy and early childhood.

1. Introduction

The prevalence of congenital hypothyroidism (CH) in the past has been approximately 1 in 3,000 to 1 in 4,000 births with a higher incidence in Hispanic individuals [1]. More recent data suggest an increased prevalence of CH in the United States, possibly reflecting changes in screening methods [2, 3]. CH is the most frequent endocrine disease in infants, and, in most cases, the disorder is permanent [1]. When diagnosed and treated promptly and adequately, children born with CH experience normal physical growth and neurological development. Here we present a 3-year-old boy diagnosed at birth with congenital hypothyroidism, with subsequent poor compliance with L-thyroxine replacement.

2. Case Presentation

J. D. is a 2 11/12-year-old male, born in Mexico and diagnosed by neonatal screening with CH. He was then treated with L-thyroxine for approximately 1 year, until his mother lost her health insurance coverage and could not purchase the medication. Shortly after his family immigrated to the United States, J. D. was taken to St. Christopher's Hospital for Children's (SCHC) Emergency Department (ED) for evaluation.

His mother described a history of developmental delay, especially affecting his motor and language skills, as well as a history of constipation. Upon physical examination (PE), J. D.'s vital signs were as follows: temperature (T) of 97.6°F, heart rate (HR) of 95 beats per minute, blood pressure (BP) of 95/54 mmHg, and respiratory rate (RR) of 20 breaths per minute. His weight and length were both below the 3rd percentile (statural age of an 8 1/2-month old). J. D. was able to sit and crawl but could not stand or walk; he could only bear weight on his legs with support. The rest of his PE was significant for coarse facial features (Figures 1 and 2), macroglossia (Figure 1), a protuberant abdomen and a small umbilical hernia (Figure 3), and dry skin. His thyroid was not palpable. The serum TSH was very elevated (1,620 mIU/L) and the free T4 and thyroglobulin undetectable (Table 1); his serum prolactin level was mildly elevated (27.9 ng/mL). On the day of presentation, J. D. was placed on 50 μg L-thyroxine daily (~5 μg/kg/day), and a follow-up evaluation was arranged.

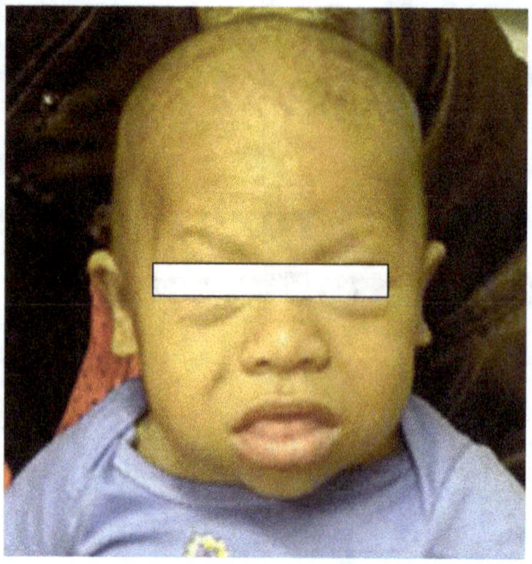

FIGURE 1: Photograph of patient demonstrating his coarse facial features and macroglossia.

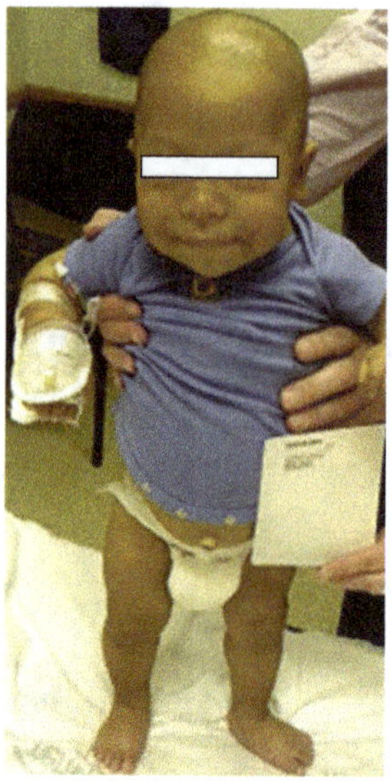

FIGURE 2: Patient stands with support. His height was significantly below the 3rd percentile (statural height of a 8 1/2-month-old male).

When evaluated at the SCHC Endocrinology Outpatient Clinic 2 weeks later, his mother reported increased activity, alertness, and appetite. In addition, his constipation had improved and he was less sleepy. His PE was virtually unchanged when compared to the one obtained in the ED. His dentition was delayed, with only 12 erupted teeth. His testicular volume was 4 cc bilaterally and he had no pubic hair.

A thyroid ultrasound revealed thyroid hypoplasia, with the right lobe measuring 5 mm anteriorly posteriorly (AP) and 6 mm in width (W), and the left lobe measuring 4 mm (AP) × 9 mm (W). Upon evaluation by a pediatric neurologist, his psychomotor developmental stage was found to be at the 18-month-old level for personal/social, fine motor/adaptive and language skills; his gross motor skills were at the 12-month-old level (by Denver's scale). His muscle tone

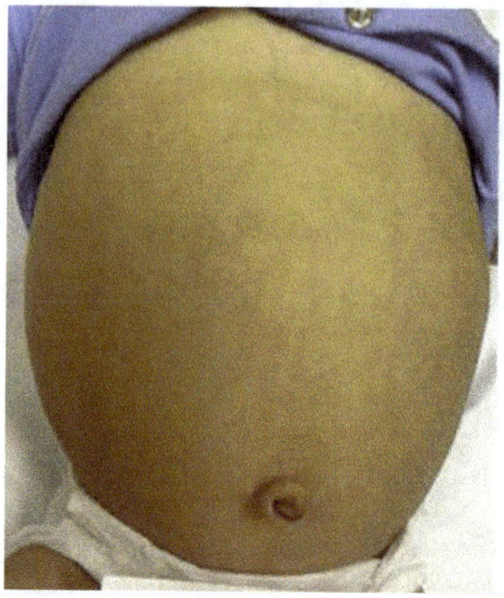

FIGURE 3: Protuberant abdomen and a small umbilical hernia.

was mildly but symmetrically decreased in all extremities, and his deep tendon reflexes were decreased.

J. D. was evaluated again at the Endocrinology Clinic 4 months after his initial visit to the ED. His mother reported that he had increased strength, which he was pulling to stand, trying to walk, and was much more active and alert. His testicular size was prepubertal. Laboratory studies revealed normal serum TSH and a free T4 (2.84 mIU/L and 1.5 ng/dL, resp.). Serum prolactin was also normal (Table 1).

After being treated with L-thyroxine for 7 months, J. D. grew 8 cm. He was enrolled in an early interventional program to improve his developmental skills. As per his mother, his vocabulary included more words and he was able to go up steps; he had also started to feed himself without help. Although his free T4 was normal (1.1 ng/dL), his TSH was found to be elevated (20.93 mIU/L).

J. D. was subsequently lost to followup for a few months because of change of insurance. Multiple attempts to contact his mother by phone and by certified mail were unsuccessful. He did not return to our clinic until 9 months later (16 months after his initial presentation): J. D. had grown 9.4 cm since his previous clinic visit (9 months prior). His maternal grandmother reported that he was a very active child who enjoyed singing and dancing. She described that his motor and language skills continued to improve: he was able to run, walk up and down stairs and he knew many words in both English and Spanish. His grandmother stated that his pediatrician at a local health center had been checking his thyroid function tests periodically. His grandmother also stated that J. D.'s dose of L-thyroxine had been increased to 75 mcg 2 months prior by his pediatrician; repeat thyroid function tests 1 month after the dose change were reported as normal. At our endocrinology clinic, thyroid function tests were obtained and a bone age study requested; a follow-up visit with his pediatric neurologist was also recommended. J. D.'s thyroid function tests revealed a normal TSH (0.79 mIU/L) and a borderline-high free T4 (1.7 ng/dL); as a result, the L-thyroxine dose was unchanged. His bone age, obtained one month after the last visit, was delayed (between 2 years

TABLE 1: Initial and follow-up laboratory studies.

	Initial	6 weeks	4 months	7 months	16 months
TSH (mIU/L)	1620	5.2	2.84	20.93	0.79
Free T4 (ng/dL)[1]	<0.10 (<1.29)	1.41 (18.15)	1.5 (19.30)	1.1 (14.16)	1.7 (21.88)
Prolactin (ng/mL)[2]	27.9 (1,213.04)	10.1 (439.13)	5.1 (221.74)	—	—
Thyroglobulin (ng/mL)[3]	<0.5 (<0.5)	—	—	—	—

Values in Systeme International (SI) units are in parentheses.
[1]To convert to pmol/L multiply by 12.87.
[2]To convert to pmol/L multiply by 43.478.
[3]To convert to μg/L multiply by 1.

8 months and 3 years at the chronological age of 4 years and 5 months).

3. Discussion

Thyroid hormones play an essential role in normal statural growth: in fact, growth failure is a known complication of congenital hypothyroidism (CH). Before the neonatal screening was initiated in the 1970s, the percentage of children with CH having a height below the 10th percentile has been shown to range from 19% to 31% [4, 5]. After the introduction of the screening, several studies have reported a normal linear growth in infancy and childhood [6–8], while others have described a slight growth deceleration early in childhood in children with severe CH at diagnosis [9–11]. With respect to the achievement of a normal final height, some studies have suggested that the adequacy of L-thyroxine replacement in the first 6 months of life may influence the adult height of children with CH detected by newborn screening [12]. In contrast, other studies have found no correlation between severity at diagnosis, etiology, or initial L-thyroxine dosage [13, 14]. The only postnatal factor consistently found to be related to adult height has been the age at the start of treatment. Interestingly, longstanding untreated CH has been associated with permanent height loss. Boersma et al. have described two children with CH, who were left untreated for several years; although they experienced a marked catch-up growth, both of them reached an adult height below their target height [15].

It is well known that CH diagnosed on clinical grounds would often lead to severe cognitive and motor delays. Studies of children diagnosed in the prescreening era have reported that 8% to 29% patients affected by CH developed intellectual disability (i.e., IQ below 70) [5, 16, 17].

In contrast, a number of longitudinal studies of cohorts of children diagnosed with CH by screening have clearly demonstrated how hypothyroidism-related mental retardation can be successfully prevented [18–20]. On the other hand, while it is evident that early and adequate treatment can avoid serious sequelae, numerous studies have reported subtle but statistically significant neurological deficits in children with CH detected by screening when compared to unaffected individuals [21–23].

The initial severity of CH may be responsible for a less than ideal outcome. Indeed, evidence from multiple follow-up studies conducted in the United States and in Europe indicate that patients with lower T4 and more delayed skeletal maturation at the time of diagnosis by screening are more likely to exhibit subnormal cognitive skills [24–26]. Less obvious appears the effects of other variables: one study has shown that the timing of treatment initiation does not affect outcome [27], while other studies have demonstrated that the age at the start of treatment is correlated with neurological outcome in children with CH even after the introduction of the neonatal screening [18–21]. In addition, another study has indicated that higher initial L-thyroxine dose and faster time to normalization of thyroid function are important in preventing neurodevelopmental impairment [28].

Another variable thought to be an important prognostic factor for intellectual outcome is compliance to L-thyroxine treatment [19, 29, 30]. In a Norwegian study, neuropsychological tests administered at the mean age of 20 years to subjects with CH diagnosed by neonatal screening program have shown that their mean serum T4 level during the second year of life was a strong predictor of their verbal IQ [21]. In a German study of patients with CH with an early onset of treatment (9 days) and high initial L-thyroxine dose (14 μg/kg/day), a decreased IQ score was correlated with poor compliance rather than with the severity of CH [31]. It appears that the discontinuation of L-thyroxine treatment experienced by our patient does not exclusively affect less affluent countries or families of low socioeconomic status. A retrospective analysis in the United States published in 2010 revealed that, by age of 3 years, the percentage of children with CH diagnosed by neonatal screening who had discontinued thyroxine replacement was 38%, and it was similar between Medicaid-enrolled and privately insured children [32]. While it is conceivable that some of these children were affected by transient hypothyroidism, many others may have been affected by permanent CH, like our patient, and thus are at risk for significant long-term sequelae especially if they are not treated adequately during the first three years of life until brain development is complete.

In conclusion, since neonatal screening for congenital hypothyroidism has been introduced, early L-thyroxine treatment has virtually eliminated hypothyroidism-related growth failure and severe neurological impairment. However, our patient demonstrates that prolonged lack of treatment due to poor compliance (despite early thyroid hormone replacement) may still be responsible for significant growth failure and psychomotor delay during childhood and possible permanent neurological deficits. This case emphasizes the importance of a consistent adherence to treatment in preventing such complications, especially in infancy and early childhood.

References

[1] S. R. Rose, R. S. Brown, T. Foley et al., "Update of newborn screening and therapy for congenital hypothyroidism," *Pediatrics*, vol. 117, no. 6, pp. 2290–2303, 2006.

[2] J. Deladoëy, J. Ruel, Y. Giguère, and G. Van Vliet, "Is the incidence of congenital hypothyroidism really increasing? A 20-year retrospective population-based study in Québec," *Journal of Clinical Endocrinology and Metabolism*, vol. 96, no. 8, pp. 2422–2429, 2011.

[3] J. P. Brosco, M. Mattingly, and L. M. Sanders, "Impact of specific medical interventions on reducing the prevalence of mental retardation," *Archives of Pediatrics and Adolescent Medicine*, vol. 160, no. 3, pp. 302–309, 2006.

[4] G. J. Frost and J. M. Parkin, "Management of patients with congenital hypothyroidism," *British Medical Journal*, vol. 290, no. 6480, pp. 1485–1489, 1985.

[5] J. A. Hulse, "Outcome for congenital hypothyroidism," *Archives of Disease in Childhood*, vol. 59, no. 1, pp. 23–29, 1984.

[6] H. Bucher, A. Prader, and R. Illig, "Head circumference, height, bone age and weight in 103 children with congenital hypothyroidism before and during thyroid hormone replacement," *Helvetica Paediatrica Acta*, vol. 40, no. 4, pp. 305–316, 1985.

[7] L. Moschini, P. Costa, E. Marinelli et al., "Longitudinal assessment of children with congenital hypothyroidism detected by neonatal screening," *Helvetica Paediatrica Acta*, vol. 41, no. 5, pp. 415–424, 1986.

[8] L. Moreno, H. Ythier, G. A. Loeuille, M. F. Lebecq, J. L. Dhondt, and J. P. Farriaux, "Etude de la croissance et de la maturation osseuse au cours de l'hypotyroidie congenitale depistee en periode neonatale. A propos de 82 observations," *Archives Francaises de Pediatrie*, vol. 46, no. 10, pp. 723–728, 1989.

[9] D. B. Grant, "Growth in early treated congenital hypothyroidism," *Archives of Disease in Childhood*, vol. 70, no. 6, pp. 464–468, 1994.

[10] R. Aronson, R. M. Ehrlich, J. D. Baily, and J. F. Rovet, "Growth in children with congenital hypothyroidism detected by neonatal screening," *Journal of Pediatrics*, vol. 116, no. 1, pp. 33–37, 1990.

[11] S. Heyerdahl, A. Ilicki, J. Karlberg, B. F. Kase, and A. Larsson, "Linear growth in early treated children with congenital hypothyroidism," *Acta Paediatrica*, vol. 86, no. 5, pp. 479–483, 1997.

[12] Z. Dickerman and L. De Vries, "Prepubertal and pubertal growth, timing and duration of puberty and attained adult height in patients with congenital hypothyroidism (CH) detected by the neonatal screening programme for CH—a longitudinal study," *Clinical Endocrinology*, vol. 47, no. 6, pp. 649–654, 1997.

[13] M. Salerno, M. Micillo, S. Di Maio et al., "Longitudinal growth, sexual maturation and final height in patients with congenital hypothyroidism detected by neonatal screening," *European Journal of Endocrinology*, vol. 145, no. 4, pp. 377–383, 2001.

[14] P. Bain and J.-E. Toublanc, "Adult height in congenital hypothyroidism: prognostic factors and the importance of compliance with treatment," *Hormone Research*, vol. 58, no. 3, pp. 136–142, 2002.

[15] B. Boersma, B. J. Otten, G. B. A. Stoelinga, and J. M. Wit, "Catch-up growth after prolonged hypothyroidism," *European Journal of Pediatrics*, vol. 155, no. 5, pp. 362–367, 1996.

[16] J. Alm, A. Larsson, and R. Zetterstrom, "Congenital hypothyroidism in Sweden. Psychomotor development in patients detected by clinical signs and symptoms," *Acta Paediatrica Scandinavica*, vol. 70, no. 6, pp. 907–912, 1981.

[17] G. J. Frost and J. M. Parkin, "A comparison between the neurological and intellectual abnormalities in children and adults with congenital hypothyroidism," *European Journal of Pediatrics*, vol. 145, no. 6, pp. 480–484, 1986.

[18] W. F. Simons, P. W. Fuggle, D. B. Grant, and I. Smith, "Intellectual development at 10 years in early treated congenital hypothyroidism," *Archives of Disease in Childhood*, vol. 71, no. 3, pp. 232–234, 1994.

[19] J. Simoneau-Roy, S. Marti, C. Deal, C. Huot, P. Robaey, and G. Van Vliet, "Cognition and behavior at school entry in children with congenital hypothyroidism treated early with high-dose levothyroxine," *Journal of Pediatrics*, vol. 144, no. 6, pp. 747–752, 2004.

[20] S. Bargagna, D. Dinetti, A. Pinchera et al., "School attainments in children with congenital hypothyroidism detected by neonatal screening and treated early in life," *European Journal of Endocrinology*, vol. 140, no. 5, pp. 407–413, 1999.

[21] B. Oerbeck, K. Sundet, B. F. Kase, and S. Heyerdahl, "Congenital hypothyroidism: influence of disease severity and L-thyroxine treatment on intellectual, motor, and school-associated outcomes in young adults," *Pediatrics*, vol. 112, no. 4, pp. 923–930, 2003.

[22] J. F. Rovet, "Long-term neuropsychological sequelae of early-treated congenital hypothyroidism: effects in adolescence," *Acta Paediatrica*, vol. 88, no. 432, pp. 88–95, 1999.

[23] J. F. Rovet, "In search of the optimal therapy for congenital hypothyroidism," *Journal of Pediatrics*, vol. 144, no. 6, pp. 698–700, 2004.

[24] G. H. Murphy, J. A. Hulse, I. Smith, and D. B. Grant, "Congenital hypothyroidism: physiological and psychological factors in early development," *Journal of Child Psychology and Psychiatry and Allied Disciplines*, vol. 31, no. 5, pp. 711–725, 1990.

[25] S. L. Tillotson, P. W. Fuggle, I. Smith, A. E. Ades, and D. B. Grant, "Relation between biochemical severity and intelligence in early treated congenital hypothyroidism: a threshold effect," *British Medical Journal*, vol. 309, no. 6952, pp. 440–445, 1994.

[26] M. J. E. Kempers, L. van der Sluijs Veer, R. W. G. Nijhuis-van der Sanden et al., "Neonatal screening for congenital hypothyroidism in The Netherlands: cognitive and motor outcome at 10 years of age," *Journal of Clinical Endocrinology and Metabolism*, vol. 92, no. 3, pp. 919–924, 2007.

[27] M. J. E. Kempers, L. van der Sluijs Veer, M. W. G. Nijhuis-van der Sanden et al., "Intellectual and motor development of young adults with congenital hypothyroidism diagnosed by neonatal screening," *Journal of Clinical Endocrinology and Metabolism*, vol. 91, no. 2, pp. 418–424, 2006.

[28] K. A. Selva, A. Harper, A. Downs, P. A. Blasco, and S. H. LaFranchi, "Neurodevelopmental outcomes in congenital hypothyroidism: comparison of initial T4 dose and time to reach target T4 and TSH," *Journal of Pediatrics*, vol. 147, no. 6, pp. 775–780, 2005.

[29] J. J. Bongers-Schokking, H. M. Koot, D. Wiersma, P. H. Verkerk, and S. M. P. F. De Keizer-Schrama, "Influence of timing and dose of thyroid hormone replacement on development in infants with congenital hypothyroidism," *Journal of Pediatrics*, vol. 136, no. 3, pp. 292–297, 2000.

[30] S. Heyerdahl, "Treatment variables as predictors of intellectual outcome in children with congenital hypothyroidism," *European Journal of Pediatrics*, vol. 155, no. 5, pp. 357–361, 1996.

[31] A. Gruters, K. P. Liesenkoetter, M. Zapico et al., "Results of the screening program for congenital hypothyroidism in Berlin (1978–1995)," *Experimental Clinical Endocrinology and Diabetes*, vol. 105, supplement 4, pp. 28–31, 1997.

[32] A. R. Kemper, L. Ouyang, and S. D. Grosse, "Discontinuation of thyroid hormone treatment among children in the United States with congenital hypothyroidism: findings from health insurance claims data," *BMC Pediatrics*, vol. 10, article 9, 2010.

15

Metastatic Papillary Thyroid Carcinoma in a Paediatric Patient

Nthabiseng Ellen Mothata,[1] **Takalani Gidion Morulana**,[2] **Nyaweleni Tshifularo**,[2] **Phumudzo Bridgett Nemutaduni**,[3] **Nozipho Elizabeth Nyakale**,[3] **and Moshawa Calvin Khaba**[1]

[1]*Department of Anatomical Pathology, Dr George Mukhari Academic Laboratory, National Health Laboratory Services, Sefako Makgatho Health Sciences University, Ga-Rankuwa, South Africa*
[2]*Department of Paediatric Surgery, Dr George Mukhari Academic Hospital, Sefako Makgatho Health Sciences University, Ga-Rankuwa, South Africa*
[3]*Department of Nuclear Medicine, Dr George Mukhari Academic Hospital, Sefako Makgatho Health Sciences University, Ga-Rankuwa, South Africa*

Correspondence should be addressed to Moshawa Calvin Khaba; ckhaba@yahoo.co.uk

Academic Editor: Mihail A. Boyanov

Papillary thyroid carcinoma is the most common endocrine cancer in the paediatric population. Although the disease is diagnosed at a later stage, the prognosis is favourable. When these patients present with lymph nodal and/or pulmonary metastases, they may be initially confused for infectious diseases such as tuberculosis. Therefore, thorough clinical assessment including radiology and microbiological and histopathological assessment is important for early and correct diagnosis. We report an 11-year-old female patient who presented with cervical lymphadenopathy and the histopathological assessment confirmed metastatic papillary thyroid carcinoma. Subsequent radiological investigation revealed further metastasis to the lung. This manuscript highlights the difficulties that might be encountered in the initial management of paediatric PTC which present atypically.

1. Introduction

Paediatric thyroid carcinomas are rare endocrine cancers, majority of which are comprised of papillary thyroid carcinoma (PTC) followed by follicular carcinoma [1]. They are associated with radiation exposure, thyroid disease such as Hashimoto's thyroiditis, and inherited condition such as familial adenomatous polyposis. They are more common in older children and adolescence with a female-to-male ratio of 5 : 1 [2, 3]. Approximately less than 3% of the patients have thyroid nodules which should raise a high index of suspicion for malignancy [1, 4]. A definite diagnosis is usually delayed due to the subtle presentation of the primary malignancy, and therefore, they may present late with metastatic disease [1]. The gold standard of diagnosis is histopathology. Surgery and radioactive iodine are the treatment of choice in these patients and are dependent on the risk groups [5]. Although they present with metastatic disease, the prognosis still remains good [2]. We present a paediatric patient who presented atypically with metastatic PTC to the cervical lymph nodes and lungs.

2. Case Presentation

An 11-year-old African female patient presented to paediatric surgery department with a 4 months' history of lump on the left side of the neck. She gave a history of a painless and slow-growing lump on the left side of the neck that was treated with antibiotics by several general practitioners with no improvement. She did not have any comorbidities; however, her mother has a thyroidectomy for nodular goiter. She appeared chronically ill without pallor, jaundice, or proptosis. Her vital signs were within normal limits. She had a lateral neck mass that measured 50 mm × 40 mm which was mobile, nontender, and hard with attachment to the skin. Other systemic examinations were unremarkable. Blood investigation was within normal limits including thyroid function tests. A neck ultrasound showed an enlarged left cervical lymph node with a normal blood flow in the right and left thyroid lobes. There was a macrolobulated lesion (TIRADS 5) with increased flow and mass effect to the internal jugular vein (Figure 1(a)). A lymph node biopsy was done and confirmed a metastatic papillary thyroid carcinoma. A subsequent staging computed tomography (CT) scan showed a distinct focal peripheral mass lesion on the inferior pole of the left thyroid lobe with calcifications, mass effect on the left internal jugular vein (Figure 1(b)), and bilateral upper lung lobe nodules. An uneventful total thyroidectomy with a modified neck dissection was done and sent for histopathological assessment.

Gross pathology showed a thyroid tumour that measured 55 × 35 × 10 mm and matted lymph nodes. The tumour was unencapsulated, hemorrhagic, and firm without necrosis.

Microscopic examination confirmed papillary variant of PTC evidenced by tumour arranged in papillae, nests, and follicles (Figures 2(a) and 2(b)). These structures were lined by follicular cells with nuclei exhibiting grooves, clearing, pseudoinclusions, overlapping, and crowding. In addition, five lymph nodes that were sampled showed metastatic disease.

An iodine-123 single photon emission computed tomography (SPECT) scan done postsurgery, under high thyrotropin stimulation (>30 mU/L), showed increased nonuniform uptake in level II, III, and IV cervical lymph nodes, mild residual uptake in the thyroid bed, and increased uptake in the lungs bilaterally (Figure 3(a)). These features confirmed metastatic disease to the lymph nodes and lungs.

A left lateral lymph node clearance was done which further confirmed metastatic papillary thyroid carcinoma. Four weeks postsurgery, the patient received 100 mCi of I-131 therapy. This was under TSH stimulation with the withdrawal of eltroxin for 4 weeks and given I^{131} under maximally stimulated TSH. Prophylactic dose of prednisone was given in conjunction with this therapy to minimize inflammatory response that may result from the radiation.

The posttherapeutic iodine-131 images (Figure 3(b)) done prior to discharge were congruent in pattern to the staging iodine-123 scan images. Thyroid function tests were low (thyroxine: 10.4 pmol/L, tri-iodo thyronine: 5.6 pmol/L, and thyroid-stimulating hormone: 0.54 mIU/L). The patient was discharged on eltroxin daily.

At the 6th month follow-up visit, she tolerated the RAI well with improved nutritional status. She was euthyroid with TSH: 4.13 mIU/L, T4: 9.4 pmol/L, T3: 6.0 pmol/L, and thyroglobulin: >300 μg/L. She was put on lifetime thyroid hormone replacement therapy.

3. Discussion

Papillary thyroid carcinoma is the leading cause of paediatric endocrine cancers with an incidence of 6% of all cancers [1]. In typical cases of PTC, patients present as multifocal involving both lobes and 50% of children present with cervical lymph node metastasis and lung metastasis. The initial evaluation of thyroid nodule or neck mass is serum TSH and T4 which in most cases is normal at presentation, followed by neck ultrasound. This is followed by a confirmatory fine-needle aspiration (FNA) [6]. Our patient presented with atypical feature, an asymptomatic neck mass on the left side of the neck; therefore, a normal workup for thyroid disease was not followed. She did not have risk factors for thyroid malignancy; hence, a clinical diagnosis of thyroid malignancy was not entertained. Whilst Hashimoto's thyroiditis (HT) is the commonest risk factor associated with paediatric PTC [7], the patient did not report any history of autoimmune disease. Furthermore, histopathological assessment of thyroid did not reveal background HT. While thyroid function tests would not have helped as they are usually normal, FNA of the mass should still be done. This helps to exclude nonmalignant and malignant disease. Clinician should always have a high index of suspicion for malignancy in children who presents with asymptomatic neck mass.

The histomorphological features of PTC in children are the same as in adults. Although it may present with varied growth patterns including papillary, follicular, and solid, amongst others, the diagnosis is based on typical nuclear features. These features include Orphan Annie eye nuclei which are optically clear. They also exhibit pseudoinclusion and grooves [8]. The diagnosis on the index patient was done based on these features.

The management of PTC involves extensive planning from staging preoperatively and deciding on approach that will benefit both the patient and family. Given the very high rate of metastatic disease in this population, preoperative neck ultrasound to identify suspicious lymph nodes and chest X-ray and/or chest CT should be considered in these patients as it will guide on the type of surgical treatment to be followed.

The latest American Thyroid Association (ATA) children's guidelines, published in 2015, recommend radioactive iodine therapy (RAI) after total thyroidectomy for intermediate- and high-risk groups who have extensive central neck lymph node involvement or locally invasive or extensive lateral neck cervical lymph nodes. The aim of RAI is to increase the response rate to surgical management. It has been reported that when radioactive iodine therapy is used in conjunction with thyroid-stimulating hormone (TSH) suppression, the rate for complete response is 47.32% and for partial response is 38.39%. Postsurgical RAI therapy is indicated in paediatric PTC due to its increased risk of bilateral (30%) or multifocal involvement (65%) [6, 8].

Lymph node dissection is recommended to reduce the risk of recurrence and increase the efficacy of RAI therapy in patients with extrathyroidal invasion or locoregional metastasis [8–10].

The index patient was in the high-risk group, and hence, a total thyroidectomy with radical neck dissection and radioactive therapy was the preferred choice of treatment.

The follow-up guidelines include serum thyroglobulin on levothyroxine every 3–6 months for 2–3 years then

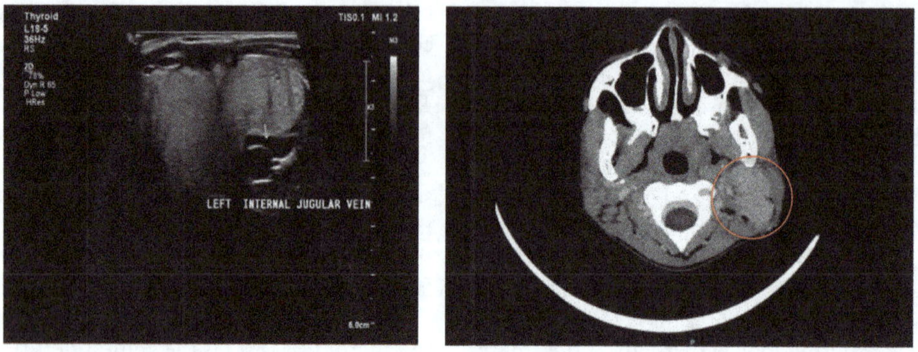

(a) (b)

FIGURE 1: (a) Neck ultrasound shows enlarged left cervical lymph node compressing on the left internal jugular vein; (b) CT scan shows mattered left cervical lymphadenopathy (○).

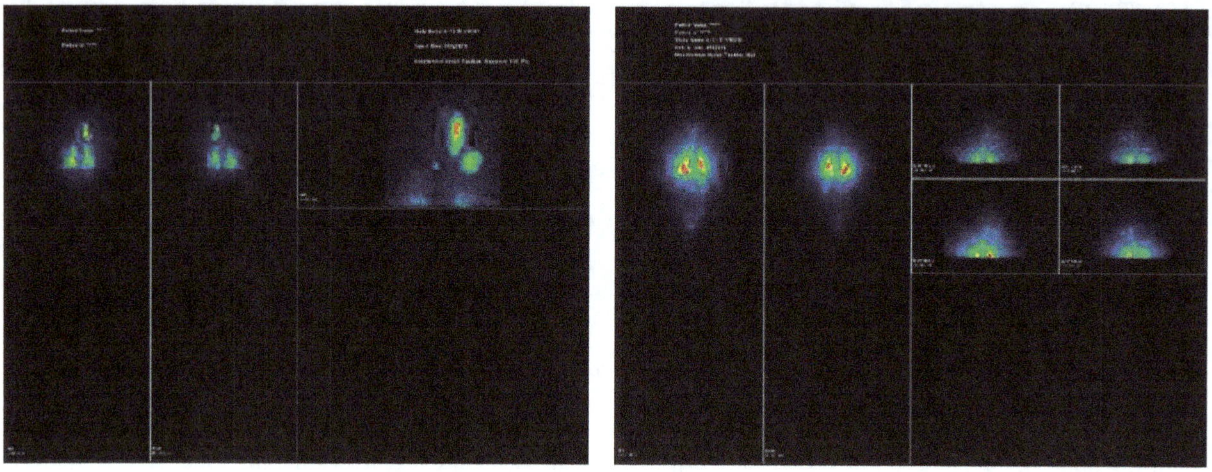

(a) (b)

FIGURE 2: (a) I^{123} and (b) I^{131} show increased nonuniform uptake in level II, III, and IV cervical lymph nodes, mild residual uptake in the thyroid bed, and increased uptake in the lungs bilaterally.

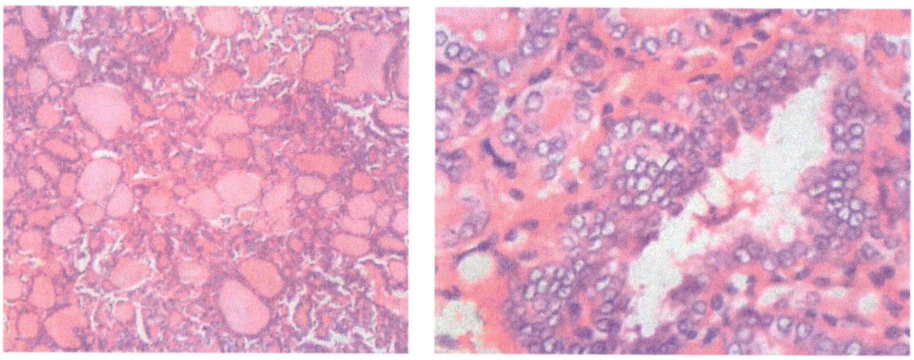

(a) (b)

FIGURE 3: (a) Thyroid tumour with papillary and follicular pattern; (b) typical nuclear features of PTC: nuclear overlapping, clearing, and occasional grooves.

annually and thyroid ultrasound including cervical lymph nodes for 6–12 months for intermediate- and high-risk groups and annually for low-risk patients. In case the thyroglobulin level is elevated, and the thyroid ultrasound is negative, then a CT scan of the chest and neck is recommended. In children, more than 98% of cases have a good survival rate at 10 years while few patients develop progressive or refractory disease not amenable to surgical intervention or resistant to radioactive therapy.

The prognosis for PTC is excellent with low mortality rate. The survival rate for different risk groups is as follows: 99% for low-risk groups, 83% for intermediate-risk groups, and 43% for high-risk groups [11].

The survivors of childhood ductal thyroid carcinoma need a follow-up for life since recurrence has been reported at 40 years after initial therapy [8].

In conclusion, fine-needle aspiration may provide early diagnosis in children with neck mass and avoid delayed management. A high index of suspicion for PTC should be maintained, regardless of risk factors. This allows for early targeted treatment with reduction in morbidity and mortality in this population. Surgical treatment with or without lymph node dissection and radiotherapy remains the cornerstone of management in paediatric PTC.

Consent

Written, informed consent was obtained from the parent of the patient for publication of this case report. A copy of the consent form is available for review.

Acknowledgments

The authors all express their gratitude to the patient's parents who gave consent for this case to be presented in this paper.

References

[1] V. A. Paulson, E. R. Rudzinski, and D. S. Hawkins, "Thyroid cancer in the pediatric population," *Genes (Basel)*, vol. 10, no. 9, p. 723, 2019.

[2] K. A. Lee, M. T. A. Sharabiani, D. Tumino et al., "Differentiated thyroid cancer in children: a UK multicentre review and review of the literature," *Clinical Oncology*, vol. 31, no. 6, pp. 385–390, 2019.

[3] J. Chen, N. Huang, Q. Ji, Y. Wang, Y. Zhu, and D. Li, "Multifocal papillary thyroid cancer in children and adolescents: 12-year experience in a single center," *Gland Surgery*, vol. 8, no. 5, pp. 507–515, 2019.

[4] A. I. Stefan, A. Piciu, A. Mester, D. Apostu, M. Badan, and C. I. Badulescu, "Pediatric thyroid cancer in Europe: an overdiagnosed condition? a literature review," *Diagnostics*, vol. 10, no. 2, p. 112, 2020.

[5] P. K. Prasad, P. Mahajan, D. S. Hawkins, S. Mostoufi-Moab, and R. Venkatramani, "Management of pediatric differentiated thyroid cancer: an overview for the pediatric oncologist," *Pediatric Blood and Cancer*, vol. 67, no. 6, p. e28141, 2020.

[6] J. D. Prescott and M. A. Zeiger, "The RET oncogene in papillary thyroid carcinoma," *Cancer*, vol. 121, no. 13, pp. 2137–2146, 2015.

[7] M. L. Sur, R. Gaga, C. Lazăr, C. Lazea, C. Aldea, and D. Sur, "Papillary thyroid carcinoma in children with Hashimoto's thyroiditis-a review of the literature between 2000 and 2020," *Journal of Pediatric Endocrinology and Metabolism*, vol. 33, no. 12, pp. 1511–1517, 2020.

[8] G. L. Francis, S. G. Waguespack, A. J. Bauer et al., "Management guidelines for children with thyroid nodules and differentiated thyroid cancer," *Thyroid*, vol. 25, no. 7, pp. 716–759, 2015.

[9] H. D. Baumgarten, A. J. Bauer, A. Isaza, S. Mostoufi-Moab, K. Kazahaya, and N. S. Adzick, "Surgical management of pediatric thyroid disease: complication rates after thyroidectomy at the children's hospital of philadelphia high-volume pediatric thyroid center," *Journal of Pediatric Surgery*, vol. 54, no. 10, pp. 1969–1975, 2019.

[10] L. Massimo, D. Zarri, and D. Caprino, "Psychosocial aspects of survivors of childhood cancer or leukemia," *Minerva pediatrica*, vol. 57, no. 6, pp. 389–397, 2005.

[11] I. D. Hay, T. Gonzalez-Losada, M. S. Reinalda, J. A. Honetschlager, M. L. Richards, and G. B. Thompson, "Long-term outcome in 215 children and adolescents with papillary thyroid cancer treated during 1940 through 2008," *World Journal of Surgery*, vol. 34, no. 6, pp. 1192–1202, 2010.

16

An Adolescent Female with Bipolar Disorder Presenting with Lithium-Induced Hyperthyroidism

Pratibha Rana,[1] Patria Alba Aponte,[1] and Ghufran Babar[2]

[1]*Children's Mercy Hospital, 3101 Broadway Blvd., Kansas City, MO 64111, USA*
[2]*Department of Pediatric Endocrinology, Children's Mercy Hospital, 3101 Broadway Blvd., Kansas City, MO 64111, USA*

Correspondence should be addressed to Ghufran Babar; gbabar@cmh.edu

Academic Editor: Lucy Mastrandrea

Lithium therapy has been associated with several endocrine disorders including thyroid dysfunction, diabetes insipidus, and hyperparathyroidism. While its suppressive effect on thyroid function is well known, it is very rare to observe lithium-induced hyperthyroidism especially in the pediatric population. Here, we describe a case of lithium-induced hyperthyroidism in an adolescent female with bipolar disorder. The patient is a 17-year-old female who was treated with lithium for bipolar disorder and presented with symptoms and laboratory findings consistent with hyperthyroidism. Since thyroid autoantibodies were negative, thyroid dysfunction was attributed to lithium toxicity. Indeed, her clinical and biochemical hyperthyroid state resolved after stopping lithium therapy. Lithium-associated hyperthyroidism can occur in the pediatric population. We propose close monitoring of thyroid hormone levels in children on lithium therapy.

1. Case Report

Bipolar disorders are common in adolescents, with a lifetime prevalence of 2.5% [1] and 0.1% in children aged 9–13 years [2]. Lithium is commonly used for the treatment of bipolar disorders in children and adolescents [3]. It has been associated with several endocrine disorders including thyroid dysfunction, diabetes insipidus, and hyperparathyroidism. Its suppressive effect on thyroid function is well known; in contrast, lithium-induced hyperthyroidism is rare with a prevalence in the range of between 1% and 1.7% in the adult population [4, 5]. The first case of thyrotoxicosis in a patient treated with lithium was reported in 1974 [6]. Hyperthyroidism in lithium-treated patients has been associated with diffuse goiter, toxic multinodular goiter, and painless thyroiditis [7]. Lithium is also implicated in granulomatous thyroiditis, and it is reported to induce auto-antibody formation and autoimmunity in susceptible individuals [8]. There have not been any cases reported about lithium-induced hyperthyroidism in pediatric population. We are presenting an adolescent girl treated with lithium who presented with hyperthyroidism.

2. Methods

Retrospective chart review of the case study was carried out. Since it is a single case report, an approval from the Institutional Review Board (IRB) and consent are not required. However, when a new patient is seen in our clinic, the family signed a consent form for treatment and possible use of any clinical finding to report anonymously.

3. Case Presentation

Our patient is a 17-year-5-month-old female with bipolar disorder who was treated with lithium. She had been placed on Concerta, Abilify, and Lamictal before being switched to lithium monotherapy due to the limited success of these initial therapies. She responded well to lithium for two years until about 3-4 weeks prior to presentation, when she developed dizziness, heat intolerance, excessive sweating, tremors, and palpitations. Due to these symptoms, she stopped taking lithium and sought medical attention at her primary care provider's (PCP's) office. The PCP ordered laboratory tests which revealed a

TABLE 1: Hormonal profile of the patient with gradual improvements of thyroid hormone levels from being hyperthyroid to euthyroid.

Timeline	TSH (0.35–5.5 mcIU/mL)	Free T4 (0.9–1.9 ng/dL)	Total T3 (55–209 ng/dL)
Initial lab work	0.01	3.5	
2 days later	<0.02	3.7	351
2 weeks later	<0.02	2.0	
1 month later	<0.02	1.5	
2 months	<0.02	0.9	188
3 months	0.39	0.8	175
5 months	2.61	1.2	172
7 months	2.62	1.1	134

`suppressed TSH (<0.02 mcIU/mL, normal range: 0.35–5.50) and an elevated free T4 (3.5 ng/dL, normal range: 0.8–1.9), both consistent with hyperthyroidism. Her lithium level at that time was <0.3 (normal range: 0.6–1.2 mmol/L), likely due to noncompliance during the past two weeks. The PCP received these results on the weekend, and the patient was referred to the emergency department (ED) where, on examination, she was tachycardic (140 bpm), afebrile, and her blood pressure was 132/84 mmHg. Her thyroid exam revealed the presence of a nontender goiter; no nodules were palpable. Repeat laboratory tests at the ED confirmed biochemical hyperthyroidism (TSH: <0.02 mcIU/mL, total T3: 351 ng/dl, normal range: 55 to 209) and an elevated free T4 (3.7 ng/dL). There was a prolonged QT interval on her EKG. Of note, our patient had no family history of autoimmunity or thyroid disease. Thyroid suppressive therapy was initiated with methimazole, 10 mg PO 3 times a day (0.46 mg/kg/day) as advised by the endocrinologist. She was also started on propranolol (60 mg/day~0.92 mg/kg/day). The ESR, CRP, CBC, and BMP were normal. Thyroid autoantibodies (antithyroid peroxidase antibody, antithyroglobulin antibody, and thyroid stimulating immunoglobulin) were all negative. She was advised not to restart lithium and consult her psychiatrist. She was seen in the endocrine clinic about two weeks later, after being off-lithium for four weeks; her hyperthyroid symptoms had improved; however, she still had palpitations and heat intolerance, while her heart rate and blood pressure were still above the age appropriate ranges (101 bpm and 133/74 mm hg, respectively). She had mild tongue fasciculation but no exophthalmos. Repeat thyroid function tests showed a lower free T4 level (2.0 ng/dl) as compared with two weeks ago, while the TSH was still suppressed. A subsequent endocrine visit two weeks later showed a normalized free T4 (1.5 ng/dl) and improved clinical hyperthyroidism. As a result, propranolol was discontinued, while methimazole treatment was maintained. By three months after her initial presentation, the methimazole dose was reduced (10 mg b.i.d.) due to a borderline-low (0.8 ng/dl, normal range of 0.8 to 1.9 ng/dL), Methimazole was eventually discontinued after five months of initial presentation. At her last follow-up in the endocrine clinic (seven months after diagnosis of hyperthyroidism and several weeks after stopping methimazole), she was clinically and biochemically euthyroid (Table 1).

4. Discussion

The prevalence of bipolar disorders in adolescence ranges between 1.8% and 2.5% [9, 10]. They are considered as the fourth leading cause of disability among adolescent worldwide. In children with bipolar disorders, lithium is the only mood stabilizer approved by the FDA for acute mania and maintenance treatment [11]. In a recent meta-analysis of studies on the effects of lithium on thyroid function, the investigators compared the prevalence of hypothyroidism in patients treated with lithium with controls. The overall odds of clinical hypothyroidism were close to six times greater in lithium-treated subjects than in controls. Conversely, this study did not find any difference between patients and controls on lithium with respect to the prevalence of increased thyroid function [4]. On the contrary, lithium-induced hyperthyroidism is rare even in adults [12]; it is estimated to have the annual incidence of 0.1% [13]. Other studies have estimated the prevalence to be in the range of 1%–1.7% [5, 14]. Only a small number of children treated with lithium present with subclinical or clinical hypothyroidism, and/or goiter [15, 16], to our knowledge, ours is the first case of a pediatric patient with lithium-induced hyperthyroidism. The possible mechanism regarding lithium-induced hyperthyroidism is thought to be due to an expansion of the intrathyroidal iodine pool, induction of autoimmune hyperthyroidism (Graves' disease), and a toxic thyroid nodule or painless thyroiditis [7, 17]. In patients with primary affective disorders, thyroid autoantibodies were detected in 8 of 40 subjects treated with lithium, and only in 3 patients were treated with other psychotropic drugs. Furthermore, the lithium-treated patients exhibited significantly reduced numbers of suppressor and or cytotoxic T cells and increased B cell activity compared to those treated with drugs other than lithium [18]. Similar to amiodarone-induced toxic thyroiditis, painless thyroiditis may also be the result of a direct toxic effect of lithium on the thyroid, which seems to be the likely mechanism in our patient, in whom results of tests for thyroid antibodies remained negative. Furthermore, it has been reported that lithium-associated silent thyroiditis occurred with an incidence rate of approximately 1.3 cases per 1000 person-years, and lithium-associated thyrotoxicosis occurred with an incidence rate of approximately 2.7 cases per 1000 person-years, higher than the reported incidence rates of silent thyroiditis (<0.03–0.28 cases per 1000 person-years) and of thyrotoxicosis (0.8–1.2 cases per 1000 person-years) in the general population and calculated the odds of lithium exposure to be 4.7-fold higher in patients with thyroiditis [7]. Recently, a meta-analysis of 52 studies showed in nine of these that were cross-sectional or cohort studies describing around 2500 patients that 2.6% patients were hypothyroid [19]. Another cross-sectional study reported just one patient (1.2%) in their lithium-treated group [20]. The histopathological features of the thyroid gland showed an immunological phenomenon with lymphoid follicles and fibrosis in affected thyroid glands [21], and this autoimmune process was not detected in other prospective studies, pre- and postlithium treatment [22, 23]. In our patient, the thyroid antibodies were negative; CBC, C-reactive protein (CRP), and sedimentation rate (ESR) were normal, suggesting that a mild silent thyroiditis may have been the cause of hyperthyroidism. Miller and Daniels described that most hyperthyroid patients had serum lithium level in the therapeutic range [7]. However, our patient's lithium level was not elevated due to discontinuation of treatment 2 weeks before the levels were checked. The duration of lithium therapy in patients who develop hyperthyroidism and lithium-associated silent thyroiditis range between 6 days and 15 years. However, in some cases, thyrotoxicosis occurred 4 days to 5 months after withdrawal of lithium therapy [24], and in our patient, the duration of lithium therapy was about 2 years. In conclusion, lithium-induced hyperthyroidism is very rarely diagnosed in adults and has never been reported in children before our case. We believe it is necessary to increase awareness of the possibility of such drug-induced thyroid dysfunction in the pediatric population, especially in children with hyperthyroidism and negative thyroid autoantibodies. The transient nature of this disorder is associated with a better prognosis compared to patients with Graves' disease. Since lithium-induced hyperthyroidism may occur even after years of lithium therapy, it is advisable to regularly monitor the thyroid function in children during the whole duration of lithium treatment.

References

[1] K. R. Merikangas, H. S. Akiskal, J. Angst et al., "Lifetime and 12-month prevalence of bipolar spectrum disorder in the national comorbidity survey replication," *Archives of General Psychiatry*, vol. 64, no. 5, pp. 543–552, 2007.

[2] E. J. Costello, A. Angold, B. J. Burns et al., "The great smoky mountains study of youth," *Archives of General Psychiatry*, vol. 53, no. 12, pp. 1129–1136, 1996.

[3] B. Grant and J. A. Salpekar, "Using lithium in children and adolescents with bipolar disorder: efficacy, tolerability, and practical considerations," *Pediatric Drugs*, vol. 20, no. 4, pp. 303–314, 2018.

[4] R. F. McKnight, M. Adida, K. Budge, S. Stockton, G. M. Goodwin, and J. R. Geddes, "Lithium toxicity profile: a systematic review and meta-analysis," *The Lancet*, vol. 379, no. 9817, pp. 721–728, 2012.

[5] B. E. W. Brownlie and J. E. Wells, "The epidemiology of thyrotoxicosis in New Zealand: incidence and geographical distribution in north canterbury, 1983-1985," *Clinical Endocrinology*, vol. 33, no. 2, pp. 249–259, 1990.

[6] L. M. Franklin, "Thyrotoxicosis developing during lithium treatment: case report," *The New Zealand Medical Journal*, vol. 79, no. 511, p. 782, 1974.

[7] K. K. Miller and G. H. Daniels, "Association between lithium use and thyrotoxicosis caused by silent thyroiditis," *Clinical Endocrinology*, vol. 55, no. 4, pp. 501–508, 2001.

[8] M. J. Sinnott, H. D. McIntyre, and S. M. Pond, "Granulomatous thyroiditis and lithium therapy," *Australian and New Zealand Journal of Medicine*, vol. 22, no. 1, p. 84, 1992.

[9] A. R. Van Meter, A. L. R. Moreira, and E. A. Youngstrom, "Meta-analysis of epidemiologic studies of pediatric bipolar disorder," *The Journal of Clinical Psychiatry*, vol. 72, no. 9, pp. 1250–1256, 2011.

[10] K. R. Merikangas, L. Cui, G. Kattan, G. A. Carlson, E. A. Youngstrom, and J. Angst, "Mania with and without depression in a community sample of US adolescents," *Archives of General Psychiatry*, vol. 69, no. 9, pp. 943–951, 2012.

[11] J. McClellan, R. Kowatch, and R. L. Findling, "Practice parameter for the assessment and treatment of children and adolescents with bipolar disorder," *Journal of the American Academy of Child & Adolescent Psychiatry*, vol. 46, no. 1, pp. 107–125, 2007.

[12] M. L. Barclay, B. E. W. Brownlie, J. G. Turner, and J. E. Wells, "Lithium associated thyrotoxicosis: a report of 14 cases, with statistical analysis of incidence," *Clinical Endocrinology*, vol. 40, no. 6, pp. 759–764, 1994.

[13] A. Bocchetta and A. Loviselli, "Lithium treatment and thyroid abnormalities," *Clinical Practice and Epidemiology in Mental Health*, vol. 2, no. 1, pp. 23–28, 2006.

[14] R. Yassa, A. Saunders, C. Nastase, and Y. Camille, "Lithium-induced thyroid disorders: a prevalence study," *The Journal of Clinical Psychiatry*, vol. 49, no. 1, pp. 14–16, 1988.

[15] R. L. Findling, A. Robb, N. K. McNamara et al., "Lithium in the acute treatment of bipolar I disorder: a double-blind, placebo controlled study," *Pediatrics*, vol. 136, no. 5, pp. 885–894, 2015.

[16] G. R. DeLong and A. L. Aldershof, "Long-term experience with lithium treatment in childhood: correlation with clinical diagnosis," *Journal of the American Academy of Child & Adolescent Psychiatry*, vol. 26, no. 3, pp. 389–394, 1987.

[17] M. T. McDermott, K. D. Burman, F. D. Hofeldt, and G. S. Kidd, "Lithium-associated thyrotoxicosis," *The American Journal of Medicine*, vol. 80, no. 6, pp. 1245–1248, 1986.

[18] R. Wilson, J. H. McKlllop, G. T. Crocket et al., "The effect of lithium therapy on parameters thought to be involved in the development of autoimmune thyroid disease," *Clinical Endocrinology*, vol. 34, no. 5, pp. 357–361, 1991.

[19] F. Fairbrother, N. Petzl, J. G. Scott, and S. Kisely, "Lithium can cause hyperthyroidism as well as hypothyroidism: a systematic review of an under-recognised association," *Australian & New Zealand Journal of Psychiatry*, vol. 53, no. 5, pp. 384–402, 2019.

[20] O. K. Tuncel, F. Akdeniz, S. S. Ozbek, G. Kavukcu, and G. U. Kocabas, "Thyroid function and ultrasonography abnormalities in lithium-treated bipolar patients: a cross-sectional study with healthy controls," *Noro Psikiyatri Arsivi*, vol. 54, no. 2, pp. 108–115, 2017.

[21] T. Kontozoglou and N. Mambo, "The histopathologic features of lithium-associated thyroiditis," *Human Pathology*, vol. 14, no. 8, pp. 737–739, 1983.
[22] D. H. Myers, R. A. Carter, B. H. Burns, A. Armond, S. B. Hussain, and V. K. Chengapa, "A prospective study of the effects of lithium on thyroid function and on the prevalence of antithyroid antibodies," *Psychological Medicine*, vol. 15, no. 1, pp. 55–61, 1985.
[23] J. R. Calabrese, A. D. Gulledge, K. Hahn, R. Skwerer, M. Kotz, and O. P. Schumacher, "Autoimmune thyroiditis in manic depressive patients treated with lithium," *American Journal of Psychiatry*, vol. 142, no. 11, pp. 1318–1321, 1985.
[24] A. H. Dang and J. M. Hershman, "Lithium-associated thyroiditis," *Endocrine Practice*, vol. 8, no. 3, pp. 232–236, 2002.

17

Genotyping of *ABCC8*, *KCNJ11* and *HADH* in Iranian Infants with Congenital Hyperinsulinism

Somayyeh Hashemian,[1] Reza Jafarzadeh Esfehani,[2] Siroos Karimdadi,[1] Nosrat Ghaemi,[1] Peyman Eshraghi,[1] Najmeh Malekzadeh Gonabadi,[3] Amirhossein Sahebkar,[4,5,6] Rahim Vakili,[1] and Mohammad Reza Abbaszadegan[7]

[1]*Department of Pediatric Diseases, Akbar Hospital, Faculty of Medicine, Mashhad University of Medical Sciences, Mashhad, Iran*
[2]*Department of Medical Genetics, Faculty of Medicine, Mashhad University of Medical Sciences, Mashhad, Iran*
[3]*Faculty of Sciences, Sistan and Baluchestan University, Zahedan, Iran*
[4]*Biotechnology Research Center, Pharmaceutical Technology Institute, Mashhad University of Medical Sciences, Mashhad, Iran*
[5]*Applied Biomedical Research Center, Mashhad University of Medical Sciences, Mashhad, Iran*
[6]*School of Pharmacy, Mashhad University of Medical Sciences, Mashhad, Iran*
[7]*Medical Genetic Research Center, Medical School, Mashhad University of Medical Sciences, Mashhad, Iran*

Correspondence should be addressed to Amirhossein Sahebkar; amir_saheb2000@yahoo.com, Rahim Vakili; vakilir@mums.ac.ir, and Mohammad Reza Abbaszadegan; abbaszadeganmr@mums.ac.ir

Academic Editor: Suat Simsek

Background. Congenital hyperinsulinism (CHI) is a heterogeneous disease with various underlying genetic causes. Among different genes considered effective in the development of CHI, *ABCC8*, *KCNJ11*, and *HADH* genes are among the important genes, especially in a population with a considerable rate of consanguineous marriage. Mutational analysis of these genes guides clinicians to better treatment and prediction of prognosis for this rare disease. The present study aimed to evaluate genetic variants in *ABCC8*, *KCNJ11*, and *HADH* genes as causative genes for CHI in the Iranian population. *Methods.* The present case series took place in Mashhad, Iran, within 11 years. Every child who had a clinical phenotype and confirmatory biochemical tests of CHI enrolled in this study. Variants in *ABCC8*, *KCNJ11*, and *HADH* genes were analyzed by the polymerase chain reaction and sequencing in our patients. *Results.* Among 20 pediatric patients, 16 of them had variants in *ABCC8*, *KCNJ11*, and *HADH* genes. The mean age of genetic diagnosis was 18.6 days. A homozygous missense (c.2041-21G > *A*) mutation in the *ABCC8* gene was seen in three infants. Other common variants were frameshift variants (c.3438dup) in the *ABCC8* gene and a missense variant (c.287-288delinsTG) in the *KCNJ11* gene. Most of the variants in our population were still categorized as variants of unknown significance and only 7 pathogenic variants were present. *Conclusion.* Most variants were located in the *ABCC8* gene in our population. Because most of the variants in our population are not previously reported, performing further functional studies is warranted.

1. Introduction

Congenital hyperinsulinism (CHI) is an important cause of hypoglycemia during the neonatal period and infancy. While transient hypoglycemia could be considered as a common metabolic abnormality among neonates, only 1% of these infants develop repetitive or persistent episodes of hypoglycemia [1]. During CHI, an increased level of insulin within the infant's blood decreases free glucose and results in neurological dysfunction. Repeated episodes of hypoglycemia can also result in neurological damage including mental retardation and developmental delay [2, 3]. Considering the heterogeneous nature of CHI, not all affected infants will have the same clinical presentation and histological findings.

CHI diagnostic algorithms start from the metabolic evaluation followed by molecular investigation and genotyping. Although genetic analysis is the most useful test in hyperinsulinism diagnostic approach, specific radiological modalities such as 18-F-DOPA positron emission tomography (PET) scan are also used to specify lesions [4]. Variants in some specific genes that regulate insulin secretion are considered to be responsible for the development of CHI. *ABCC8* and *KCNJ11* are among the most common genes involved in CHI [5, 6]. These genes encode subunits of ATP sensitive K^+ (KATP) channels in beta cells. *ABCC8* and *KCNJ11* gene variants impair the function of these channels resulting in disrupted membrane depolarization and dysregulated entry of calcium ion ending up in insulin release into plasma [2, 7]. Both of these genes are located on the chromosome 11p15.1 and separated by a few kilobases. *HADH* is the other well-known causative gene for CHI and variants in this gene cause enzymatic defects. *HADH* gene-inactivating variants have been described in CHI patients, resulting in decreased enzymatic activity of L-3-hydroxyacyl-CoA-dehydrogenase [8, 9]. Different types of variants including missense, nonsense, frameshift, and insertions or deletions inactivate these three genes. Determination of such variants in candidate genes is useful in various ways including choosing the best treatment approach [5]. Diazoxide is a KATP channel agonist and the first line of therapy in most of the CHI patients. Those patients who are not responsive to diazoxide may use octreotide as an alternative treatment. Surgical therapy might be used for those CHI patients who are not responsive to pharmacological therapies. Recessive variants in *ABCC8* and *KCNJ11* genes are usually considered to be less responsive to some therapies including diazoxide while compound heterozygotes may have better treatment responses [5, 10]. In contrast to recessive variants, dominant mutations will have a better treatment response [5]. Many case reports and case series have reported new variants in *ABCC8* and *KCNJ11* genes in different populations. We have previously demonstrated rare genetic variants in these two genes in an Iranian population and also demonstrated the clinical efficacy of sirolimus therapy in CHI patients [11]. The prevalence of specific variants in each population seems to be unique and genotyping for CHI has not been widely reported in the Iranian population. Other alternative diagnostic options for CHI include PET scan that helps identifying localization of focal lesions. In the present report, we explored the variants in *ABCC8* and *KCNJ11* genes as the most common genes involved in CHI. Hence, we aimed to evaluate value of genotyping in the diagnostic process, which is a crucial step in CHI treatment.

2. Material and Methods

2.1. Subjects. The present case series was approved by the Mashhad University of Medical Sciences Ethics Committee and included pediatric patients who were referred to the pediatric ward of the Imam Reza Hospital (Mashhad, Iran) from 2008 to 2017. Every neonate/child who had clinical and laboratory features of persistent hypoglycemia underwent assessment of "critical" sample in hypoglycemic state (with hypoglycemia defined as plasma glucose less than 50 mg/dL). Cases who had (1) hyperinsulinemia (defined as plasma insulin greater than 2 μU/mL), or (2) hypofatty acidemia (plasma free fatty acids less than 1.5 mmol/L), or (3) hypoketonemia (defined as plasma beta-hydroxybutyrate less than 2 mmol/L), or (4) inappropriate glycemic response to 1 mg intravenous glucagon (changes in plasma glucose greater than 40 mg/dL) were defined to have hyperinsulinism, and treatment with dextrose fluid therapy, diazoxide, and then octreotide were administered if needed [10]. All patients who had confirmed diagnosis of hyperinsulinism underwent genetic evaluation and were enrolled in the present study if their parents filled an informed consent form. Patients underwent molecular diagnosis for hyperinsulinemic hypoglycemia after genetic counseling. Because of the limitations, genetic testing was limited to the most common genes involved in CHI. Moreover, PET-CT data and surgical specimens of all patients were not available. Among the study population, only six patients were previously reported in the literature and their genotypes and clinical data are considered in the present study as well. Some of them had closed follow-up with PET scan study or surgery, which has been reported previously (Table 1) [11].

2.2. Sampling and DNA Extraction. To perform molecular tests, venous blood (3 mL) was taken from all subjects and their parents in EDTA tubes. Genomic DNA was extracted using the salting-out method. DNA samples' quality and quantity were examined using nano-drop and gel-electrophoresis and stored in the freezer at −70°C.

2.3. PCR Sequencing. Mutational analysis of coding and flanking intronic regions of the *KCNJ11, HADH,* and *ABCC8* genes was performed using Sanger sequencing following PCR fragment amplification. Interpretation of the pathogenicity of the genetic variants in these genes was checked by VarSome software based on the American College of Medical Genetics (ACMG) instructions [12, 13]. Molecular genetic analysis was performed in the genetic lab of the Mashad University of Medical Sciences and/or genetic lab of the Exeter University in UK.

3. Results

Twenty patients were enrolled in the present study. Among this population, four infants did not have genetic variants in *ABCC8, KCNJ11,* or *HADH* gene. Among the other 16 infants, 11 patients were female and five were male. The mean age of genetic diagnosis was 18.6 days in those who had *ABCC8* or *KCNJ11* variants (except one case who had delay in the diagnosis of CHI). Most of the infants had their genetic tests few weeks after birth. The patient with the most delayed genetic diagnosis was the one who was diagnosed at the age of 3.5 years. Most of the patients had variants in the *ABCC8* gene (Table 1). A missense and aberrant splicing variants in the *ABCC8* gene (c.2041-21G > A) were seen in three infants. Other common variants were frameshift variants (c.3438dup) in the *ABCC8* gene and a missense variant (c.287-288delinsTG) in the *KCNJ11* gene. According

TABLE 1: Genotypes and pathogenicity prediction by using online prediction tools and the clinical significance according to Varsome.

Gene	Gender	Birth weight (gr)	Symptom onset	BS-INS at diagnosis	molecular diagnosis	Variant	Zygosity	GnomAD allele frequency	Iranome allele frequency	Clinical significance (varsome.com)	Family history	Surgery	Response to Diazoxide	Clinical Comments (patients did not response to diazoxide underwent surgery or other drugs)
ABCC8	F	4200	4D	27–47	1M	c.331G>A p.Gly111Arg	Hom^	0.000008	—	Pathogenic	—	50D	—	Received diazoxide and octreotide before surgery and sirolimus for 3 months after surgery #
	F	2600	1D	34–63	2.5M	c.2809C>T p.Leu937=	Hom^	—	—	Pathogenic	—	30D	—	Received diazoxide and sirolimus after surgery # histologic features: diffused islet hyperplasia
	F	4350	3D	22–53	1M	c.1671+1G>A	Hom^	—	—	Pathogenic	—	57D	—	—
	F	3400	3D	20–57	3M,6D						+~	—	+	Received octreotide plus diazoxide in some weeks infancy,continued with diazoxide
	M	4000	2D	25–33	1M,4D	c.2041-21G>A	Hom^	0.00002	—	Likely Pathogenic	+~	2M	—	PET scan: no uptake in pancreas He died because of sepsis following the surgery
	M	4200	1D	18–27	1M						+~~	—	—	Received diazoxide plus octreotide but lost follow up
	F	3100	2D	28–69	4M	c.3438dup p.Thr1147HisfsTer48	Het (pat)*	—	—	Pathogenic	—	2M	—	—
	F	3000	4D	40–12	5M,22D	c.1109G>C p.Arg370Thr	Het (de novo)	—	—	Uncertain Significance	—	—	+	—
	F	2800	3D	25–38	6Y,9M	c.3438dup p.Thr1147HisfsTer48	Het (pat)*	—	—	Pathogenic	—	55D	—	Received insulin after surgery because of hyperglycemia
	F	4200	1D	12–28	1M,2D	c.3151dup p.Cys1051LeufsTer64	Hom^	—	—	Pathogenic	—	—	—	Received diazoxide plus octreotide but lost follow up
	M	3150	4D	32–54	1M	c.96C>G p.Asn32Lys c.2041-21G>A	Comp-Het	— 0.00002	—	Uncertain Significance Uncertain Significance	—	—	—	Received sirolimus and responded to sirolimus therapy #
	M	2300	5D	44–34.6	3.5Y	c.3446G>A p.Cys1149Ty	Hom^	—	—	Likely Pathogenic	—	3.5Y	—	Received sirolimus plus diazoxide after surgery PET scan: avid lesion in the head of pancreas histologic features: islet cell hyperplasia

Table 1: Continued.

Gene	Gender	Birth weight (gr)	Symptom onset	BS-INS at diagnosis	molecular diagnosis	Variant	Zygosity	GnomAD allele frequency	Iranome allele frequency	Clinical significance (varsome.com)	Family history	Surgery	Response to Diazoxide	Clinical Comments (patients did not response to diazoxide underwent surgery or other drugs)
KCNJ11	F	3800	3D	28–44	1M,19D	c.287-288delinsTG p.Ala96Val	Hom^	—	—	Uncertain Significance	—	2M	—	—
	F	3500	2D	36–65	2M	c.370T>A p.Ser124Thr	Hom^	—	—	Uncertain Significance	—	2M	—	Received sirulimus ,octreotide and diazoxide before surgery. Continued with low doses of diazoxide after surgery #
	F	4100	1D	28–28	22D	c.362T>G p.Phe121Cys	Hom^	—	—	Uncertain Significance	+~~	—	—	Pet Scan :a mild uptake in the head of pancreas Did not responded to diazoxide alone , continued with octreotide and sirolimus #
HADH	M	3100	15D	38–14	1M	c.706C>T p.Arg236Ter	Hom^	0.00001	—	Pathogenic	—	—	+	PET scan: Uptake in the head of pancreas .Followed by pancreatectomy with no attacks of hypoglycemia

BS: Blood sugar (mg/dl); INS: insulin (IU/ml); D: day; M: Month; Y: year; Pat: paternal; Comp-Het: Compound heterozygote. # The patient previously reported from our center. ^The mother and father are heterozygote for the variant. * The mother did not have any variant in the three genes and the father was asymptomatic and carrying the variant. ~ The patients are first cousins. ~~ The family had child with similar clinical manifestations but without genetic workups.

to the ACMG guideline, most of the genetic variants in our population were reported as variants with uncertain significance.

4. Discussion

According to the results of this study, more than half of the study population with a clinical diagnosis of CHI had variants in the *ABCC8* gene. Additionally, most of these patients had variants with uncertain significance in *ABCC8* or *KCNJ11* genes.

Recurrent or persistent hypoglycemia is the first clue for the diagnosis of CHI. The presentation of CHI usually begins during the neonatal period and some types of CHI including focal CHI can present later in life. Less than half of the children with CHI have the genetic form of this disease [7]. At least variants in nine genes have been reported to be related to CHI. Among these genes, *ABCC8* and *KCNJ11* carry most of the mutations that cause CHI and other mutations are common in specific populations. HADH gene is among the other genes that have been reported to be common in countries with considerable consanguinity including Iran [14]. Variants in both *KCNJ11* and *ABCC8* genes, which are located on chromosome 11p15.1, are characterized by defective Kir6.2 and SUR1 subunits of ATP-dependent K channels in B-cells [6]. KATP channel variants result in various degrees of dysfunction ranging from partial to complete loss of channel function in B-cells [15]. Recessive and dominant variants in both of these genes can cause CHI [7].

Many studies from around the world have evaluated the heterogeneous genotypes of CHI patients. It is noteworthy to mention that even in the same country, a wide range of variants in *ABCC8* and *KCNJ11* genes are present. As summarized in Table 1, only a small number of variants have been previously reported in the literature. Only a few studies from Iran evaluated the genotype of CHI patients. Recently, a study from Iran evaluated six patients with CHI and the only similar variants to our study were the c.96 C *G* variants in the *ABCC8* gene [14]. Alaei et al. [14] reported that one of their patients had this variant in homozygous form while our patient had this variant in compound heterozygous form. Another study from Iran evaluated 23 patients with hyperinsulinemic hypoglycemia [16]. The authors demonstrated that after screening for *ABCC8, HADH, HNF4A, KCNJ11, GLUD1*, and *GCK*, only 4 patients did not show any variant in these genes. Most of their patients had variants in the *HADH* gene and the *ABCC8* gene was the next gene with frequent variants. The only similar variants between this study and the present one are the splicing variants in the *ABCC8* gene (c.2041-21G > *A*) [16]. They reported that their female heterozygous patient had died at the age of 3 months. In our population, we reported a compound heterozygous male with this variant and three homozygous infants. The c.2041-21G > *A* variants were the most common variants in our population.

Other genetic variants were slightly similar to studies from other countries. Kapoor et al. demonstrated that among a CHI population who were referred to a children hospital in England, c.331 G > *A* variant in the *ABCC8* gene was one of the most common variants [2]. Another study from England provided the same results. Among their 53 CHI patients in a 13-year period, only the c.331 G > *A* variant was similar to our study [17]. The c.331 G > *A* variants in *ABCC8* gene were also the only similar variants between our study and a retrospective Chinese study [18].

In our studied population, only one compound heterozygous variant was found. Compound heterozygous status has been reported in other studies while Senniappan et al. have previously reported the same heterozygous variants in the Iranian population [16, 19]. Their patient was a female child who died at 3 months of age [16]. Similar to the Senniappan et al.'s study, Mohnike et al. also demonstrated a case of paternally heterozygous child with c.2041-21G > *A* variant in the *ABCC8* gene and focal CHI [20]. Their patient has undergone surgery but the outcome was not mentioned [20]. Sousa-Santos et al. reported that even patients with the same compound heterozygous variants in the *ABCC8* gene (c.3576delG and c.742 C *T*) can have different phenotypes [21]. Moreover, a combination of heterozygous variants in *ABCC8* and *KCNJ11* genes has been reported to be responsible for CHI [22].

Although genetic analysis can be applied as an important tool for diagnostic and management purposes in some patients, genotyping in our population showed that most of the variants were still categorized as variants of unknown significance (VUS) in *ABCC8* or *KCNJ11* genes. However, further genetic studies are needed to unravel molecular basis of CHI.

4.1. Limitations. In the present study, we used Sanger sequencing for the genotyping of all patients, and therefore, some other possible genetic variants including copy number variations might have been undetectable by using this technique. Moreover, all of our patients did not undergo other diagnostic workups including PET scan. Only six patients with closed follow-up have been reported previously [11]. The high cost of these imaging and other molecular techniques including using multiplex ligation-dependent probe amplification or gene panel analysis by next generation sequencing might have limited the interpretation of the results of our research in its present form. Furthermore, we did not have histological specimens of our patients. Finally, we evaluated a particular gene panel as causative genes for CHI in the Iranian population and we were not able to investigate other genes.

5. Conclusion

The present study evaluated genetic variants in *ABCC8, KCNJ11*, and *HADH* genes in 20 children. Approximately, 75% of children with CHI phenotype had variants in *ABCC8* and *KCNJ11* genes. According to the present results, c.2041-21G > *A* missense variant in the *ABCC8* gene was the most common variant in our Iranian population. Most of the variants in our population were variants with unknown significance and only seven patients had pathogenic variants.

Authors' Contributions

Somayyeh Hashemian and Reza Jafarzadeh Esfehani equally contributed as co-first authors.

Acknowledgments

The authors would like to thank Dr. Mehri Tafazoli in Sadra Lab, Mashhad, Iran, and Dr. Hanieh Yaghootkar in the University of Exeter, UK, for collecting and performing molecular genetic assessments for some of their patients. This study was financially supported by the Mashhad University of Medical Sciences, Mashhad, Iran.

References

[1] P. Goel and S. R. Choudhury, "Persistent hyperinsulinemic hypoglycemia of infancy: an overview of current concepts," *Journal of Indian Association of Pediatric Surgeons*, vol. 17, no. 3, pp. 99–103, 2012.

[2] R. R. Kapoor, S. E. Flanagan, V. B. Arya, J. P. Shield, S. Ellard, and K. Hussain, "Clinical and molecular characterisation of 300 patients with congenital hyperinsulinism," *European Journal of Endocrinology*, vol. 168, no. 4, pp. 557–564, 2013.

[3] E. C. McNay and V. E. Cotero, "Mini-review: impact of recurrent hypoglycemia on cognitive and brain function," *Physiology & Behavior*, vol. 100, no. 3, pp. 234–238, 2010.

[4] A. Casertano, A. De Matteis, E. Mozzillo et al., "Diagnosis of congenital Hyperinsulinism can occur not only in infancy but also in later age: a new flow chart from a single center experience," *Italian Journal of Pediatrics*, vol. 46, no. 1, pp. 1–7, 2020.

[5] C. James, R. R. Kapoor, D. Ismail, and K. Hussain, "The genetic basis of congenital hyperinsulinism," *Journal of Medical Genetics*, vol. 46, no. 5, pp. 289–299, 2008.

[6] S. Galcheva, H. Demirbilek, S. Al-Khawaga, and K. Hussain, "The genetic and molecular mechanisms of congenital hyperinsulinism," *Frontiers in Endocrinology*, vol. 10, p. 111, 2019.

[7] I. Banerjee, M. Salomon-Estebanez, P. Shah, J. Nicholson, K. E. Cosgrove, and M. J. Dunne, "Therapies and outcomes of congenital hyperinsulinism-induced hypoglycaemia," *Diabetic Medicine*, vol. 36, no. 1, pp. 9–21, 2019.

[8] S. Galcheva, H. Demirbilek, S. Al-Khawaga, and K. Hussain, *The Genetic and Molecular Mechanisms of Congenital Hyperinsulinism*, vol. 10, no. 111, 2019.

[9] P. T. Clayton, S. Eaton, A. Aynsley-Green et al., "Hyperinsulinism in short-chain L-3-hydroxyacyl-CoA dehydrogenase deficiency reveals the importance of β-oxidation in insulin secretion," *Journal of Clinical Investigation*, vol. 108, no. 3, pp. 457–465, 2001.

[10] B. Dekel, D. Lubin, D. Modan-Moses, J. Quint, B. Glaser, and J. Meyerovitch, "Compound heterozygosity for the common sulfonylurea receptor mutations can cause mild diazoxide-sensitive hyperinsulinism," *Clinical Pediatrics*, vol. 41, no. 3, pp. 183–186, 2002.

[11] S. Hashemian, R. Jafarzadeh Esfehani, S. Karimdadi, R. Vakili, D. Zamanfar, and A. Sahebkar, "Clinical efficacy evaluation of sirolimus in congenital hyperinsulinism," *International Journal of Endocrinology*, vol. 2020, Article ID 7250406, 6 pages, 2020.

[12] C. Kopanos, V. Tsiolkas, A. Kouris et al., "VarSome: the human genomic variant search engine," *Bioinformatics*, vol. 35, no. 11, pp. 1978–1980, 2019.

[13] S. Richards, N. Aziz, N. Aziz et al., "Standards and guidelines for the interpretation of sequence variants: a joint consensus recommendation of the American College of medical genetics and genomics and the association for molecular pathology," *Genetics in Medicine*, vol. 17, no. 5, pp. 405–423, 2015.

[14] M. R. Alaei, S. Akbaroghli, M. Keramatipour, and A. Alaei, "A case series: congenital hyperinsulinism," *International Journal of Endocrinology and Metabolism*, vol. 14, no. 4, Article ID e37311, 2016.

[15] F.-F. Yan, Y.-W. Lin, C. MacMullen, A. Ganguly, C. A. Stanley, and S.-L. Shyng, "Congenital hyperinsulinism associated ABCC8 mutations that cause defective trafficking of ATP-sensitive K+ channels: identification and rescue," *Diabetes*, vol. 56, no. 9, pp. 2339–2348, 2007.

[16] S. Senniappan, A. Sadeghizadeh, S. E. Flanagan et al., "Genotype and phenotype correlations in Iranian patients with hyperinsulinaemic hypoglycaemia," *BMC Research Notes*, vol. 8, p. 350, 2015.

[17] V. B. Arya, M. Guemes, A. Nessa et al., "Clinical and histological heterogeneity of congenital hyperinsulinism due to paternally inherited heterozygous ABCC8/KCNJ11 mutations," *European Journal of Endocrinology*, vol. 171, no. 6, pp. 685–695, 2014.

[18] W.-Y. Wang, Y. Sun, W.-T. Zhao et al., "Congenital hyperinsulinism in China: a review of Chinese literature over the past 15 years," *Journal of Clinical Research in Pediatric Endocrinology*, vol. 9, no. 3, pp. 194–201, 2017.

[19] B. H. Lee, J. Lee, J.-M. Kim et al., "Three novel pathogenic mutations in KATP channel genes and somatic imprinting alterations of the 11p15 region in pancreatic tissue in patients with congenital hyperinsulinism," *Hormone Research in Paediatrics*, vol. 83, no. 3, pp. 204–210, 2015.

[20] K. Mohnike, I. Wieland, W. Barthlen et al., "Clinical and genetic evaluation of patients with KATPChannel mutations from the German registry for congenital hyperinsulinism," *Hormone Research in Paediatrics*, vol. 81, no. 3, pp. 156–168, 2014.

[21] F. Sousa-Santos, H. Simões, L. Castro-Feijóo et al., "Congenital hyperinsulinism in two siblings with ABCC8 mutation: same genotype, different phenotypes," *Archives of Endocrinology and Metabolism*, vol. 62, no. 5, pp. 560–565, 2018.

[22] K. Rozenkova, A. Nessa, B. Obermannova et al., "Could a combination of heterozygous ABCC8 and KCNJ11 mutations cause congenital hyperinsulinism?" *Journal of Pediatric Endocrinology & Metabolism: JPEM*, vol. 30, no. 12, pp. 1311–1315, 2017.

18

Case of Hypercalcemia Secondary to Hypervitaminosis A in a 6-Year-Old Boy with Autism

Arpita Kalla Vyas and Neil H. White

Division of Pediatric Endocrinology and Diabetes, Department of Pediatrics, Washington University in Saint Louis and Saint Louis Children's Hospital, Saint Louis, MO 63110, USA

Correspondence should be addressed to Neil H. White, white_n@kids.wustl.edu

Academic Editors: H. G. Dorr and G. Nijpels

Vitamin A intoxication secondary to over-the-counter nutritional supplements and from its use in acne treatment has been described. However, there have been very few case reports of chronic hypervitaminosis A leading to hypercalcemia in the pediatric population. This paper describes a boy with hypercalcemia secondary to chronic vitamin A intoxication in the context of vitamin A usage for therapy of autism. In addition to discontinuation of vitamin A, hyperhydration, and furosemide, the hypercalcemia in this patient required the use of prednisone and pamidronate to normalize the calcium.

1. Introduction

Hypercalcemia is an infrequent occurrence in children except during the initial newborn period. The various etiologies of hypercalcemia are also relatively rare in children. In this paper, we describe a 6-year-old autistic boy who developed hypercalcemia secondary to hypervitaminosis A, and we review the literature related to hypervitaminosis A and hypercalcemia.

2. Case Report

A 6-year-old boy presented to our emergency room because of vomiting and abdominal pain. His parents reported that he had a 3-day history of low-grade fever together with abdominal pain, emesis, and constipation. There was no history of altered mental status, coryzal symptoms, or headaches. He was reported to have "autism", and four weeks earlier he had been placed on a "specific carbohydrate diet" including "egg protein shakes." Two days later, he developed "hives", and the egg protein shakes were discontinued. However, pruritus continued and he developed excoriated and dry lips over the next few days. These latter symptoms continued until his presentation to our emergency room.

His past medical history was significant for premature birth at 30 weeks gestation, nocturnal enuresis for the past 8 months with some recent improvement using a bed alarm, and an inguinal hernia repair at the age of 3 years. He had been diagnosed with pervasive behavioral/developmental disorder attributed to autism. In an attempt to manage his behavior, he was started on a casein- and gluten-free "specific carbohydrate diet" (eggs, fruits, vegetables without complex carbohydrates) together with protein shakes. These had been discontinued two weeks prior to admission because of the development of a skin rash and pruritis. He had also been placed on multiple dietary and vitamin supplements as part of the management of his autism. These included 6 drops/day of vitamin A (equivalent to 30,000 IU per day) added to his diet for the past 4 months, Vitamin B12 shots twice per week, a custom-made multivitamin, Vitamin E Drops, Coenzyme Q and Omega-3 fatty acids.

Family history revealed that his father had a history of kidney stones as a young adult, which had not been further evaluated and have not recurred. Maternal grandmother had thyroid surgery for an "overactive thyroid." There was no family history of hyperparathyroidism, thyroid neoplasms, pheochromocytomas, pituitary tumors, or islet cell tumors.

On examination when he was initially seen in the emergency unit, his weight was 21.6 kg (50th percentile)

TABLE 1: Course of calcium levels during first hospital stay.

Day	Time	Total calcium	Comments
1	19:37	13.7	IV hydration 3.0 L/m^2/day + furosemide 1 mg/kg IV
2	04:01	13.1	
2	17:14	12.7	
2	23:14	11.5	IV hydration reduced to 1.5 L/m^2/day
3	05:00	11.4	Oral rehydration started
3	17:55	10.6	
4	05:21	10.0	
4	17:43	10.2	
5	11:38	10.9	Discharged home

TABLE 2: Course of calcium levels during second hospital stay.

Day	Time	Total Calcium	Comments
1	15.47	12.6	IV hydration 3.0 L/m^2/day + Prednisone 2 mg/kg/day + Furosemide 1 mg/kg BID
2	08:00	12.5	
2	23:00	14.7	Pamidronate 0.5 mg/kg IV IV hydration 3.5 L/m^2/day
3	06:24	13.4	
4	16:30	11.4	Oral rehydration started
4	22:15	10.8	
5	08:05	9.8	
6	10:00	9.5	
7	10:00	8.4	Discharged home

and height 123.5 cm (80th percentile). He was sleepy and in discomfort complaining of abdominal pain. He was mildly dehydrated. He was noted to have cheilitis and a blanching erythematous rash on his face. He had symmetric hyperreflexia in all four limbs with normal muscle tone. Funduscopic examination was within normal limits. HEENT, abdominal, cardiovascular, and respiratory exam were all within normal limits. There was no evidence of thyromegaly, and thyroid gland was nontender. Sexual maturation was Tanner Stage 1.

On initial presentation, he had a normal basic metabolic profile except that the total calcium was 13.7 mg/dL (normal range: 8.6–10.3). Serum creatinine was 0.6 mg/dL and BUN 26 mg/dL indicative of his mild dehydration. Intravenous hydration was initiated, and he was hospitalized for evaluation and treatment of hypercalcemia. He was initially treated with intravenous hydration using 0.9% saline at 3 L/m^2/day. He also received a single dose of intravenous furosemide 1 mg/kg. His calcium stabilized with hydration and furosemide therapy within 48 hours and remained stable (though still near or slightly above the upper limits of normal) off IV fluids for 24 hours (see Table 1).

Supplemental vitamin A was discontinued on admission. During his initial hospitalization, serum phosphorus was 4.0 mg/dL (normal: 3.0–6.0 mg/dL), intact PTH <3 pg/mL (normal: 14–72), 25-hydroxy-vitamin D 22.3 ng/mL (normal: 10–55), and 1,25 dihydroxy-vitamin D 16 pg/mL (normal: 22–67). TSH 2.29 mcIU/mL (normal: 0.35–5.5), Free T4 0.95 ng/dL (normal: 0.9–1.8 ng/dL), alkaline phosphatase 209 IU/L (normal: 140–420), AST 76 IU/L (normal: 10–60), and ALT 34 IU/L (normal: 10–35). EKG showed normal sinus rhythm. A urinary calcium/creatinine fractional excretion ratio was 0.03, and calcium/creatinine ratio was 0.9 at the time when serum calcium was 13.1 mg/dl. Both parents had normal serum calcium and phosphorous levels. Serum vitamin A level was 1738 mcg/L (normal: 360–1200 mcg/L).

He was discharged home on the fifth hospital day with instructions for oral fluid intake of at least 1.5 L/m^2/day. His total serum calcium on the day of discharge was 10.9 mg/dL. Serum calcium was to be checked by his primary physician daily and was stable for two days. Three days after discharge, he presented again to the emergency unit with recurrence of abdominal pain, vomiting, and generally not feeling well. He had not been able to keep up with the recommended oral hydration plan of at least 1.5 L/m^2/day. At this point in time, mother also gave a history of hair loss since discharge. He had lost 2 kg in weight. He had marked blanching erythema on the cheeks and rest of the body together with cheilosis. Total calcium at this time was 12.6 mg/dL. He had not received any vitamin A since the initial admission seven days earlier. He was hospitalized once again and started on 3.0 L/m^2/day normal saline hydration, 2 mg/kg/day of prednisone, and furosemide 1 mg/kg BID. Despite these measures, his calcium rose to 14.7 mg/dL during the next 24 hours (Table 2) at which point he was given a single dose of pamidronate 0.5 mg/kg IV.

Calcium came down to 9.8 mg/dL over the next two days and to 8.4 mg/dL five days after pamidronate. He was changed to oral hydration, and serum calcium remained normal over the next few days. He was discharged home after six days to continue oral hydration and close followup. During this second admission, he had a skeletal survey that was remarkable only for a bilateral coxa valga deformity and mild generalized osteopenia. His serum vitamin A level was 2668 mcg/L. Tuberculin test was negative, and a chest X-ray and renal ultrasound were normal. Parathyroid hormone-related peptide (PTHrP) was 0.3 pmol/L (normal: <2 pmol/L). He also had a normal bone scan. After discharged home, he remained stable without additional hypercalcemia. His serum Vitamin A level 30 days after discontinuation of vitamin A was at 1201 mcg/L and serum calcium of 8.9 mg/dL.

3. Discussion

Hypercalcemia is an uncommon finding in children. Although uncommon, hyperparathryoidism can cause hypercalcemia in the pediatric age group [1]. In addition to hyperparathryoidism, the differential diagnosis of hypercalcemia includes malignancy, hypervitaminosis D, granulomatous diseases, medications, other endocrine disorders,

Table 3: Causes of hypercalcemia.

Parathyroid hormone-related
Primary hyperparathyroidism
Sporadic
Familial
MENI or MENII
Tertiary hyperparathyroidism
Associated with renal insufficiency
Vitamin D-related
Vitamin D intoxication
Granulomatous disease
Malignancy
Humoral hypercalcemia of malignancy
(Associated with PTHrP)
Solid tumors
Medications
Thiazide diuretics
Lithium
Milk-alkali syndrome
Vitamin A intoxication
Other endocrine disorders
Hyperthyroidism
Adrenal insufficiency
Acromegaly
Pheochromocytoma
Familial hypocalciuric hypercalcemia (FHH):
(Mutation in calcium-sensing receptor)

and familial hypocalciuric hypercalcemia. The causes of the hypercalcemia are summarized in Table 3.

Our patient presented with nausea, abdominal pain, constipation, vomiting, and lethargy, all typical symptoms of hypercalcemia and his serum total calcium was 13.7 mg/dL. He underwent an extensive evaluation including careful history, family history, physical examination, and lab work to exclude possible causes of hypercalcemia. Serum phosphorus was normal, and plasma intact PTH was appropriately suppressed, ruling out hyperparathyroidism. 25-hydroxy vitamin D and 1,25-dihydroxy vitamin D levels were not elevated ruling out hypervitaminosis D. The low 1,25-dihydroxy-vitamin D probably reflects a reduced activity of the renal 1-hydroxylase enzyme activity in the face of suppressed PTH; PTH is required for activation of the 1-hydroxylase enzyme. Tuberculin test, chest X-ray, and bone survey were normal ruling out a granulomatous process (tuberculosis or sarcoidosis). Bone scan was normal and PTHrP were low, thus making malignancy-related hypercalcemia unlikely. Free T4 and TSH were normal, ruling out hyperthyroidism, and there were no signs or symptoms suggestive of adrenal insufficiency, acromegaly, or pheochromocytoma. Both parents had normal calcium and phosphorus and our patient's urinary calcium : creatinine ratio was high (0.9), thus ruling out familial hypocalciuric hypercalcemia (FHH). FHH results from heterozygous mutations in the calcium sensing receptor gene (*CASR*) and is inherited in autosomal dominant fashion. Clinically, patients with FHH have relative hypocalcuria (<4 mg/kg/day) and inappropriately normal PTH in the face of persistent mild hypercalcemia, none of which our patient had. He was not taking any medications known to cause hypercalcemia other then Vitamin A that he was receiving as part of his treatment for autism. Considering his history of excessive vitamin A intake (30,000 IU/day), his elevated vitamin A levels, and a complete evaluation to rule out other causes of hypercalcemia, this boy would appear to represent a case of hypercalcemia secondary to vitamin A intoxication. In addition, our patient had other signs of vitamin A intoxication, including alopecia, excoriation of skin, cheilosis and mild elevation in AST.

Hypercalcemia as a complication of vitamin A therapy was first described in 1953 by Shaw and Niccoli [2]. We are aware of only 11 reported cases with this unique association of hypercalcemia as a complication of vitamin A toxicity. These reported cases fit into four general categories: (1) those receiving all-*trans* retinoic acid (ATRA) therapy for treatment of acute promyelocytic leukaemia [3]; (2) hemodialysis patients who consume nutritional supplements containing a pharmacological dosage of vitamin A [4]; (3) those who ingest massive dosage of vitamin A [5–10]; (4) those who become hypercalcemic secondary to vitamin A toxicity occurring during commercially available tube feeds [11]. To best of our knowledge, there has only been one other case report to date of a child with hypercalcemia secondary to vitamin A supplementation as part of a plan to improve the behavioral aspects of autism [12].

Vitamin A has a long biological half-life and accumulates in adipose tissue. The combination of relatively rapid absorption with slow clearance can produce acute toxicity after a high dose and chronic toxicity after prolonged intake of substantially smaller doses. Children are particularly sensitive to vitamin A and can become intoxicated with lower doses than those required to cause toxicity in adults. The toxic effects of vitamin A involve multiple organs. These organs include the bone, brain, liver, and the skin. Symptoms and signs include alopecia, anorexia, bone pain and tenderness, bulging fontanelles and craniotabes (in infants), fissuring of lip corners (cheilosis), hepatomegaly, hyperostosis, photophobia, pruritis, pseudotumour cerebri, skin desquamation, and skin erythema [13]. Prolonged vitamin A intoxication may cause premature epiphyseal closure. Our patient had many of these findings, including alopecia, anorexia, cheilosis, pruritis, skin desquamation and skin erythema.

It is not clear how vitamin A causes hypercalcemia and influences bone metabolism. Binkley and Krueger [14] reported hypercalcemia, elevated alkaline phosphatase, and an increased incidence of spontaneous bone fractures associated with hypervitaminosis A. Bélanger and Clark [15] found increased osteoblastic activity with an increase in periosteal bone apposition in rats fed large doses of vitamin A. This new bone was entirely cancellous. It was also noted that osteocytes matured rapidly in this new bone tissue compared to bone that had been previously laid down. Various degrees of enhanced osteolysis were recorded on α-radiographs. They concluded that under the influence of hypervitaminosis A, new bone was deposited and at the same time, greater resorption occurred. Fell and Mellanby [16] added pure vitamin A acetate (1000–3000 IU/100 mL) *in vitro* to tibia, fibulae, radii, and ulnae from 17- to 20-day old fetal mice and found that the matrix of terminal cartilage softened, shrank, and almost or completely disappeared whilst cartilage cells remained normal in appearance. This action was thought to be provoked by the release of bound protease and altered permeability of the lysosomes by the vitamin A. Though less dramatic than *in vitro*, these effects were confirmed *in vivo* [17]. In addition it is known that receptors for retinoic acid are located on both osteoclast and osteoblast [17]. All these findings suggest a direct effect of vitamin A on bone.

The general goals for treatment of hypercalcemia include stabilization and reduction of the calcium level with adequate hydration, increasing urinary calcium excretion, inhibition of osteoclast activity in the bone, and treatment of the underlying cause (when possible). Specific therapeutic approaches include hydration, loop diuretics, glucocorticoids, calcitonin, and bisphosphonates. In cases of hypercalcemia secondary to vitamin A intoxication, several modes of therapy have been reported. Hydration with normal saline and diuresis with furosemide are common initial treatments. Glucocorticoids are often helpful. Wieland et al. (1971) [5] described use of prednisone 20 mg/kg to resolve hypercalcemia secondary to vitamin A toxicity (vitamin A level of 934) in a 16-year-old girl who had consumed 100,000 IU/day for 6 months. Frame et al. in 1974 [7] also described steroid use in a 46-year-old salesman with hypercalcemia and kidney stones who had a vitamin A level of 625 after consuming >75000 IU vitamin A per day. Prednisone 40 mg/day stabilized the calcium over one week; hypercalcemia recurred once the prednisone was stopped. Successful treatment of hypercalcemia secondary to hypervitaminosis A may require a combination of approaches and a treatment course that extends beyond the initial normalization of the calcium. This was true in our patient who promptly relapsed back to being hypercalcemic after the initial treatment appeared to have been successful.

Two cases have been reported of use of pamidronate in patients with vitamin A-induced hypercalcemia. Bhalla et al. [11] described a case of hypercalcemia secondary to excess vitamin A from enteral feeding. This patient was initially treated using aggressive hydration with normal saline and furosemide but as the serum calcium was persistently elevated, intravenous pamidronate was instituted and the hypercalcemia resolved. Sakamoto et al. [3] reported the case of an 11-year-old patient with known acute promyelocytic leukaemia who developed hypercalcemia after ATRA treatment. Pamidronate was used to treat the hypercalcemia.

We report here a case of hypercalcemia secondary to vitamin A intoxication occurring during management of Autism. Autism is a spectrum disorder defined by DSM 4 criteria characterized by delay in language development, impairment of social interaction, and the use of restrictive stereotype behavioral patterns prior to three years of age. No single approach has proven effective in treating autism, and professionals and families have found that a combination of treatments may be effective in treating symptoms and behaviors that make it hard for individuals with autism to function. These may include psychosocial and pharmacological interventions. While there are no drugs, vitamins or special diets that have been clearly shown to correct the underlying neurological problems that seem to cause autism, changes to diet and the addition of certain vitamins or minerals are thought by some to help with behavioral issues. Over the past 10 years, there have been claims that adding essential vitamins such as B6 and B12 and removing gluten and casein from a child's diet may improve digestion, allergies, and sociability. Not all investigators and experts agree as to whether these therapies are effective or scientifically valid. It is also speculated that autism may be linked to a G-protein defect that affects the retinoid receptors in the brain. Therefore, vitamin A has been suggested as a possible intervention to improve visual and sensory perception, language processing, and attention [18]. In this paper, our patient was receiving 30,000 IU of vitamin A per day for 4 months; this is nearly ten times the recommended daily allowance (RDA) for vitamin A. Published literature states that RDA for vitamin A is 3000 IU in the pediatric age group and 5000 IU in adults [7]. There are no published data regarding the recommended dosage of vitamin A for treatment of autistic patients to help with the behavioral and neurological aspect of the condition.

Hypercalcemia is a potentially serious side effect of vitamin A supplementation or retinoic acid treatment for various disorders. In cases of hypercalcemia, it is important to obtain a careful dietary and medication history to assist in identifying the underlying etiology. In addition, patients treated with vitamin A, retinoic acid, or their analogs should be monitored for serum calcium levels at regular intervals. When hypercalcemia complicates the therapy, consideration should be given to discontinuing vitamin A supplementation or retinoic acid treatments unless clear benefit of such treatments has been observed.

Acknowledgments

The authors wish to thank Ana Maria Arbelaez and Rebecca Green for their advice and critical review in the preparation of this paper.

References

[1] J. Kollars, A. E. Zarroug, J. Van Heerden et al., "Primary hyperparathyroidism in pediatric patients," *Pediatrics*, vol. 115, no. 4, pp. 974–980, 2005.

[2] E. W. Shaw and J. Z. Niccoli, "Hypervitaminosis A: report of a case in an adult male," *Annals of internal medicine*, vol. 39, no. 1, pp. 131–134, 1953.

[3] O. Sakamoto, M. Yoshinari, T. Rikiishi et al., "Hypercalcemia due to all-trans retinoic acid therapy for acute promyelocytic leukemia: a case report of effective treatment with bisphosphonate," *Pediatrics International*, vol. 43, no. 6, pp. 688–690, 2001.

[4] S. Fishbane, G. L. Frei, M. Finger, R. Dressler, and S. Silbiger, "Hypervitaminosis A in two hemodialysis patients," *American Journal of Kidney Diseases*, vol. 25, no. 2, pp. 346–349, 1995.

[5] R. G. Wieland, F. H. Hendricks, F. Amat y Leon, L. Gutierrez, and J. C. Jones, "Hypervitaminosis A with hypercalcaemia," *Lancet*, vol. 1, no. 7701, p. 698, 1971.

[6] C. M. Katz and M. Tzagournis, "Chronic adult hypervitaminosis A with hypercalcemia," *Metabolism*, vol. 21, no. 12, pp. 1171–1176, 1972.

[7] B. Frame, C. E. Jackson, W. A. Reynolds, and J. E. Umphrey, "Hypercalcemia and skeletal effects in chronic hypervitaminosis A," *Annals of Internal Medicine*, vol. 80, no. 1, pp. 44–48, 1974.

[8] G. Fisher and P. G. Skillern, "Hypercalcemia due to hypervitaminosis A," *Journal of the American Medical Association*, vol. 227, no. 12, pp. 1413–1414, 1974.

[9] V. V. Ragavan, J. E. Smith, and J. P. Bilezikian, "Vitamin A toxicity and hypercalcemia," *American Journal of the Medical Sciences*, vol. 283, no. 3, pp. 161–164, 1982.

[10] S. C. Baxi and G. E. Dailey, "Hypervitaminosis A. A cause of hypercalcemia," *Western Journal of Medicine*, vol. 137, no. 5, pp. 429–431, 1982.

[11] K. Bhalla, D. M. Ennis, and E. D. Ennis, "Hypercalcemia caused by iatrogenic hypervitaminosis A," *Journal of the American Dietetic Association*, vol. 105, no. 1, pp. 119–121, 2005.

[12] A. Kimmoun, B. Leheup, F. Feillet, F. Dubois, and A. Morali, "Hypercalcemia revealing iatrogenic hypervitaminosis A in a child with autistic troubles," *Archives de Pediatrie*, vol. 15, no. 1, pp. 29–32, 2008.

[13] K. L. Penniston and S. A. Tanumihardjo, "The acute and chronic toxic effects of vitamin A," *American Journal of Clinical Nutrition*, vol. 83, no. 2, pp. 191–201, 2006.

[14] N. Binkley and D. Krueger, "Hypervitaminosis A and bone," *Nutrition Reviews*, vol. 58, no. 5, pp. 138–144, 2000.

[15] L. F. Bélanger and I. Clark, "Alpharadiographic and histological observations on the skeletal effects of hypervitaminoses A and D in the rat," *Anatomical Record*, vol. 158, no. 4, pp. 443–451, 1967.

[16] H. B. Fell and E. Mellanby, "Effects of hypervitaminosis A on foetal mouse bones cultivated in vitro; preliminary communication," *British Medical Journal*, vol. 2, no. 4678, pp. 535–539, 1950.

[17] C. M. Rohde and H. DeLuca, "Bone resorption activity of all-trans retinoic acid is independent of vitamin D in rats," *Journal of Nutrition*, vol. 133, no. 3, pp. 777–783, 2003.

[18] M. N. Megson, "Is autism a G-alpha protein defect reversible with natural vitamin A?" *Medical Hypotheses*, vol. 54, no. 6, pp. 979–983, 2000.

19

DKA with Severe Hypertriglyceridemia and Cerebral Edema in an Adolescent Boy: A Case Study and Review of the Literature

Tansit Saengkaew, Taninee Sahakitrungruang, Suttipong Wacharasindhu, and Vichit Supornsilchai

Division of Endocrinology, Department of Pediatrics, Faculty of Medicine, Chulalongkorn University, Bangkok 10330, Thailand

Correspondence should be addressed to Tansit Saengkaew; tansitpedpsu@gmail.com

Academic Editor: Wayne V. Moore

A 13-year-old adolescent boy with type 1 diabetes mellitus (1b) presented with diabetic ketoacidosis (DKA) and cerebral edema. Grossly lipemic serum and lipemia retinals due to extremely high triglyceride (TG) level were observed without evidence of xanthoma or xanthelasma. Cerebral edema was treated by appropriate ventilation and mannitol administration. Normal saline was carefully given and regular insulin was titrated according to blood sugar levels. Triglyceride levels were reduced from 9,800 mg/dL to normal range within 9 days after conventional treatment was commenced without antilipid medication. Based on our review of the literature, this is the first reported case of confirmed pediatric DKA with severe hypertriglyceridemia and cerebral edema. In patients with DKA and hypertriglyceridemia, clinicians should be mindful of the possibility of associated acute pancreatitis and cerebral edema.

1. Introduction

Diabetic ketoacidosis (DKA) is a common presentation of type 1 diabetes mellitus that requires urgent treatment. Diagnostic criteria for DKA include hyperglycemia (BS > 200 mg/dL), ketosis, and metabolic acidosis. The most serious complication in delayed diagnosis of DKA is cerebral edema, a complication that increases patient morbidity and mortality. Acute pancreatitis (AP), peripheral venous thrombosis, pulmonary edema, and rhabdomyolysis are only rarely found in patients with DKA [1].

Severe hypertriglyceridemia (TG > 1,000 mg/dL) is another rare complication found in DKA patients. Severe hypertriglyceridemia can increase risk of acute pancreatitis, especially in patients with TG levels higher than 1,000–1,772 mg/dL [2, 3]. Prevalence of severe hypertriglyceridemia was found in about 8% of adults with DKA [4], but few data have been reported in children with severity ranging from asymptomatic to severe acute pancreatitis. The mechanism of hypertriglyceridemia in DKA that has been proposed involves increased free fatty acid (FFA) secretion from adipocytes by counterregulatory hormone stimulation, which results in decreased clearance of VLDL-TG [5]. Recommended treatment includes intravenous fluid and insulin administration appropriated to DKA treatment guidelines. Plasmapheresis or heparinization was used in some reported cases to decrease triglyceride level in adults [6–13]. The objective of this report is to present and describe the clinical features, laboratory investigations, case management, and natural course of hypertriglyceridemia in a 13-year-old adolescent boy with DKA. A review of the literature relating to hypertriglyceridemia and its manifestations in children with DKA was performed and is included in this report for purposes of comparison with our patient.

We searched all English articles that were published and shown in PubMed, MEDLINE, and Web of Science up to August 2015. The keywords were DKA, hypertriglyceridemia, cerebral edema, and acute pancreatitis. We selected only publications (retrospective cohort studies and case reports) about children, adolescents, and young adults who presented with DKA and hypertriglyceridemia. All clinical and laboratory data including age at presentation, initial TG level, diagnosis and treatment of acute pancreatitis, and duration of TG return to normal range were reviewed and summarized.

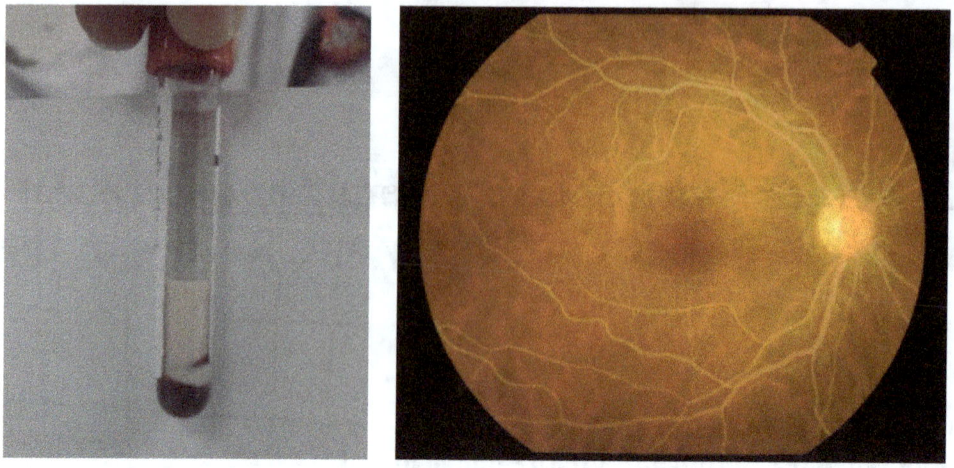

(a) (b)

FIGURE 1: Images describing lipemic serum (a) and lipemia retinals, whitish, creamy vessels of retina (b).

2. Case Presentation

A 13-year-old boy with type 1 diabetes mellitus (T1DM) presented at the Emergency Department of King Chulalongkorn Memorial Hospital (Bangkok, Thailand) with Kussmaul breathing and confusion, after having malaise and polyuria for one month and epigastric pain for 2 days. He was diagnosed with T1DM at another hospital one year earlier and was being treated with insulin, metformin, and glipizide. Our patient reported having discontinued all medications for 6 months prior to this admission. His maternal grandmother was diagnosed with type 2 diabetes mellitus at the age of 40 and her condition was reported as being effectively controlled with oral hypoglycemic drugs. No family history of dyslipidemia was reported. On admission, our patient was confused, agitated, and disoriented regarding time, place, and persons. Vital signs revealed body temperature of 38.5°C, pulse rate 128, respiratory rate 26/min with Kussmaul pattern, and blood pressure 156/102 mmHg. Anthropometric measurements showed weight of 43 kg, height 152 cm, and body mass index (BMI) 18.61 kg/m^2. There was no eruptive or tuberous xanthoma or xanthelasma at the skin. Ophthalmologic examination revealed presence of whitish, creamy vessels of retinas, called lipemia retinals (Figure 1(a)). No focal neurologic deficit was noted.

At presentation, our patient was found to have DKA, with initial BS of 513 mg/dL, venous blood gas with pH 7.062, pCO_2 22.4 mmHg, HCO_3 6.4, and BE −21.7 mEq/L, and serum ketone 3.2 mmol/L. His blood demonstrated a grossly lipemic appearance (Figure 1(b)) and his lipemic condition disturbed the results of other biochemical blood investigations. Cerebral edema was diagnosed according to 1 major criterion (alteration and fluctuation of consciousness) and 2 minor criteria (lethargy and diastolic blood pressure >90 mmHg). CT of the brain was not performed due to the unstable clinical condition of our patient. He was intubated due to deterioration of consciousness and cerebral edema. Mannitol (0.5 mg/kg) was subsequently administered and 3% NaCl was given intravenously to maintain a hypernatremic state for purposes of decreasing intracranial pressure. Normal saline was carefully given and regular insulin was then started and titrated to 0.2 units/kg/hr according to patient blood sugar levels. He was out of DKA as defined by pH > 7.3, bicarbonate > 15 mmol/L, and serum ketone negative, within 24 hours. Lipid profiles were analyzed on the second day of admission, with results revealing triglyceride of 9,810 mg/dL, cholesterol 705 mg/dL, LDL 254 mg/dL, and HDL 6 mg/dL. Patient had no abdominal pain and serum amylase was 57 IU/L. Therefore, acute pancreatitis was excluded. Triglyceride level was reduced to 377 mg/dL within 9 days of admission (Figure 2) without the use of antilipid medication. Our patient was extubated within 2 days of admission after recovery from DKA and cerebral edema. His father's lipid profiles showed cholesterol of 215 mg/dL, triglyceride 111 mg/dL, LDL 144 mg/dL, and HDL 50 mg/dL. His mother's lipid profiles showed cholesterol of 167 mg/dL, triglyceride 75 mg/dL, LDL 101 mg/dL, and HDL 47 mg/dL.

After discharge from the hospital, T1DM treatment with basal-bolus insulin regimen was commenced. Our patient continued to have HbA1c-related complications (10–15%) due to poor self-treatment compliance. Although he developed DKA twice as a result, his TG levels remained within normal range.

3. Discussion

Two large series reported data in adult DKA with severe hypertriglyceridemia [4, 19]. Fulop and Eder found that 15 of 136 (11%) DKA patients had severe hypertriglyceridemia (TG > 1,000 mg/dL), but only one patient developed acute pancreatitis [19]. Incidence of severe hypertriglyceridemia was similarly found in 8 of 100 (12.5%) adult DKA patients in the other of the two studies, with half of the patients developing acute pancreatitis [4]. In children, most cases were individually presented in patient case reports (Table 1). All reported cases had TG levels higher than 1,000 mg/dL,

TABLE 1: Literature review of pediatric DKA patients with hypertriglyceridemia.

Patients	Age (year)	Peak TG (mg/dL)	Acute pancreatitis	Cerebral edema	Treatment with antilipid medication	Time to normalized TG level (days, (TG level))
Cywinski et al., 1965 [14]	12.5	>1,000	Yes	Suspected	No	7 (232)
Blackett et al., 1986 [6]	13	14,461	No	Suspected	No	7 (122)
Slyper et al., 1994 [15]	14	3,119	Yes	Suspected	No	NA
Kadota-Shinozaki et al., 1997 [16]	19	3,386	Yes	No	No	2 (483)
Hahn et al., 2010 [10]	20	15,000	Yes	No	No	3 (506)
Williamson et al., 2012 [12]	8	10,852	No	No	No	17 (NA)
Lutfi et al., 2012 [11]	10	16,334	Yes	No	Fenofibrate, plasmapheresis	1.5 (1,100)
Kota et al., 2012 [17]	12	1,020	Yes	No	No	3 (340)
Aboulhosn and Arnason, 2013 [13]	18	1,724	Yes	No	No	NA
Wolfgram and Macdonald, 2013 [18]	10	8,300	Yes	No	No	NA
Our case	**13**	**9,810**	**No**	**Yes**	**No**	**9 (377)**

NA, not available.

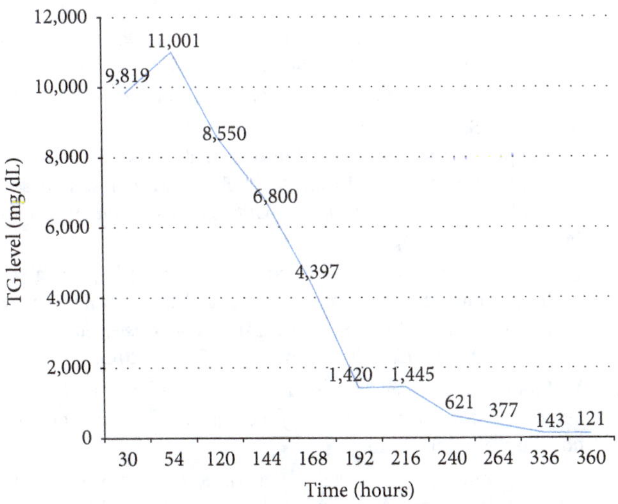

FIGURE 2: Triglyceride levels after DKA treatment.

supporting the hypothesis that elevated TG (>1,000 mg/dL) is a risk factor for acute pancreatitis [2, 3]. However, 3 out of 11 patients (2.8%) did not develop acute pancreatitis. One pediatric patient did not develop acute pancreatitis, even though he had extremely high TG level (14,461 mg/dL) [6]. As such, other risk factors for this condition need to be identified. Accordingly, clinical investigations for acute pancreatitis should be routine in all cases presenting with TG level higher than 1,000 mg/dL to ensure early and proper management.

The postulated mechanism of hypertriglyceridemia in DKA patients centers on lack of insulin action, which activates lipolysis in adipose tissue that then results in free fatty acid (FFA) formation and increases in VLDL formation by the liver [19]. In addition, insulin normally inhibits ApoC-III expression, which plays a major role in inhibiting lipoprotein lipase (LPL) and hepatic lipase (HL). This results in decreased hydrolysis and delayed VLDL-TG clearances from plasma. As a result, ApoC-III increases in an insulin-deficient state, with a subsequent increase in plasma TG level [5]. Severe hypertriglyceridemia-induced pancreatitis develops as a result of increased FFA levels that are produced from triglyceride hydrolysis by pancreatic lipase and insulin deficiency. High FFA levels cause acute pancreatitis as a result of capillary endothelium and pancreatic acinar cell destruction [14, 20].

Appropriate management of DKA with hypertriglyceridemia includes intravenous fluid and insulin administration according to DKA guideline, because the major mechanism of hypertriglyceridemia is insulin deficiency. Plasma TG level was gradually reduced to less than 500 mg/dL within 3–17 days in most cases. However, 9 of 15 patients reviewed by Fulop and Eder had normal plasma TG concentrations for up to 6 months without any lipid-lowering agent [19]. One patient reported by Lutfi et al. who had extremely high TG level (16,334 mg/dL) with renal insufficiency and who failed with conservative treatment was successfully treated by plasmapheresis [11]. TG levels were reduced from 5,093 to 1,157 mg/dL in that study. Heparinization was also reported as an alternative treatment for hypertriglyceridemia in adult DKA patients, together with fluid and insulin administration [8]. In that study, TG levels were reduced from 8,701 mg/dL to normal range within 2 days of treatment without abnormal bleeding.

Cerebral edema was suspected in 3 pediatric cases from the literature review and one case from the present report. All 3 cases from the literature had abnormal pupillary reflex with unconsciousness, but all had spontaneous recovery without treatment by mannitol or hypertonic saline. To our knowledge and based on our review of the literature, the association between severe hypertriglyceridemia and cerebral edema is unclear. The hypothesized mechanism is that hyperviscosity due to extremely high TG level likely causes decreased cerebral blood flow, which may correlate with cerebral edema [21]. Yuen et al. found that severe dehydration and hypertriglyceridemia aggravated cerebral hypoperfusion, which had the effect of worsening cerebral edema.

The weakness of our case was that serum lipase test was not done and contrast enhanced CT of the abdomen was not performed. Even though the patient had no abdominal pain and normal amylase level, acute pancreatitis could not be absolutely excluded.

In this case report, we presented a pediatric DKA patient with cerebral edema and severe hypertriglyceridemia. In patients with DKA and hypertriglyceridemia caused by severe insulin deficiency, clinicians should be mindful of the possibility of associated acute pancreatitis and cerebral edema. Triglyceride levels were gradually decreased to normal range within 9 days after standard intravenous fluid and insulin administration was commenced.

Acknowledgments

The authors gratefully acknowledge all pediatric residents and nurses at King Chulalongkorn Memorial Hospital for providing exceptional patient care.

References

[1] J. I. Wolfsdorf, J. Allgrove, M. E. Craig et al., "Ispad clinical practice consensus guidelines 2014. Diabetic ketoacidosis and hyperglycemic hyperosmolar state," *Pediatric Diabetes*, vol. 15, supplement 20, pp. 154–179, 2014.

[2] V. G. Athyros, O. I. Giouleme, N. L. Nikolaidis et al., "Long-term follow-up of patients with acute hypertriglyceridemia-induced pancreatitis," *Journal of Clinical Gastroenterology*, vol. 34, no. 4, pp. 472–475, 2002.

[3] S. Sandhu, A. Al-Sarraf, C. Taraboanta, J. Frohlich, and G. A. Francis, "Incidence of pancreatitis, secondary causes, and treatment of patients referred to a specialty lipid clinic with severe hypertriglyceridemia: a retrospective cohort study," *Lipids in Health and Disease*, vol. 10, article 157, 2011.

[4] S. Nair, D. Yadav, and C. S. Pitchumoni, "Association of diabetic ketoacidosis and acute pancreatitis: observations in 100 consecutive episodes of DKA," *American Journal of Gastroenterology*, vol. 95, no. 10, pp. 2795–2800, 2000.

[5] S. Qu, T. Zhang, and H. H. Dong, "Effect of hepatic insulin expression on lipid metabolism in diabetic mice," *Journal of Diabetes*, 2015.

[6] P. R. Blackett, J. H. Holcombe, P. Alaupovic, and J. D. Fesmire, "Plasma lipids and apolipoproteins in a 13-year-old boy with diabetic ketoacidosis and extreme hyperlipidemia," *The American Journal of the Medical Sciences*, vol. 291, no. 5, pp. 342–346, 1986.

[7] M. J. Rumbak, T. A. Hughes, and A. E. Kitabchi, "Pseudonormoglycemia in diabetic ketoacidosis with elevated triglycerides," *American Journal of Emergency Medicine*, vol. 9, no. 1, pp. 61–63, 1991.

[8] R. P. Cole, "Heparin treatment for severe hypertriglyceridemia in diabetic ketoacidosis," *Archives of Internal Medicine*, vol. 169, no. 15, pp. 1439–1441, 2009.

[9] J. Wolfsdorf, M. E. Craig, D. Daneman et al., "Diabetic ketoacidosis in children and adolescents with diabetes," *Pediatric Diabetes*, vol. 10, supplement 12, pp. 118–133, 2009.

[10] S. J. Hahn, J.-H. Park, J. H. Lee, J. K. Lee, and K.-A. Kim, "Severe hypertriglyceridemia in diabetic ketoacidosis accompanied by acute pancreatitis: case report," *Journal of Korean Medical Science*, vol. 25, no. 9, pp. 1375–1378, 2010.

[11] R. Lutfi, J. Huang, and H. R. Wong, "Plasmapheresis to treat hypertriglyceridemia in a child with diabetic ketoacidosis and pancreatitis," *Pediatrics*, vol. 129, no. 1, pp. e195–e198, 2012.

[12] S. Williamson, V. Alexander, and S. A. Greene, "Severe hyperlipidaemia complicating diabetic ketoacidosis," *Archives of Disease in Childhood*, vol. 97, no. 8, p. 735, 2012.

[13] K. Aboulhosn and T. Arnason, "Acute pancreatitis and severe hypertriglyceridaemia masking unsuspected underlying diabetic ketoacidosis," *BMJ Case Reports*, vol. 2013, 2013.

[14] J. S. Cywinski, F. A. Walker, H. White, and H. S. Traisman, "Juvenile diabetes mellitus associated with acute pancreatitis," *Acta paediatrica Scandinavica*, vol. 54, no. 6, pp. 597–602, 1965.

[15] A. H. Slyper, D. T. Wyatt, and C. W. Brown, "Clinical and/or biochemical pancreatitis in diabetic ketoacidosis," *Journal of Pediatric Endocrinology*, vol. 7, no. 3, pp. 261–264, 1994.

[16] A. Kadota-Shinozaki, T.-A. Nakamura, H. Hidaka et al., "Diabetic lipemia with maturity-onset diabetes of the young," *Internal Medicine*, vol. 36, no. 8, pp. 571–574, 1997.

[17] S. K. Kota, S. Jammula, S. K. Kota, L. K. Meher, and K. D. Modi, "Acute pancreatitis in association with diabetic ketoacidosis in a newly diagnosed type 1 diabetes mellitus patient; case based review," *International Journal of Clinical Cases and Investigations*, vol. 4, no. 1, pp. 54–60, 2012.

[18] P. M. Wolfgram and M. J. Macdonald, "Severe hypertriglyceridemia causing acute pancreatitis in a child with new onset type i diabetes mellitus presenting in ketoacidosis," *Journal of Pediatric Intensive Care*, vol. 2, no. 2, pp. 77–80, 2013.

[19] M. Fulop and H. Eder, "Severe hypertriglyceridemia in diabetic ketosis," *The American Journal of the Medical Sciences*, vol. 300, no. 6, pp. 361–365, 1990.

[20] A. Chait and J. D. Brunzell, "Chylomicronemia syndrome," *Advances in Internal Medicine*, vol. 37, pp. 249–273, 1992.

[21] N. Yuen, S. E. Anderson, N. Glaser, D. J. Tancredi, and M. E. O'Donnell, "Cerebral blood flow and cerebral edema in rats with diabetic ketoacidosis," *Diabetes*, vol. 57, no. 10, pp. 2588–2594, 2008.

20

Type 2 Diabetes Mellitus, a Sequel of Untreated Childhood Onset Growth Hormone Deficiency Developing in a 17-Year-Old Patient

Rohan K. Henry[1] **and Ram K. Menon**[2]

[1] *Division of Endocrinology, Department of Pediatrics, Nationwide Children's Hospital, The Ohio State University College of Medicine, Columbus, OH 43205, USA*
[2] *Division of Endocrinology, Department of Pediatrics, C.S. Mott Children's Hospital, Michigan Medicine, University of Michigan Medical School, Ann Arbor, MI 48109, USA*

Correspondence should be addressed to Rohan K. Henry; rohan.henry@nationwidechildrens.org

Academic Editor: Lucy Mastrandrea

In a seminal report, a 17-year-old boy with panhypopituitarism had fatty liver (FL) amelioration with growth hormone (GH). By extension, since hepatic insulin resistance (IR) is key to FL and type 2 diabetes mellitus (T2DM), GH then may ameliorate the IR of T2DM. We present a 17-year-old nonobese female with untreated childhood onset growth hormone deficiency (CO-GHD) who developed type 2 diabetes mellitus (T2DM) and steatohepatitis with bridging fibrosis. Based on height z-score of – 3.1 and a history of radiation therapy as treatment for a medulloblastoma at 7 years of age, GHD was quite likely. GH therapy was, however, not initiated at 15 years of age (when growth was concerning) based on full skeletal maturity. After she developed T2DM, GHD was confirmed and GH was initiated. With its initiation, though insulin dose decreased from 2.9 (~155 units) to 1.9 units/kg/day (~ 100 units), her T2DM was, however, not fully reversed. This illustrates the natural history of untreated CO-GHD and shows that though hepatic IR can be ameliorated by GH, full reversal of T2DM may be prevented with irreversible hepatic changes (fibrosis). Clinicians caring for pediatric patients and otherwise should remember that, even in patients beyond the cessation of linear growth, GH can have a crucial role in both glucose and lipid metabolism.

1. Introduction

The role of growth hormone (GH) in growth promotion is well known by clinicians, however, less appreciated is its effect on metabolism in the well state. In 1936, Bernardo Houssay, M.D. in the New England Journal of Medicine, proposed that the anterior pituitary gland after the liver and pancreas plays a key role in glucose metabolism. That key role was later shown to be due in part to GH [1].

The effect of GH on glucose metabolism involves two phases: an initial phase which involves a decrease in glucose (an insulin-like effect) and a second phase which includes its effects on gluconeogenesis and fat mobilization [2]. In both states of growth hormone deficiency and excess, these effects on glucose metabolism will be altered.

Altered glucose and fat metabolism are important components of fatty liver (FL) and type 2 diabetes (T2DM), both states of hepatic insulin resistance (IR). In fact, a seminal case of fatty liver (FL) resolution with GH administration in a 17-year-old patient with panhypopituitarism treated initially with levothyroxine and hydrocortisone alone was reported by *Takano* et al. in 1997 [3]. This suggests that GH treatment of T2DM which may be associated with GHD has the potential to reduce the IR which may be present.

We outline a case of untreated childhood onset growth hormone deficiency (CO-GHD) who presented with type 2 diabetes mellitus (T2DM) and also steatohepatitis. We discuss her management and evidence from the basic sciences and clinical studies which show that her presentation with T2DM and steatohepatitis was likely associated with untreated GHD

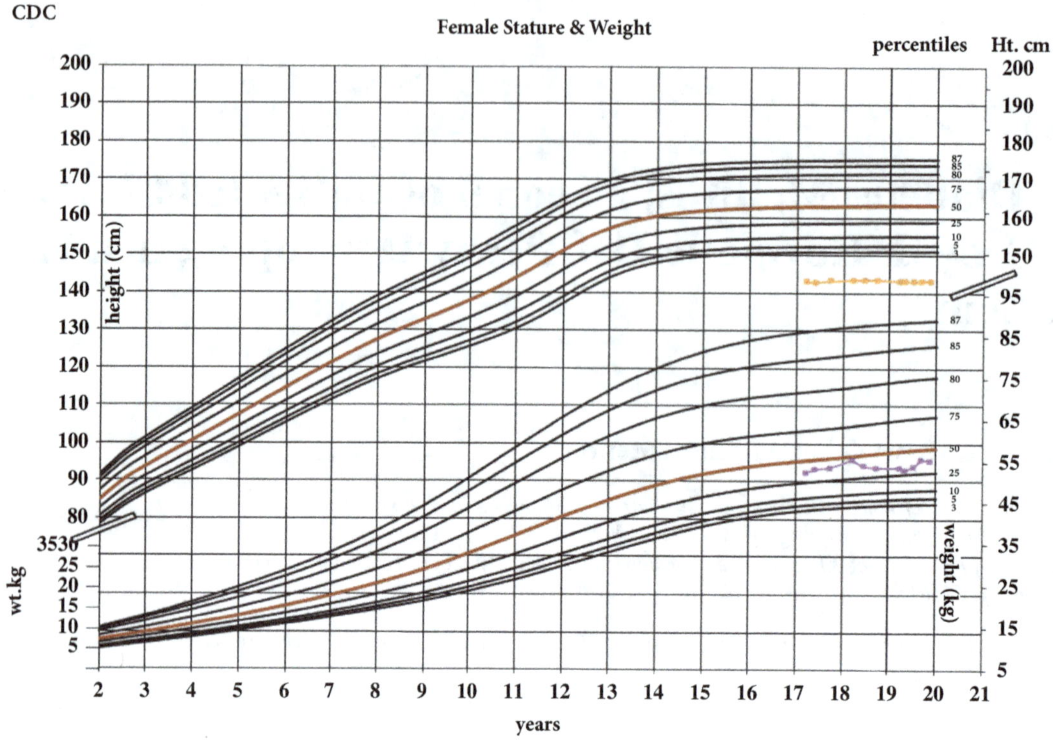

FIGURE 1: Patient's weight for age and height for age on CDC growth charts after being 17 years old.

and that with GH supplementation her condition was ameliorated. Lastly, we discuss the implications of this case.

2. Case Presentation

A 17-year-old nonobese Caucasian female who had a history of a medulloblastoma diagnosed at 7 years of age was treated with radiation therapy. She subsequently developed TSH and GnRH deficiencies. Though GHD was suspected based on height (z-score of – 3.1; see Figure 1), treatment had not been initiated based on the initial management focus being to treat her medulloblastoma. At 15 years of age when her bone age showed full skeletal maturity, her parents were informed that GH therapy could not be pursued because her linear growth was complete.

On presentation, the patient's height was 141.3 cm (z= - 3.1) and weight was 53 kgs (36th percentile for age). Body mass index was 25.8 kg/m^{-2} (86th percentile for age). Surveillance labs done at the oncology clinic showed glucosuria. Further testing showed HbA1c of 9.6% and on another day her fasting glucose was 277 mg/dL. Based on these results, diabetes mellitus was diagnosed.

When glutamic acid decarboxylase (GAD-65; Esoterix), islet-cell (Esoterix), insulin (Esoterix), and zinc transporter 8 (ARUP Laboratories) antibodies as well as DNA panel for maturity onset diabetes of youth (MODY) genes (HNF4α, GCK, IPF1, HNF1α, and HNF1β, [Athena Diagnostics]) returned all negative along with an elevated fasting C-peptide level of 3 ng/mL (normal: 0.4 - 2.1), T2DM was diagnosed. With the initiation of traditional basal/bolus insulin therapy using conventional dosing, a rapid escalation to peak total daily insulin dose of 2.9 units/kg/day (~ 155 units/day) was required to treat her refractory hyperglycemia. Treatment nonadherence was thought to be the unlikely cause of her increased insulin requirements based on the agreement between her insulin dosing and prescription refill data.

A comprehensive evaluation for conditions associated with IR was negative. However, based on Arginine/Clonidine stimulation testing showing peak GH level of 0.8 (normal: ≥ 10 ng/mL), a diagnosis of GHD was made. GH supplementation was initiated at 0.3 mgs daily and titrated based on IGF-1 levels.

After GH was started, her systolic and diastolic blood pressures (BP) which were mildly elevated between 124-136 and 77-89, respectively, became more normal. Despite this, lisinopril 5 mgs once daily was added for microalbuminuria.

With the diagnosis of T2DM and our patient having a significant family history of adverse cardiovascular risk factors, she was started on atorvastatin 10 mgs once daily. Within 2 months of therapy, her LDL cholesterol (LDL-C) decreased to 74 mg/dL. Table 1 shows serial lipid profiles.

Though her diabetes was not fully reversed with GH, her HbA1c decreased to 5.9% and 5.8% at 6 and 19 months, respectively. Her insulin therapy requirement decreased to 1.9 units/kg/day (~ 100 units) at 12 months after the start of GH.

Magnetic Resonance Imaging (MRI) of the brain and abdomen indicated a small anterior pituitary gland and liver masses, respectively. Liver biopsy showed steatohepatitis with bridging fibrosis (Figure 2). With GH therapy, her liver transaminases trended to normalcy (Table 1). Repeat MRI abdomen at 20 months after the start of GH showed stability of the liver lesions when compared to that done at 14 months.

Table 1: Some of the patient's lab tests with reference to growth hormone start.

TEST	RESULT			REFERENCE RANGE
	Baseline	**12 mths**	**22 mths**	
Aspartate aminotransferase	92	36	33	< 40 U/L
Alanine aminotransferase	87	24	56	15- 50 U//L
Total Cholesterol	247	99	132	95- 195 mg/dL
HDL Cholesterol	32	27	43	40- 58 ng/dL
LDL Cholesterol	171	57	65	73- 117 mg/dL
Triglyceride	267	70	120	20-200 mg/dL
IGF-1	74	146	294	121-566 ng/mL

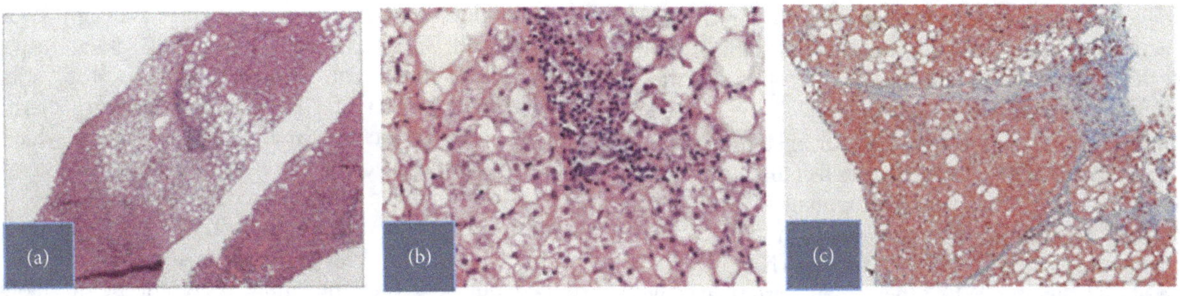

Figure 2: Slides from the patient's liver biopsy. **(a)** Low power liver section, **(b)** ballooning hepatocyte degeneration, a feature of hepatic cell death, and **(c)** intervening fibrous tissue seen as a terminal stage of liver injury. These all constitute steatohepatis with moderate steatosis.

These hyperintense lesions like the initial ones were located in the liver's parenchyma and the appearance of the liver was otherwise normal.

With GH therapy, the patient's stamina improved. She was now able to work for 20 hours weekly without becoming fully exhausted and her Quality of Life-Assessment of Growth Hormone Deficiency in Adults (QoL-AGHDA) and Quality of Life Satisfaction (QLS) scores, both questionnaire-based, improved (Figure 3).

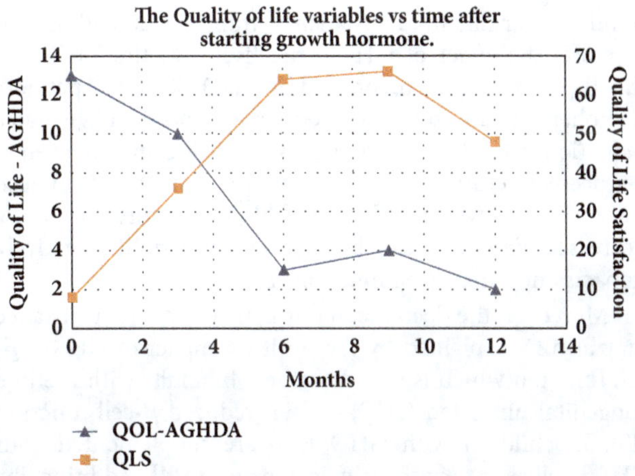

Figure 3: The patient's Quality of Life (QoL) scores with time. QoL-AGHDA: Quality of Life-Assessment of Growth Hormone Deficiency in Adults. QLS: Quality of Life Satisfaction. $_1$A decrease in score for QoL-AGHDA indicates an improvement in QoL-AGHDA, whereas an increase in QLS indicates an improvement while taking GH therapy.

3. Discussion

This case demonstrates that GH supplementation in an adolescent with CO-GHD led to improvements in transaminases, insulin requirements, and glucose control.

Several mouse models have corroborated the association of GHD with IR. In mice with liver GH receptor (GH-R) knockout, metabolic syndrome (MetS), steatohepatitis, increased inflammation, liver fibrosis, and hepatic tumor develop [4]. Additionally, a similar mouse model resulted in hyperinsulinemia, hyperglycemia, and IR. With the restoration of the liver's IGF-1 expression, there was an improvement in both insulin sensitivity and serum lipid profile. This, however, did not protect against hepatic inflammation induced by steatosis. This shows that GH and not IGF-1 directly affects lipid uptake and lipogenesis [5]. Also in a prior study again involving a liver specific GH receptor knockout mice, de novo lipogenesis was increased; however, this increase was not associated with the classic insulin mediated pathway [6]. So, our patient's IR and hepatic steatosis can be explained by her GHD based on data from some studies as well as the effect of GH in inhibiting this.

Evidence for the association of hepatic steatosis with GHD is also provided by the abnormalities involving the downstream pathway of GH signal transduction. Mice with hepatocyte-specific deletion of Janus kinase 2 (JAK2L), involved in the postreceptor phase of GH signaling, were lean but had FL. They also showed increased levels of GH, triglycerides, and plasma free fatty acids. Since GH in some instances can cause lipolysis, GH-deficient *little* mice which were crossed to JAK2L mice had both a rescuing of the FL and an increased expression of a fatty acid transporter [7]. Though this provides a mechanism for the FL observed with the liver specific disruption of GH signaling, in the same mice, elevated GH levels occurring as a consequence of disrupted signaling can cause an increase in resting energy expenditure [8]. In this situation, steatohepatitis is prevented based on increased fatty acid utilization. So the putative lipolytic action of GH can be offset by hyperinsulinemia; hence, the action of GH is variable and depends on the physiological context.

Additionally, mice with signal transducer and activator of transcription (STAT) 5 mutations, another downstream signal from GH, also develop steatohepatitis [9]. Since pathologies involving the downstream pathways in GH signal transduction are associated with steatohepatitis, this supports the role of GH in lipid metabolism and the notion that the FL changes in our patient may be due to GHD.

Clinical reports about Laron syndrome, primary GH insensitivity involving a molecular defect in human GH-R, have also documented the development of FL, IR, and T2DM [10]. In addition, men with hypopituitarism have a high prevalence of nonalcoholic FL disease (NAFLD) in the absence of GH therapy. When these men were treated with GH, there was histological improvement in the liver. This demonstrates that NAFLD is predominantly attributable to GH [11].

Though a follow-up liver biopsy was not done, the trend to normal in our patient's transaminases (Table 1) supports the effect of GH on the liver and the likelihood that these changes were induced by GHD. Since our patient's steatohepatitis improved with GH treatment, she likely had a reduction in her hepatic IR. The evidence for this was seen in her decreased insulin requirements. This reduction in IR also was associated with her decreased blood pressures and these decreased pressures can be explained since IR negatively impacts endothelial cell function [12].

Moreover, the decrease in our patient's insulin resistance may also be explained by the positive impact of GH on β-cell function which is well described. In adults with lifetime congenital untreated GHD, there is reduced β-cell function [13]. In children with GHD who are supplemented with GH, β-cell secretory capacity is enhanced [14]. Additionally, studies in mice have shown that, with isolated GHD, β-cell function deteriorates. This deterioration is not due to changes in β-cell mass [15]. Studies by *Nielsen* et al. have shown that GH stimulates β-cell proliferation, glucose induced insulin release, and insulin gene expression *in vitro* [16]. These also provide a possible mechanism for the decrease in our patient's IR.

Atorvastatin was added to our patient's treatment because although an amelioration of her LDL-C was expected with GH therapy, this did not happen. Plausible explanations for this include a genetic basis for her hyperlipidemia. This could have been superimposed on an accumulated adverse CV risk profile which developed based on the time period of her untreated CO-GHD [17]. Atorvastatin was also added to her treatment as well since based on her history of T2DM, her LDL-C levels needed improvement.

Based on the points discussed, with evidence from adult studies, clinical reports, and, more recently, mouse models (even with the lack of pediatric studies, especially long-term ones) explaining the important contribution of GH to normal lipid and glucose metabolism, there is enough data to reinforce the benefits of treating GHD even when linear growth is completed.

Pediatric clinicians should highlight and reinforce that GH supplementation has the potential to prevent adverse metabolic consequences in untreated states of severe deficiency. Also important is the fact that, even with growth cessation, supplementation with GH may improve QoL-AGHDA and QLS scores [18]. These questionnaire-based scores address the impact of GHD on issues of relevance to patients with GHD and can be useful for tracking the patient's response to treatment. The QoL-AGHDA tool addresses the general impact of GHD on each patient whereas the QLS score accounts for the level of importance which each individual may place on the issues affecting his/her life and gives a summarized weighted score based on these.

In conclusion, this case illustrates not only that both NAFLD and T2DM are potential associations of untreated GHD but also that they may represent points along the natural history of hepatic IR secondary to untreated GHD. Furthermore, clinicians should ensure that patients with CO-GHD are not only treated in childhood but also appropriately transitioned to adult GH dosing after growth has ceased. This is important as GH can have a crucial role beyond the period of linear growth. With delayed GH initiation, it is possible that, with irreversible hepatic injury (such as bridging fibrosis in this patient), there may not be total amelioration of the metabolic manifestations seen in patients with GHD.

Additional Points

Learning Points. (i) Growth hormone is integral to both glucose and lipid metabolism even after the period of linear growth. (ii) Insulin resistance (IR) can be a feature of untreated growth hormone deficiency (GHD). (iii) Hepatic steatosis and type 2 diabetes mellitus (T2DM) being both hepatic IR states could be a feature of the natural history of untreated GHD. (iv) While growth hormone supplementation may ameliorate IR seen in the setting of T2DM and GHD, it is likely that delayed supplementation may not fully ameliorate IR if simple steatosis progresses to steatohepatitis with fibrosis.

Consent

Consent was obtained from the patient prior to the submission of this publication.

Authors' Contributions

Rohan K. Henry and Ram K. Menon contributed to drafting the article. Rohan K. Henry contributed to the critical revision of the article. All authors approved the final version of the article to be published.

Acknowledgments

The authors would like to thank Robert Hoffman, M.D., for his critical review of this manuscript.

References

[1] B. A. Houssay, "Carbohydrate Metabolism," *The New England Journal of Medicine*, vol. 214, no. 20, pp. 971–986, 1936.

[2] S. Melmed, "Medical progress: acromegaly," *The New England Journal of Medicine*, vol. 355, no. 24, pp. 2558–2573, 2006.

[3] S. Takanoj, S. Kanzaki, M. Sato, T. Kubo, and Y. Seino, "Effect of growth hormone on fatty liver in panhypopituitarism," *Archives of Disease in Childhood*, vol. 76, no. 6, pp. 537-538, 1997.

[4] Y. Fan, X. Fang, A. Tajima et al., "Evolution of Hepatic Steatosis to Fibrosis and Adenoma Formation in Liver-Specific Growth Hormone Receptor Knockout Mice," *Frontiers in Endocrinology*, vol. 5, 2014.

[5] Z. Liu, J. Cordoba-Chacon, R. D. Kineman et al., "Growth hormone control of hepatic lipid metabolism," *Diabetes*, vol. 65, no. 12, pp. 3598–3609, 2016.

[6] J. Cordoba-Chacon, N. Majumdar, E. O. List et al., "Growth hormone inhibits hepatic de novo lipogenesis in adult mice," *Diabetes*, vol. 64, no. 9, pp. 3093–3103, 2015.

[7] B. C. Sos, C. Harris, S. M. Nordstrom et al., "Abrogation of growth hormone secretion rescues fatty liver in mice with hepatocyte-specific deletion of JAK2," *The Journal of Clinical Investigation*, vol. 121, no. 4, pp. 1412–1423, 2011.

[8] S. Y. Shi, R. García Martin, R. E. Duncan et al., "Hepatocyte-specific deletion of Janus kinase 2 (JAK2) protects against diet-induced steatohepatitis and glucose intolerance," *The Journal of Biological Chemistry*, vol. 287, no. 13, pp. 10277–10288, 2012.

[9] Y. Cui, A. Hosui, R. Sun et al., "Loss of signal transducer and activator of transcription 5 leads to hepatosteatosis and impaired liver regeneration," *Hepatology*, vol. 46, no. 2, pp. 504–513, 2007.

[10] Z. Laron, "Lessons from 50 years of study of laron syndrome," *Endocrine Practice*, vol. 21, no. 12, pp. 1395–1402, 2015.

[11] H. Nishizawa, G. Iguchi, A. Murawaki et al., "Nonalcoholic fatty liver disease in adult hypopituitary patients with GH deficiency and the impact of GH replacement therapy," *European Journal of Endocrinology*, vol. 167, no. 1, pp. 67–74, 2012.

[12] E. Cersosimo and R. A. DeFronzo, "Insulin resistance and endothelial dysfunction: The road map to cardiovascular diseases," *Diabetes/Metabolism Research and Reviews*, vol. 22, no. 6, pp. 423–436, 2006.

[13] C. R. Oliveira et al., "Insulin sensitivity and beta-cell function in adults with lifetime, untreated isolated growth hormone deficiency," *The Journal of Clinical Endocrinology & Metabolism*, vol. 97, no. 3, pp. 1013–1019, 2012.

[14] F. Baronio, L. Mazzanti, Y. Girtler et al., "The influence of growth hormone treatment on glucose homeostasis in growthhormone-deficient children: A six-year follow-up study," *Hormone Research in Paediatrics*, vol. 86, no. 3, pp. 196–200, 2016.

[15] J. Cordoba-Chacon, M. D. Gahete, N. K. Pokala et al., "Long-But Not Short-Term Adult-Onset, Isolated GH Deficiency in Male Mice Leads to Deterioration of β-Cell Function, Which Cannot Be Accounted for by Changes in β-Cell Mass," *Endocrinology*, vol. 155, no. 3, pp. 726–735, 2014.

[16] J. H. Nielsen, E. D. Galsgaard, A. M ldrup et al., "Regulation of beta-cell mass by hormones and growth factors," *Diabetes*, vol. 50, no. Supplement 1, pp. S25–S29, 2001.

[17] G. Johannsson, K. Albertsson-Wikland, B.-Å. Bengtsson et al., "Discontinuation of growth hormone (GH) treatment: Metabolic effects in GH-deficient and GH-sufficient adolescent patients compared with control subjects," *The Journal of Clinical Endocrinology & Metabolism*, vol. 84, no. 12, pp. 4516–4524, 1999.

[18] S. M. Webb, "Measurements of quality of life in patients with growth hormone deficiency," *Journal of Endocrinological Investigation*, vol. 31, Suppl 9, pp. 52–55, 2008.

21

Unrecognized Pseudohypoparathyroidism Type 1A as a Cause of Hypocalcemia and Seizures in a 64-Year-Old Woman

Patrizia Del Monte[1] **Carla Micaela Cuttica,**[1] **Alessandro Marugo,**[1] **Luca Foppiani**[2] **Daniela Audenino,**[3] **Tomasz Tadeusz Godowicz,**[4] **Francesca Marta Elli,**[5] **Giovanna Mantovani**[5] **and Emilio Di Maria**[6]

[1]*Endocrine Unit, Galliera Hospital, Genoa, Italy*
[2]*Internal Medicine Unit, Galliera Hospital, Genoa, Italy*
[3]*Neurology Unit, Galliera Hospital, Genoa, Italy*
[4]*Neurosurgery Unit, Galliera Hospital, Genoa, Italy*
[5]*Fondazione IRCCS Ca' Granda Ospedale Maggiore Policlinico, Endocrinology and Diabetology Unit, Department of Clinical Sciences and Community Health, University of Milan, Milan, Italy*
[6]*Department of Health Sciences, University of Genoa; Medical Genetics Unit, Galliera Hospital, Genoa, Italy*

Correspondence should be addressed to Patrizia Del Monte; patrizia.del.monte@galliera.it

Academic Editor: Eli Hershkovitz

Pseudohypoparathyroidism type 1A (PHP1A) is usually diagnosed in childhood or early adulthood. We describe the case of a 64-year-old woman admitted to the Neurological Unit for recurrent episodes of loss of consciousness and seizures. Glycemia and ECG were normal, while hypocalcemia was noted. Clinical history revealed carpo-pedal spasm since the age of 30 years, cognitive impairment, hypothyroidism since early adulthood, and menopause at 30 years. She was taking oral calcium and cholecalciferol for chronic hypocalcemia. Physical features suggested Albright's osteodystrophy. Blood calcium was confirmed low, with increased parathyroid hormone, moderate 25OH-vitamin D deficiency, and normal creatinine. Brain CT scan revealed calcifications of the basal ganglia, cortical and subcortical white matter, and cerebellum. Therapy was switched to oral calcitriol, with normalization of calcium levels; levetiracetam was started and no further seizures occurred. The clinical diagnosis of PHP1A was confirmed by molecular analysis, which demonstrated the heterozygous c.568_571del mutation of the *GNAS* gene. Our report illustrates the natural history of a patient with PHP1A, which went undiagnosed until the age of 64 years, with multi-hormonal resistance and clinical sequelae evolving throughout life, and underlines the importance of diagnosing this rare disease, which has a great impact on patients and their family life.

1. Introduction

Pseudohypoparathyroidism (PHP) is a rare congenital disorder, its estimated prevalence being 0.34 - 1.1 in 100.000; it is characterized by impairment of the parathyroid hormone (PTH) signaling pathway, with target organ resistance to the action of PTH [1, 2]. The term PHP comprises several related and highly heterogeneous diseases with genetic/epigenetic causes [3, 4]. PTH exerts its actions by binding to a transmembrane G-protein-coupled receptor, activating cAMP formation. The classical form of PHP, pseudohypoparathyroidism type 1A (PHP1A), which is associated with Albright's hereditary osteodystrophy (AHO), is caused by *de novo* or autosomal dominantly inherited inactivating mutations within the $G_{s\alpha}$-coding *GNAS* gene (20q13.3; OMIM #139320) [5]. The maternal allele is the predominant source of $G_{s\alpha}$-expression in the proximal renal tubule, thyroid, pituitary, and gonads, since paternal $G_{s\alpha}$ expression is silenced in these tissues; in other tissues, however, $G_{s\alpha}$ expression is biallelic. Therefore, an inactivating $G_{s\alpha}$ mutation causes

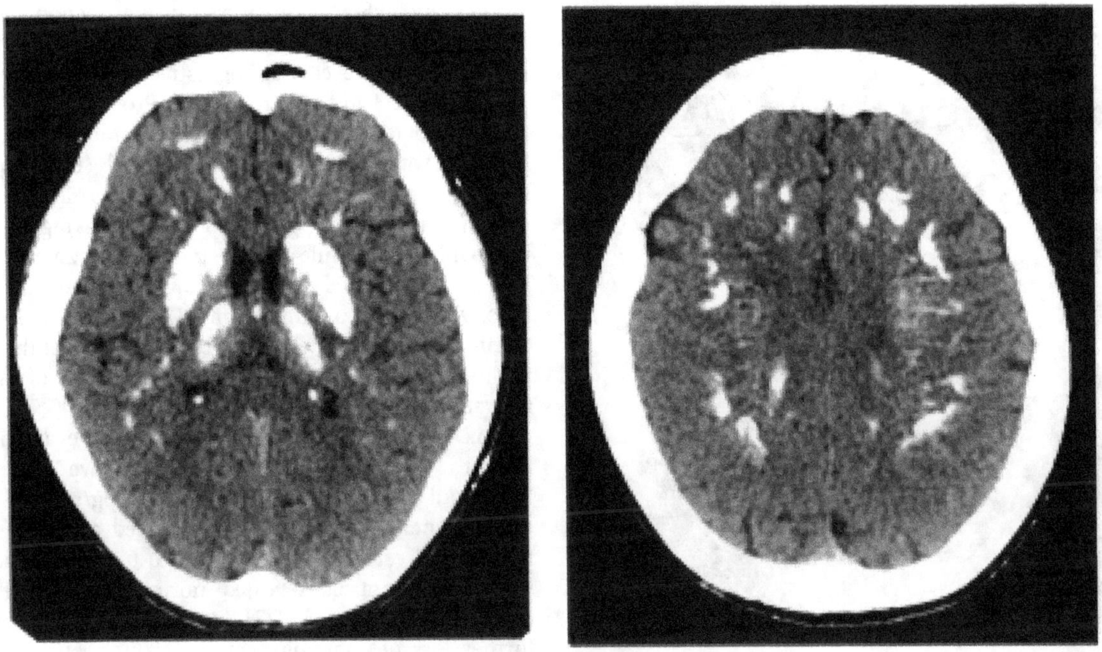

(a) (b)

FIGURE 1: Basal ganglia (a) and subcortical (b) calcifications (CT scan).

PHP1A (AHO clinical features and hormone resistance) in the case of maternal inheritance, while the same mutation on the paternal allele results in AHO clinical features only, a condition known as pseudo-pseudo-hypoparathyroidism (PPHP).

PHP1A patients often develop target-organ resistance to other hormones that act through $G_{s\alpha}$-coupled receptors, particularly TSH; resistance to gonadotrophins and GHRH is also reported.

The disease is usually diagnosed in childhood or early adulthood age, and few studies have addressed its natural history, in which its features evolve during the subject's lifetime. Moreover, to our knowledge, no diagnoses have been made after 60 years of age in patients not studied for known familial disease.

2. Clinical Case

A 64-year-old woman was admitted to the Neurological Unit of our hospital for recent recurrent episodes of loss of consciousness and seizures. Glycemia and ECG were normal, while hypocalcemia was present.

She has a normal brother and both her parents died in old age; her mother had cognitive impairment. Her clinical history evidenced carpo-pedal spasm since the age of 30 years, cognitive impairment, hypothyroidism diagnosed in early adulthood, spontaneous menarche, and oligomenorrhea followed by amenorrhea at the age of 30, which was diagnosed as precocious menopause. She was unmarried and had no pregnancy. She underwent bilateral hip arthroprosthesis at 45 and 50 years of age.

She was taking oral calcium (600 mg daily) and cholecalciferol (400 IU daily) for chronic hypocalcemia, diagnosed about 30 years earlier. She was also on therapy with perindopril for hypertension, atorvastatin for hypercholesterolemia, and L-thyroxine.

Physical examination revealed short stature (145 cm), slight overweight: 52 Kg (BMI: 25 Kg/m^2), round facies, enlarged base of the nose, and brachydactyly. Her blood chemistry evidenced hypocalcemia (7.7 mg/dl, n.v. 8.2-10.2) with increased PTH levels (169 pg/ml, n.v. 15-65 pg/ml, intact PTH immunoassay), moderate 25OH vitamin D deficiency (22 ng/ml; n.v. ≥ 30), normal creatinine (1 mg/dl), and albumin (3.9 g/dl).

Brain computed tomography (CT) revealed calcifications of the basal ganglia, the cortical and subcortical white matter, and the cerebellum (dentate nuclei); subcutaneous pericranial ectopic calcifications were also present (Figures 1, 2, and 3). Hand radiography confirmed shortness of the metacarpal bones and scapho-trapezoidal fusion (not shown). Bone mineral density of the spine and femoral bone was normal. Abdominal ultrasonography did not reveal kidney stones. The clinical picture was suggestive of PHP1A. The patient was therefore promptly switched to 1,25 $(OH)_2$ vitamin D (calcitriol 0.75 mcg daily, in 3 split doses) associated with oral calcium supplementation (1000 mg daily in 2 split doses, after lunch and dinner), with normalization of calcemia (9.2 mg/dl) and a decrease in PTH level (36 pg/ml). Serum phosphate was normal on therapy (4.3 mg/dl), while 24-hour urinary calcium on therapy was above the normal range (321 mg/24 h, n.v. <4 mg/kg/body weight); we do not have a clear explanation for this, since urinary calcium excretion is not normally increased in this condition. However, a

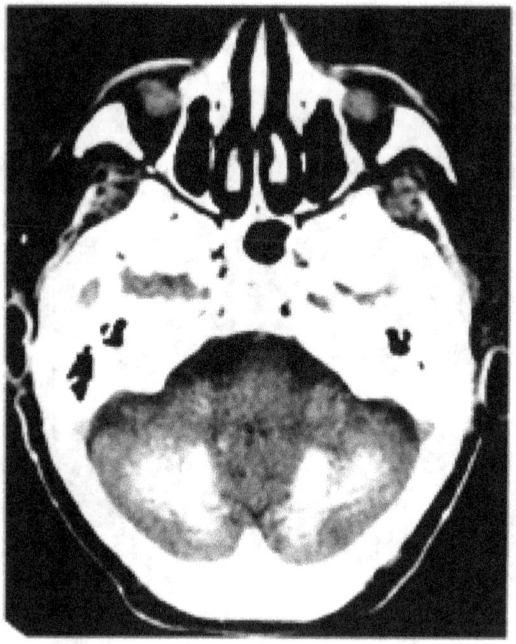

FIGURE 2: Cerebellar calcifications (CT scan).

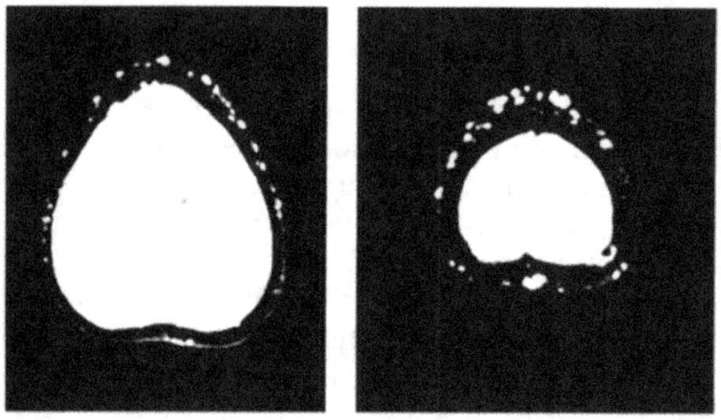

FIGURE 3: Extracranial subcutaneous ectopic calcifications (CT scan).

laboratory assay pitfall or an incorrect urine collection by the patient cannot be ruled out. A further urinary calcium control one month later, however, proved normal (200 mg/24 h). In addition, therapy with levetiracetam (1000 mg daily in 2 split doses) was started, and no further seizures or muscle spasms occurred.

The patient and her family underwent a genetic counseling session and gave informed consent to genetic analysis. Mutation analysis of the *GNAS* gene was performed on DNA extracted from a blood sample by means of Sanger sequencing and MLPA according to standard methods. The analyses revealed a heterozygous c.568_571del (p.Asp190Metfs*13) frameshift mutation. The combination of physical, biochemical, and genetic findings led to the diagnosis of PHP1A.

FT4 and TSH levels were normal during substitutive treatment with L-tiroxine (75 mcg daily). Anti-thyroperoxidase and anti-thyroglobulin antibodies were negative and thyroid ultrasonography was normal, suggesting that TSH resistance was the cause of her hypothyroidism.

LH and FSH levels were in the menopausal range (FSH: 47 mU/ml, LH: 26 mU/ml); the history of premature menopause, however, was suggestive of the development of progressive LH and FSH resistance. Prolactin, basal cortisol, and ACTH levels were in the normal range. Basal growth hormone was 0.63 ng/ml, with IGF-1 levels (129 ng/ml) in the normal range for age. Calcitonin levels were increased (range: 44-92 pg/ml, n.v. <10 pg/ml) (she was not taking any proton-pump inhibitor), while carcinoembryonic antigen (CEA) was normal. Abdominal ultrasonography was normal, as were chest-X-ray and mammography. Our interpretation is that calcitonin resistance was also present, as part of the patient's multi-hormonal resistance due to impairment of the cAMP activation pathway [6, 7].

Six months later, during follow-up evaluation, the patient's calcium level was seen to have increased to 10.6 mg/dl and PTH had decreased to 32 pg/ml; oral calcium supplementation was gradually reduced and then discontinued, and calcitriol was reduced to 0.25 mcg twice daily; subsequent controls revealed normal calcium (10 mg/dl) and slightly increased PTH (72 pg/ml) levels. She had no further loss of consciousness or seizures; on neurological examinations, levetiracetam treatment was confirmed, also on account of the frailty of the patient.

3. Discussion

This is an unusual case of the first diagnosis of PHP type 1 A in a 64-year-old woman, who presented with hypocalcemia and recent recurrent episodes of loss of consciousness and seizures. Combined evaluation of her clinical history, physical features, blood chemistry, and radiological findings suggested this diagnosis. A retrospective interpretation of her history showed how the disease had evolved during the patient's lifetime: in early adulthood, she developed PTH resistance-related hypocalcemia, carpo-pedal spasm, and hypothyroidism due to TSH resistance; around the age of 30 years, she suffered ovarian failure due to FSH and LH resistance; this was followed by bilateral hip disease requiring arthroprosthesis at 45 and 50 years and worsening hypocalcemia, which was unresponsive to cholecalciferol and oral calcium supplementation; finally, recurrent seizures recently ensued. Calcitonin resistance was also present, while IGF-1 was normal. She had no kidney stones; this is in keeping with the observation that urinary calcium levels are not markedly increased in these patients, as the action of PTH is maintained in the distal renal tubule, where GNAS gene expression is biallelic. Switching to calcitriol treatment promptly corrected the woman's hypocalcemia, and she had neither muscle spasms nor seizures on anti-epileptic medication. Both hypocalcemia and the development of multiple cortical and subcortical calcifications could have contributed to the development of seizures.

Based on the patient's clinical characterization, the targeted mutation analysis of the *GNAS* gene identified a known mutation already associated with PHP1A [8], thus allowing the clinical diagnosis to be confirmed. The mutation was presumably inherited from the mother, who was referred to as having cognitive impairment. However, as no sample was available, this hypothesis was not formally confirmed.

In accordance with the recommendations of the recently published first consensus statement on the diagnosis and management of pseudohypoparathyroidism-related disorders [7], the diagnosis should be based on clinical and biochemical characteristics, which will vary according to the age of the patient. The diagnosis of AHO should be based on the presence of major criteria (brachydactyly due to premature fusion of the epiphyses and short stature by adulthood) and additional criteria (stocky build, round facies, and ectopic ossifications). Obesity, dental manifestations, and cognitive impairment are present in a subgroup of patients. In the majority of PHP patients, the main clinical manifestations are symptoms of hypocalcemia due to PTH resistance. In patients with PHP1A, resistance to PTH is usually absent at birth and evolves over time (from the neonatal period to 22 years); the first biochemical abnormalities to appear are increased serum PTH and phosphorous levels, whereas hypocalcemia develops gradually 4-5 years later. Other associated endocrine features that support the diagnosis are as follows: early-onset hypothyroidism due to TSH resistance, which is the most common associated endocrine alteration, being present in nearly 100% of PHP1A patients; hypogonadism (due to FSH and LH resistance); hypercalcitoninemia (due to calcitonin resistance); GH deficiency (due to GHRH resistance).

Owing to the important implications for clinical management, early screening for associated conditions and genetic counselling, the molecular cause of PHP should be promptly identified, in order to confirm the diagnosis and characterize the subtype of the disease. Conversely, no genotype-phenotype correlation can be inferred based on mutation analysis [9]. In a large series, the recurrent c.568_571del mutation detected in our patient was found associated with a wide spectrum of phenotypical features. Namely, PTH levels and serum calcium ranged from 57 to 653 pg/ml (reference range 15-55) and from 1.3 to 2.7 mmol/l (reference range 2.1-2.6), respectively [10].

Few studies have focused on the natural history of this disease and on the outcome of its management. The clinical management of hypocalcemia in PHP patients is based on the administration of the active metabolite of vitamin D calcitriol ($1,25(OH)_2$ vitamin D) as in the case of our patient, who was previously on therapy with cholecalciferol.

Indeed, owing to PTH resistance, 25OH vitamin D cannot be converted by the renal tubule into its biologically active form, $1,25\ (OH)_2$ vitamin D, by PTH-dependent renal 1α-hydroxylase. The goal is to maintain normocalcemia and to keep serum PTH levels in the upper portion of the reference range, thereby avoiding PTH suppression, which can be associated with hypercalciuria and renal calcification. On the other hand, long-term and excessive secondary hyperparathyroidism can result in osteitis fibrosa cystica and dislocation of the femoral capital epiphysis (as may have occurred in our patient, who underwent bilateral hip replacement in adult age). PTH, calcium, and phosphorus should be evaluated every six months during treatment in asymptomatic patients, and more frequently when clinically indicated. Patients and families should be instructed with regard to the symptoms of hypo- and hypercalcemia.

The present case underlines the importance of early diagnosis of pseudohypoparathyroidism, as this is crucial to the appropriate treatment and lifelong management of the disease and its complications, which have a great impact on patients and their families. Appropriate genetic counselling is essential in order to establish effective communication with the family, which in turn allows relevant information to be exchanged and genetic testing to be framed within an integrated clinical path. This is in line with the recent consensus statement [7], which recommends a multidisciplinary approach addressing all aspects of the disease and its potential complications.

Consent

Informed consent was obtained from the patient and her brother.

Acknowledgments

The authors would like to thank Dr. Antonio Castaldi, Neuroradiology Unit, Galliera Hospital, Genoa, Italy, for neuroradiological images.

References

[1] M. Bastepe and H. Jüppner, "Pseudohypoparathyroidism, Albright's hereditary osteodystrophy, and progressive osseous heteroplasia: disorders caused by inactivating GNAS mutations," in *Endocrinology Adult and Pediatric*, L. Jameson and L. De Groot, Eds., pp. 1147–1159, Elsevier, 7th, chapter 66 edition, 2016.

[2] G. Mantovani, "Pseudohypoparathyroidism: Diagnosis and treatment," *The Journal of Clinical Endocrinology & Metabolism*, vol. 96, no. 10, pp. 3020–3030, 2011.

[3] S. Thiele, G. Mantovani, A. Barlier et al., "From pseudohypoparathyroidism to inactivating PTH/PTHrP signalling disorder (iPPSD), a novel classification proposed by the EuroPHP network," *European Journal of Endocrinology*, vol. 175, no. 6, pp. 1–17, 2016.

[4] O. Tafaj and H. Jüppner, "Pseudohypoparathyroidism: one gene, several syndromes," *Journal of Endocrinological Investigation*, vol. 40, no. 4, pp. 347–356, 2017.

[5] G. Mantovani, A. Linglart, I. Garin, C. Silve, F. M. Elli, and G. P. De Nanclares, "Clinical utility gene card for: Pseudohypoparathyroidism," *European Journal of Human Genetics*, vol. 21, no. 6, pp. 698–702, 2013.

[6] V. Vlaeminck-Guillem, M. D'Herbomez, P. Pigny et al., "Pseudohypoparathyroidism Ia and hypercalcitoninemia," *The Journal of Clinical Endocrinology & Metabolism*, vol. 86, no. 7, pp. 3091–3096, 2001.

[7] G. Mantovani, M. Bastepe, D. Monk et al., "Diagnosis and management of pseudohypoparathyroidism and related disorders: first international Consensus Statement," *Nature Reviews Endocrinology*, vol. 14, no. 8, pp. 476–500, 2018.

[8] L. S. Weinstein, P. V. Gejman, P. de Mazancourt, N. American, and A. M. Spiegel, "A heterozygous 4-bp deletion mutation in the Gsα gene (GNASl) in a patient with albright hereditary osteodystrophy," *Genomics*, vol. 13, no. 4, pp. 1319–1321, 1992.

[9] F. M. Elli, L. deSanctis, B. Ceoloni et al., "Pseudohypoparathyroidism Type Ia and Pseudo-Pseudohypoparathyroidism: The Growing Spectrum of GNAS Inactivating Mutations," *Human Mutation*, vol. 34, no. 3, pp. 411–416, 2013.

[10] S. Thiele, R. Werner, J. Grötzinger et al., "A positive genotype-phenotype correlation in a large cohort of patients with Pseudohypoparathyroidism Type Ia and Pseudo-pseudohypoparathyroidism and 33 newly identified mutations in the GNAS gene," *Molecular Genetics & Genomic Medicine*, vol. 3, no. 2, pp. 111–120, 2015.

22

Kocher-Debre-Semelaigne Syndrome: Hypothyroid Muscular Pseudohypertrophy—A Rare Report of Two Cases

Chandan Shaw[1] and Prachi Shaw[2]

[1] *Department of Pediatrics, Sri Manakula Vinayagar Medical College and Hospital, Kalitheerthalkuppam, Madagadipet, Pondicherry 605 107, India*
[2] *Department of Microbiology, Sri Manakula Vinayagar Medical College and Hospital, Kalitheerthalkuppam, Madagadipet, Pondicherry 605 107, India*

Correspondence should be addressed to Chandan Shaw, chandan.1974@gmail.com

Academic Editors: G. Aimaretti, T. Cheetham, and K. Kasagi

Kocher-Debre-Semelaigne syndrome (KDSS) is a rare association of muscular pseudohypertrophy and long-standing moderate-to-severe hypothyroidism in the pediatric age group. It may be confused with primary muscle disorders, lest one is cautious enough to investigate for hypothyroidism. The striking clinical features, availability of a simple treatment and a good prognosis for the condition makes it worthwhile to report the case so that all practitioners be aware of the condition and its management.

1. Introduction

Kocher-Debre-Semelaigne syndrome (KDSS) is a rare association of muscular pseudohypertrophy and long-standing moderate-to-severe hypothyroidism in the pediatric age group. The condition is rare in countries with screening programmes for hypothyroidism at birth. However, they are not uncommon in the countries where such routine screening programmes are not available, the diagnosis of hypothyroidism may be delayed—which may account for the higher incidence of the said condition.

2. Case Report

A 9-year-old girl, hailing from Senji, a village in Pondicherry, India, presented with lassitude, lethargy, mental slowing, and growth failure to the Department of Pediatrics, Sri Manakula Vinayaga Medical College and Hospital, Pondicherry. The child was apparently asymptomatic till 5 years of age, when the parents started noticing progressive weakness and lethargy along with deteriorating academic performance. She had difficulty in memorising lessons and performing mathematical calculations. There was no history of any neck swelling at any point in the history. There was no major illness reported prior to the onset of these symptoms. The milestones were achieved in the normal periods and no regression was noted. There was no similar illness, consanguinity or a history of neck swelling in the family and the dietary history was insignificant. On examination she was found to be grossly short statured [height = 100 cms against expected of 132.5 cms (75.5%)] with prominent muscular build but with infantile proportions (Figure 1). She had hoarseness of voice, a dry texture of hair and skin, and infantile facies with macroglossia and pouting lips (Figure 2). Her systemic examination revealed low intelligence quotient with psychomotor retardation, decreased power in all four limbs involving both proximal and distal muscles (grade 3/5 to 4/5), hung-up knee jerk, and a ejection systolic murmur at the base of the heart. On investigation, she was found to have hypothyroidism [TSH = 115.6 IU/L (0.2–6.0 IU/L), total T_4 = 0.12 μg/dL (5–12.5 μg/dL), T_3 = 4.4 ng/dL (60–180 ng/dL)]. The creatinine phosphokinase (CPK), serum aspartate transaminase (AST), and the lactate dehydrogenase (LDH) levels were elevated. Muscle biopsy (light microscopy/H and E staining) revealed degenerative changes with hyalinization, vacuolization, and fragmentation of fibres without any

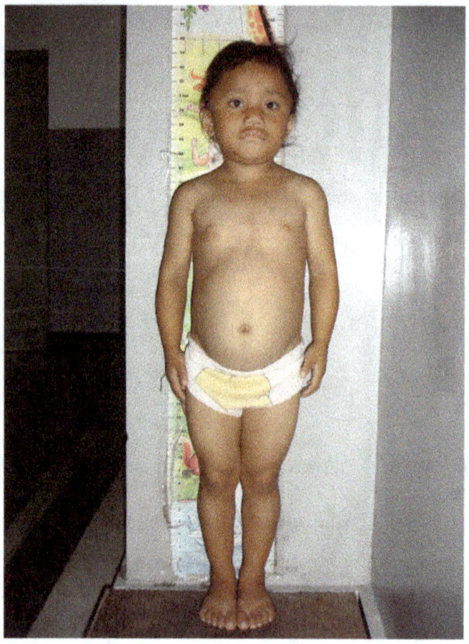

FIGURE 1: A 9-year-old girl with pseudomuscular hypertrophy in Kocher-Debre-Semelaigne syndrome.

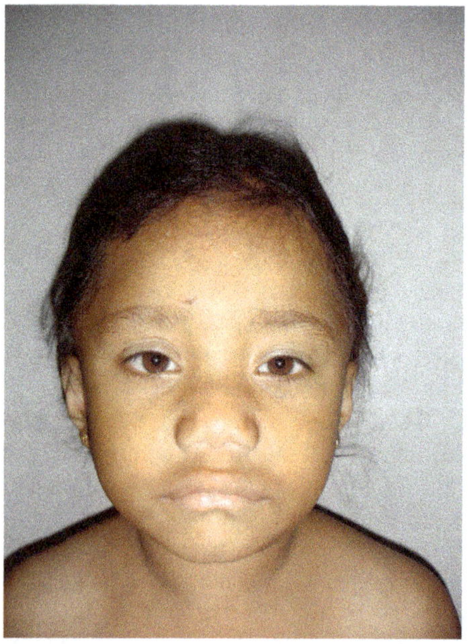

FIGURE 2: Facial features in the same girl with Kocher-Debre-Semelaigne syndrome.

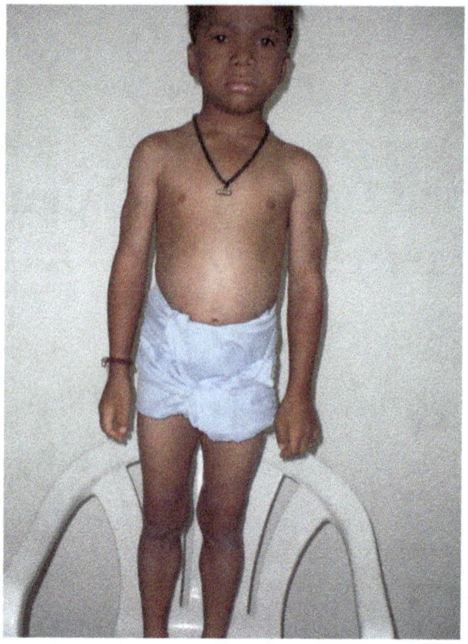

FIGURE 3: A ten-year-old boy with pseudomuscular hypertrophy in Kocher-Debre-Semelaigne syndrome.

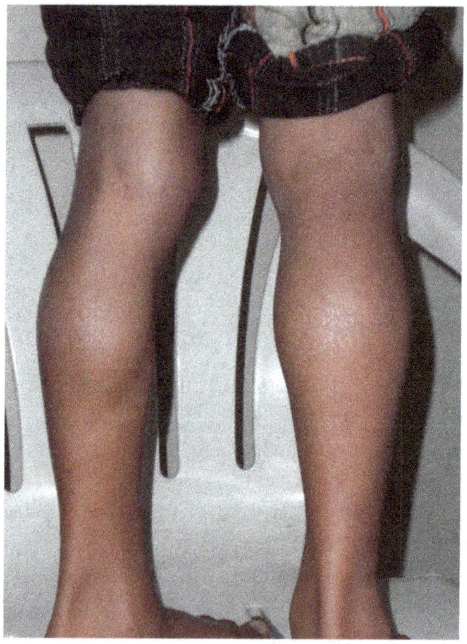

FIGURE 4: Calf pseudohypertrophy in the same boy with Kocher-Debre-Semelaigne syndrome.

inflammatory infiltrate suggestive of myopathy. Echocardiography revealed no cardiac abnormality. A diagnosis of KDSS was made on the basis of the above mentioned findings, and the child was started on levothyroxine supplementation, 50 μg/day, three months following which the child was found to be euthyroid [TSH = 2.7 IU/L, T_3 = 75 ng/dL, and T_4 = 8.6 μg/dL], and the symptoms of hypothyroidism had regressed but the muscular hypertrophy still persists after one year of thyroxine supplementation.

Another case is a ten-year-old boy hailing from Narketpally (Andhra Pradesh, India) with similar symptoms and signs (Figures 3 and 4) presented to our unit. The child had been symptomatic with symptoms like lethargy, cold intolerance, and dry skin coarse facial features for the last 6 years. The thyroid function tests were suggestive of hypothyroidism [TSH = 95.6 IU/L (0.2–6.0 IU/L), total T_4 = 0.16 μg/dL (5–12.5 μg/dL), and T_3 = 19.4 ng/dL (60–180 ng/dL)]. The CPK, AST, and muscle biopsy showed similar changes as the first child. The child was started on levothyroxine (50 μg/day), and within one month the symptoms resolved though the muscular hypertrophy still persists after nine months of thyroxine supplementation. The child was euthyroid after 3 months [TSH = 4.7 IU/L, T_3 = 65 ng/dL, T_4 = 6.6 μg/dL] Both the children are under followup.

3. Discussion

The syndrome was initially reported by Emil Theodore Kocher in 1892, while the coexistence of the muscular pseudohypertrophy was emphasized by Robert Debre and Georges Semelaigne only later in 1935 [1]. The pathogenesis of muscular pseudohypertrophy remains obscure and is believed to be due to the long-standing effects of hypo-thyroidism on the muscle fibres. The histology is nonspecific. The light microcopic features are similar to that seen in the index case; additionally one may find variation of fibre size and abortive spiral annulets [2, 3]. KDSS is usually seen in the age group 3 to 10 years [1–4]; however, there have been anecdotal reports of cases presenting as early as in the neonatal period [5] and 15 months [4]. The underlying thyroid effect may vary from both congenital (athyreosis, enzyme synthesis defects) or acquired (autoimmune) forms of hypothyroidism [1, 6]. In either of the cases reported by us, the exact cause of hypothyroidism was not ascertained, though the ultrasonography of neck and aspiration cytology of the thyroid gland was normal, thus, ruling out athyreosis. The child usually has florid symptoms of hypothyroidism and severity of the latter usually correlates directly with the muscle pseudohypertrophy and muscle cramps. This is in stark contrast to the thyroid myopathy seen in hyper- or hypothyroid state in the adults wherein wasting and atrophy are more common. The smaller body proportions in children, lower fat content and myxedema impart an athletic or Herculean semblance [1–3]. The pseudohypertrophy is most striking in the limbs, tongue, and the facial muscles as seen in the reported case [1, 4]. One may be misled by a diagnosis of a primary muscle disorder but for the biochemical evidence of hypothyroidism. The elevation of CPK levels [7] are also to mild degree and not in the proportion seen in muscular dystrophies, which are the closest clinical differentials to the syndrome considering the age group. Besides, the dystrophic changes are not seen in biopsy. The electromyography shows a myogenic lesion [8]. An association of KDSS with congenital nystagmus has been reported in the literature, which was not seen in our case. The signs and symptoms of hypothyroidism as well as the muscular pseudohypertrophy revert [3, 7] back to normal in due course of time after initiation of thyroxine supplementation, except for the fact that the final height may still be short. A well-planned and graded physiotherapy programme may be beneficial in getting rid of the muscle stiffness and achieving full potential for the muscle strength [7].

4. Conclusion

KDSS is a rare case which may be confused with primary muscle disorders, lest one is cautious enough to investigate for hypothyroidism. The striking clinical features, availability of a simple treatment, and a good prognosis for the condition makes it worthwhile to report the case so that all practitioners are aware of the condition and its management.

Acknowledgment

This paper was supported by Sri Manakula Vinayaga Medical College and Hospital, Pondicherry, India.

References

[1] M. P. Bhide, M. D. Khare, A. V. Jaykar, A. Y. Ranade, and P. N. Patnekar, "Kocher-Debre-Semelaigne syndrome," *Indian Pediatrics*, vol. 26, no. 10, pp. 1049–1052, 1989.

[2] A. Virmani, A. Gambhir, and P. U. Iyer, "Kocher Debre Semelaigne syndrome mimicking primary muscle disease," *Indian Pediatrics*, vol. 27, no. 1, pp. 88–89, 1990.

[3] P. Mehrotra, M. Chandra, and M. K. Mitra, "Kocher Debre Semelaigne syndrome: regression of pesudohypertrophy of muscles on thyroxine," *Archives of Disease in Childhood*, vol. 86, no. 3, article 224, 2002.

[4] M. S. Tullu, V. S. Udgirkar, M. N. Muranjan, S. A. Sathe, and J. R. Kamat, "Kocher-Debre-Semelaigne syndrome: hypothyroidism with muscle pseudohypertrophy," *Indian Journal of Pediatrics*, vol. 70, no. 8, pp. 671–673, 2003.

[5] J. B. Ghosh, "Kocher Debre Semelaigne syndrome in a neonate," *Indian Pediatrics*, vol. 25, no. 10, pp. 1018–1019, 1988.

[6] K. Unachak and P. Dejkhamron, "Primary congenital hypothyroidism: clinical characteristics and etiological study," *Journal of the Medical Association of Thailand*, vol. 87, no. 6, pp. 612–617, 2004.

[7] D. M. Echeverry and D. Kendlaya, "Hypothyroid myopathy," E. A. Molberg-Wolff, F. Talavera, K. Kolaski, K. L. Allen, and D. I. Campagndo, Eds., http://www.emedicine.com/pmr/topic57.htm.

[8] A. K. Affifi, S. S. Najjar, J. Mire-Salman, and R. A. Bergman, "The myopathy of the Kocher-Debre-Semelaigne syndrome: electromyography, light- and electron-microscopic study," *Journal of the Neurological Sciences*, vol. 22, pp. 445–470, 1974.

23

Myxedema Coma Associated with Macroprolactinoma: Case Report and Review of the Literature

Elizabeth Jasola Omoniyi[1,2] **and Richard J. Robbins**[1,2]

[1]*From the Division of Endocrinology, Diabetes and Metabolism, Department of Medicine, Houston Methodist Hospital, Houston, TX, USA*
[2]*Weill Cornell Medical College, New York, NY, USA*

Correspondence should be addressed to Richard J. Robbins; rjrobbins@houstonmethodist.org

Academic Editor: Toshihiro Kita

Myxedema coma is a rare life-threatening presentation of severe hypothyroidism associated with a high mortality rate. Although most cases are due to primary thyroid failure, a minority have central hypothyroidism as the underlying cause. We report the case of a 69-year-old man who presented with obtundation, hypoglycemia, and hyponatremia. The patient's initial thyroid-stimulating hormone (TSH) was within normal limits. Subsequent evaluation revealed critical anterior pituitary insufficiency due to a macroprolactinoma and a diagnosis of myxedema coma after appropriate workup The finding of a normal serum TSH should not eliminate the possibility of myxedema coma.

1. Introduction

We report a very unusual case of myxedema coma (MC). Severe hypothyroidism meeting the definition of MC is associated with a significant mortality rate (30–50%), even with standard therapy [1, 2]. The underlying causes of myxedema coma vary but usually involve a primary pathological process in the thyroid gland. Commonly, a patient with primary hypothyroidism either stops taking or stops absorbing their thyroid supplements for some time, resulting in fatigue and confusion. Mental status can gradually deteriorate; however, if precipitated by a severe infection, trauma, central nervous system depressants, or a sudden cardiovascular event, rapid onset of stupor or obtundation may ensue, termed myxedema coma. MC has also been reported rarely in patients with central hypothyroidism due to hypothalamic or pituitary diseases. We report a case of myxedema coma with central hypothyroidism associated with a macroprolactinoma.

2. Case Report

Following a rare series of three winter storms affecting Houston, TX, at the end of February 2021, there was widespread loss of power and water, and daily temperatures stayed below 0 degrees Celsius for 17 days. An estimated 250–700 Texans died from cold exposure during this period.

A 69-year-old male was brought to the emergency department in early March 2021 for evaluation of deteriorating mental status leading to disorientation and unresponsiveness. Initial laboratory tests revealed a blood glucose of 45 mg/dl and a serum sodium of 120 mEq/L. His lactic acid level was elevated at 4.2 mmol/L. He was started on intravenous 10% dextrose with no improvement of mental status, though his serum glucose rose to 102 mg/dl. A chest CT revealed a large area of infiltration in the right upper lung consistent with pneumonia. A CT scan of the head revealed calcification of the basal ganglia, thalamus, and cerebral hemispheres bilaterally. A 2 cm mass arising from the sella turcica was also noted (Figure 1). Additional laboratory studies on the day of admission (when he was hypoglycemic) revealed a serum insulin of 1.4 mU/L with normal C-peptide, IGF-2, and proinsulin levels.

He also had a significant medical history of hypertension and iron deficiency anemia that required frequent erythropoietin injections. He also had a history of daily tobacco use but had discontinued that two years prior. There was no history of illicit drug use. His only home medication was lisinopril 20 mg daily. His family reported that he had been increasingly confused and lethargic for one week prior to his emergency room presentation. His family also reported that he had not complained of headaches, nausea, vomiting, or any visual impairment.

Clinically, he was obtunded and only partially responsive to auditory stimuli. His skin was very dry and flaking off; he had generalized edema and macroglossia, but he did not have expressible galactorrhea or gynecomastia. He was variably hypothermic, with body temperature ranging from 94.8–96.1 degrees Fahrenheit. His heart rate ranged from 75 to 86 bpm. An ECG revealed a first-degree AV block. On 2 liters of nasal oxygen, his arterial pO2 was 95 mm·Hg, and his pCO2 was elevated at 48 mm·Hg. In previous medical visits, he had never been diagnosed with thyroid dysfunction, hyponatremia, or hypoglycemia. He had no prior brain imaging.

Given the newly found pituitary lesion and the patient's clinical presentation, pituitary function labs were ordered for further evaluation. His prolactin level was 1,033 ng/ml (4–15 ng/ml); free T4 was 0.2 ng/dl (0.9–1.7 ng/dl); total T3 was low at 35 ng/dl (80–200 ng/dl) with an inappropriately normal thyroid-stimulating hormone (TSH) of 2.35 uIU/ml (0.27–4.2 uIU/ml). His initial (2 PM) serum cortisol was 5 ug/dl with an ACTH of 9.6 pg/ml (7.2–63.3 pg/ml). Following intravenous cosyntropin, his cortisol rose to 10 ug/dl at 30 minutes and 11 ug/dl at 60 minutes. There was no notable change in his mental status after the cosyntropin administration. His IGF-2 was normal at 206 ng/ml (180–580 ng/ml). His initial serum parathyroid hormone level was low at 9 pg/ml.

The patient's serum follicle-stimulating hormone (FSH) was 1.0 mIU/mL (1.6–8.0 mIU/ml), and his serum luteinizing hormone (LH) was 0.3 mIU/ml (1.6–15.2 mIU/ml). An MRI of the brain confirmed a sellar and suprasellar enhancing mass, likely a pituitary adenoma, measuring 1.2 × 1.8 × 2.3 cm, with no sphenoid or cavernous sinus invasion.

The patient's total score of 85 on the widely accepted Popoveniuc et al. diagnostic scoring system [3] confirmed the diagnosis of myxedema coma. He would have received 7 points on Chiong's screening tool [4], making myxedema coma "Likely." His clinical presentation, history, and multiple laboratory and imaging findings were consistent with myxedema coma and hypopituitarism, likely secondary to a macroprolactinoma.

3. Discussion and Literature Review

We report the case of a man who had underlying central hypopituitarism, including partial TSH deficiency, as the cause of his hypothyroidism. He then developed myxedema coma, possibly due to a combination of cold exposure and pneumonia. The cause of his hypopituitarism was most likely a macroprolactinoma. As far as we can determine, this is the first documented case of myxedema coma due in part to a macroprolactinoma. We found no other case reports of this phenomenon in our literature review.

There are many potential underlying causes of MC. Two of the most common are autoimmune thyroid failure (e.g., Hashimoto thyroiditis) and post-thyroidectomy hypothyroidism. Reports of MC due to hypopituitarism with secondary hypothyroidism are quite rare and have been estimated to account for much less than 5% of all MC cases [2]. The earliest case of MC due to central hypothyroidism that we found in our literature review was reported in 1940 by Means, Hertz, and Herman, who reported MC due to Sheehan's disease hypopituitarism. An autopsy revealed atrophy of the pituitary, thyroid, adrenals, and ovaries [5]. In a 1991 literature review, Pinchera et al. estimated that hypothyroidism arising solely from hypopituitarism accounted for approximately 0.005% of all cases of hypothyroidism [6].

The most common precipitating factors in MC are hypothermia, cessation of thyroid supplements, severe infections, anesthetics, tranquilizers, respiratory failure, and stroke [1, 7]. In 2008, Dutta et al. reported on 29 cases of MC. Four (17%) likely had underlying central hypothyroidism, three of which were due to Sheehan syndrome and the last of which was due to a nonfunctioning pituitary adenoma. The precipitating cause of MC was pneumonia in three of the four patients and cold exposure in the fourth patient [8].

Several well-documented cases of MC associated with hypopituitarism have been reported in PubMed over the past 60 years [9–16]. A case with both Hashimoto thyroiditis and Sheehan syndrome leading to MC has also been reported [17], as has a case with Hashimoto thyroiditis and TSH deficiency [18]. In pediatric medicine, Thompson and Henry reported a rare case of MC due to central hypothyroidism in a 7-year-old boy with a chromosome 1q deletion [19].

Given that the vast majority (>95%) of MC cases are due to primary hypothyroidism, it can be difficult to diagnose MC when TSH is not elevated. In patients with MC due to central hypothyroidism, the TSH is typically low or normal, and these patients often have other features of hypopituitarism [8]. Additionally, given that a small but significant percentage of thyroid hormone production from the thyroid gland is TSH-independent (10–15%), these patients often also present with free T4 levels that are higher than in patients with primary hypothyroidism [8].

Although patients with MC due to central hypothyroidism typically present with altered mental status as the first symptom, their neurological impairments may be more subtle than MC due to primary hypothyroidism, in part because there is some minimal TSH-independent T4 production in central hypothyroidism. However, the mortality rate for MC appears to be similar in both central and primary hypothyroidism [8, 20].

Notably, patients with macroprolactinomas have various patterns of hypopituitarism. In a large retrospective review

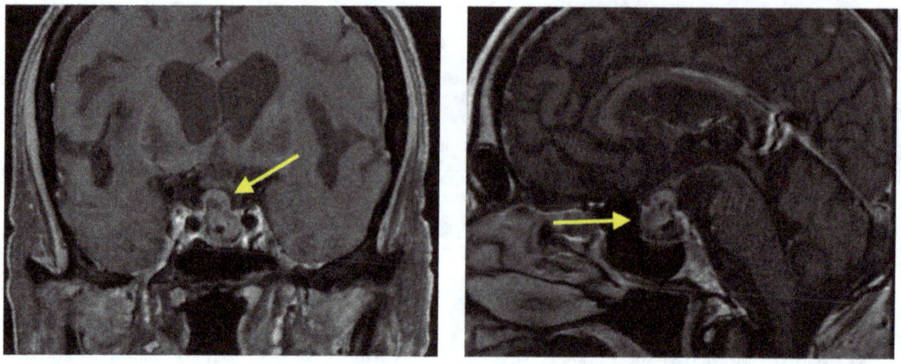

(a) (b)

FIGURE 1: (a) Coronal and (b) sagittal views of the 2 cm pituitary adenoma.

of men with macroprolactinomas (between 20–39 mm in size), 93% had central hypogonadism, 7% had central hypoadrenalism, and 18% had central hypothyroidism [21, 22]. Hyperprolactinemia is commonly associated with diminished or absent pulsatile LH and FSH secretion, likely due to endocrine inhibition of GnRH pulses [23]; however, there is no evidence that it suppresses TSH secretion in men. By contrast, dopamine agonists, which are often used to treat hyperprolactinemia, have been shown to suppress TSH [24].

Regardless of the etiology of the MC, management with high-dose intravenous levothyroxine as a loading dose, followed by a weight-based daily dose, remains the gold standard for therapy to help reverse the severe hypometabolic state in MC patients. Intravenous hydrocortisone should also be administered initially or concurrently, as patients with MC often have relative adrenocortical deficiency, which can worsen as the replacement thyroid hormone increases the metabolic rate [1].

4. Conclusion

Myxedema coma is an endocrine emergency that requires a high index of suspicion given its high mortality rate. Unusual underlying causes, such as tumoral hypopituitarism, can impede diagnosis due to the lack of elevated TSH levels. This can potentially delay time-sensitive management therapies. From our literature review and to the best of our knowledge, this is the first report of macroprolactinoma associated with MC and is worth noting, as it highlights the extensive range of complications that can arise from pituitary tumors. Overall, this case highlights the critical importance of careful and thorough clinical assessment in patients with seemingly incongruent clinical and laboratory findings.

References

[1] K. D. Burman and L. Wartofsky, "Myxedema coma," in *Werner and Ingbar's the Thyroid*, L. E. Braverman, D. S. Cooper, and P. Kopp, Eds., Wolters Kluwer, Alphen aan den Rijn, Netherlands, 2020.

[2] L. Wartofsky, "Myxedema coma," *Endocrinology and Metabolism Clinics of North America*, vol. 35, no. 4, pp. 687–698, 2006.

[3] G. Popoveniuc, T. Chandra, A. Sud et al., "A diagnostic scoring system for myxedema coma," *Endocrine Practice*, vol. 20, no. 8, pp. 808–817, 2014.

[4] Y. V. Chiong, E. Bammerlin, and C. N. Mariash, "Development of an objective tool for the diagnosis of myxedema coma," *Translational Research*, vol. 166, no. 3, pp. 233–243, 2015.

[5] J. H. Means, S. Hertz, and J. Lerman, "The pituitary type of myxedema or Simmond's disease masquerading as myxedema," *Transactions of the Association of American Physicians*, vol. 55, no. 32, 1940.

[6] A. Pinchera, E. Martino, and G. Faglia, "Central hypothyroidism," in *The Thyroid. A Fundamental and Clinical Text*, L. E. Braverman and R. D. Utiger, Eds., pp. 968–984, Lippincott Company, JB Lippincott Company, Philadelphia, PA, USA, 1991.

[7] V. Mathew, R. A. Misgar, S. Ghosh et al., "Myxedema coma: a new look into an old crisis," *Journal of Thyroid Research*, vol. 2011, Article ID 493462, 7 pages, 2011.

[8] P. Dutta, A. Bhansali, S. Masoodi, S. Bhadada, N. Sharma, and R. Rajput, "Predictors of outcome in myxoedema coma: A study from a tertiary care centre," *Critical Care*, vol. 12, no. 1, 2008.

[9] S. Bhogal, N. Patel, K. Mawa, V. Ramu, and T. Paul, "A rare case of myxedema coma presenting as bradycardia and hypotension secondary to pituitary apoplexy," *Cureus*, vol. 13, no. 5, Article ID e15196, 2021.

[10] M. J. Cullen, P. D. Mayne, and I. Sliney, "Myxoedema coma," *Irish Journal of Medical Science*, vol. 148, no. 1, pp. 201–206, 1979.

[11] S. Fischli, C. Stettler, and E. Christ, "Kardiogener Schock und psychotisches Zustandsbild seltener Ursache," *DMW—Deutsche Medizinische Wochenschrift*, vol. 131, no. 42, pp. 2333–2336, 2006.

[12] R. Hanslik, L. Kaspar, A. Kroiss, and J. Slany, "Myxödem als Ursache eines QT-Syndroms und rezidivierender Kammertachykardien [Myxedema as a cause of QT syndrome and recurring ventricular tachycardia]," *Zeitschrift für Kardiologie*, vol. 76, no. 1, pp. 58–61, 1987.

[13] L. Langeron, L. Croccel, G. Routier, and P. Choteau, "Myxedematous coma, thyroid involution and eosinophilic adenoma of the hypophysis," *Annales d'Endocrinologie*, vol. 20, pp. 490–493, 1959.

[14] T. Murase, A. Mukoyama, N. Ohsawa, S. Nagataki, T. Yamaji, and T. Tsushima, "A survival case of myxedema coma of pituitary origin," *Endocrinologia Japonica*, vol. 20, no. 3, pp. 331–334, 1973.

[15] M. Perlmutter and H. Cohn, "Myxedema crisis of pituitary or thyroid origin," *The American Journal of Medicine*, vol. 36, no. 6, pp. 883–892, 1964.

[16] W. Reinhardt and K. Mann, "Häufigkeit klinisches Bild und Behandlung des hypothyreoten Komas," *Medizinische Klinik*, vol. 92, no. 9, pp. 521–524, 1997.

[17] S. Benvenga, S. Squadrito, F. Saporito, A. Cimino, F. Arrigo, and F. Trimarchi, "Myxedema coma of both primary and secondary origin with non-classic presentation and extremely elevated creatine kinase," *Hormone and Metabolic Research*, vol. 32, no. 09, pp. 364–366, 2000.

[18] K. Iida, Y. Hino, T. Ohara, and K. Chihara, "A case of myxedema coma caused by isolated thyrotropin stimulating hormone deficiency and Hashimoto's thyroiditis," *Endocrine Journal*, vol. 58, no. 2, pp. 143–148, 2011.

[19] M. D. Thompson and R. K. Henry, "Myxedema coma secondary to central hypothyroidism: a rare but real cause of altered mental status in pediatrics," *Hormone Research in Paediatrics*, vol. 87, no. 5, pp. 350–353, 2017.

[20] I. Rodriguez, E. Fluiters, L. Perez-Mendez, R. Luna, C. Paramo, and R. Garcia-Mayor, "Factors associated with mortality of patients with myxoedema coma: Prospective study in 11 cases treated in a single institution," *Journal of Endocrinology*, vol. 180, no. 2, pp. 347–350, 2004.

[21] P. Iglesias and J. J. Diez, "Macroprolactinoma: A diagnostic and therapeutic update," *An International Journal of Medicine*, vol. 106, no. 6, pp. 495–504, 2013.

[22] A. Tirosh, C. Benbassat, A. Lifshitz, and I. Shimon, "Hypopituitarism patterns and prevalence among men with macroprolactinomas," *Pituitary*, vol. 18, no. 1, pp. 108–115, 2015.

[23] G. Page-Wilson, P. C. Smith, and C. K. Welt, "Prolactin suppresses GnRH but not TSH secretion," *Hormone Research in Paediatrics*, vol. 65, no. 1, pp. 31–38, 2006.

[24] B. R. Haugen, "Drugs that suppress TSH or cause central hypothyroidism," *Best Practice and Research Clinical Endocrinology and Metabolism*, vol. 23, no. 6, pp. 793–800, 2009.

24

Possible Iodine-Induced Thyrotoxicosis in a Previously Healthy Adolescent following Administration of Iodinated Contrast Media

Jennifer Apsan and Zoltan Antal

Department of Pediatrics, Division of Endocrinology Weill Cornell Medicine, New York Presbyterian Hospital, New York, NY, USA

Correspondence should be addressed to Jennifer Apsan; jea9136@nyp.org

Academic Editor: Lucy Mastrandrea

Introduction. Jod-Basedow Syndrome refers to a paradoxical phenomenon in which large loads of iodine can cause hyperthyroidism. It is most commonly seen in populations already at risk for thyroid disease or those with underlying kidney disease. *Case Presentation.* We present a case of an acutely ill 17-year-old boy with symptomatic hyperthyroidism following an iodinated contrast CT scan to rule out appendicitis. *Discussion/Conclusion.* This case underscores the importance of recognizing this phenomenon even in the pediatric population and in those with no preexisting history of thyroid disease. Course complications including bronchospasm, hypertension, transaminitis, and bilateral palmar desquamating rash are rare and highlight the complexities involved in the disease state and in managing side effect profiles of treatment.

1. Introduction

Iodine is an essential mineral, necessary for optimal thyroid function. Iodine is commonly found in a variety of foods, such as iodized salt and seafood, and in routinely utilized household items, including nutritional supplements and skin cleaners. In medical settings, iodine is a component of various medications (amiodarone and expectorants), iodine-based swabs used for skin cleaning prior to invasive procedures, and iodinated contrast media (ICM). ICM is an increasingly common source of potential iodine toxicity as CT scans have become an increasingly popular imaging modality in the United States [1]. Recommended adult daily iodine intake is typically set at about 150 μg per day by the Institute of Medicine, United Nations Children's Fund (UNICEF), World Health Organization, and the International Council for the Control of Iodine Deficiency Disorders (ICCIDD) [2]. Contrast media is known to contain about 13,500 μg of free iodine and 15–60 g of bound iodine [3, 4]. Typically, the physiological response to these large iodine loads is a transient hypothyroid state, induced by inhibiting the thyroid peroxidase enzyme involved in thyroglobulin iodination in a phenomenon known as the Wolff–Chaikoff effect. Eventually, equilibrium ensues as downregulation of the Na-I transporters which permit less iodine into the thyroid gland, thus allowing the gland to return to normal function by escaping the Wolff–Chaikoff effect. The escape or adaptation phenomenon can occur in as quickly as 48 hours and allows for adaptation to a high iodide environment without risk of thyroid dysfunction [5, 6]. Inability to escape from this inhibitory effect of large iodine doses can result in clinical or subclinical hypothyroidism. This has been described largely in fetuses, newborns, patients with underlying chronic disease, patients with autoimmune thyroiditis, or in those previously treated with radioimmunoassay (RAI), surgery, or antithyroid drugs, but has also been described in some with no known underlying conditions [7, 8]. In some people, a paradoxical hyperthyroid state is induced after administration of a large iodine load. Typically, this is seen in those with autoimmune thyroiditis, prior thyroid surgical history, prior goiter formation, Graves' disease, or kidney disease, which can impact iodine excretion.

Mainstays of treatment for hyperthyroidism include withdrawal of the offending agent, antithyroid drugs, beta blockade to decrease sympathetic tone, and steroids [5]. Multiple cases of iodine-induced hyperthyroidism are described in the adult population. Many of these patients have underlying thyroid or kidney disease which can predispose them to a state of iodine-induced hyperthyroidism [9–11]. This phenomenon is not described well in the pediatric population. Here, we describe the presentation, diagnosis, and management of a 17-year-old boy with presumed iodine-induced hyperthyroidism.

2. Case Presentation

A previously healthy 17-year-old adolescent presented to the emergency department with 3-4 days of acute and chronic right lower quadrant abdominal pain. He was sent for a protocoled contrast CT scan (78 ml Omnipaque 300) that was suggestive of acute appendicitis. He was taken to the operating room, on postcontrast day 1, where his appendix was removed. Intraoperatively, he experienced a brief episode of bronchospasm with complete resolution and successful extubation following epinephrine administration. The patient was found to be positive for rhinovirus/enterovirus at that time. On postoperative day 2, the patient had an acute episode of flushing, fatigue, fevers, and tachycardia. Infectious workup was pursued, and antibiotics were started. On postoperative day 4, flushing and tachycardia (HR 100–110 bpm) persisted, and further laboratory evaluation was notable for an elevated serum free T4 level of 4.1 ng/dL (reference values: 0.9–1.8 ng/dL) and a serum TSH level of <0.0008 uiu/ml (reference values: 0.6–4.8 uiu/ml), confirming a diagnosis of hyperthyroidism. Burch–Wartofsky score at the time of symptoms was 15, indicating a low risk for thyroid storm. Physical exam revealed that the patient was extremely fatigued, weak, and tremulous. There was no exophthalmos or lid lag, and no palpable thyromegaly or thyroid nodules. Further evaluations revealed negative thyroid stimulating immunoglobulin (TSI), antithyroglobulin, and antithyroperoxidase antibody levels. A significantly elevated serum thyroglobulin level was noted, 274 ng/ml (reference values: 0.8–29.4 ng/ml). Thyroid ultrasound was normal with no evidence of thyroid enlargement, hyperemia, or heterogeneity of the gland. Thyroid scintigraphy was considered but deferred secondary to the recent iodine load given for CT scan.

Methimazole therapy was initiated but appeared to be inadequate as a monotherapy despite increasing dosing, as there was a rapid worsening of clinical symptoms and biochemical hyperthyroidism (Table 1/Figure 1). A mild transient transaminitis was also noted, raising concerns over increasing the methimazole dose. Steroids and propranolol were added to the regimen on postcontrast day 9 which resulted in a rapid and steady decline of serum thyroxine levels over the next 7 days. One week after discharge and 12 days after the initiation of therapy, methimazole was weaned and discontinued secondary to a significant worsening transaminitis and bilateral palmar desquamating rash. Steroid therapy was also stopped after 8 days of treatment due to episodic hypertension. Further evaluation of the potential cause of transaminitis revealed an acute EBV infection. The transaminitis significantly improved within the subsequent 10 days, and thyroid function continued to remain within normal limits. Three months later, transaminitis fully resolved.

Serum iodine studies were obtained during the hospitalization. After contrast day 10, serum iodine levels were found to be 181 ug/L (reference values: 90–92 ug/L), which fully normalized to 79 ug/L (reference values: 52–109 ug/L) on postcontrast day 22, at which time thyroid function tests normalized as well.

3. Discussion/Conclusion

Our patient's clinical and laboratory data confirmed a diagnosis of acute, transient hyperthyroidism. The differential for transient thyroiditis in an adolescent includes Hashitoxicosis (hyperthyroidism caused by inflammation associated with Hashimoto's thyroiditis) and subacute thyroiditis in the setting of acute inflammation secondary to trauma or viral infection. Although autoimmune thyroiditis is the most common underlying cause of acute hyperthyroidism, our patient's autoantibody titers were negative, and thyroid ultrasound findings were not consistent with a diagnosis of autoimmune thyroiditis. He also had no evidence of inflammation, enlargement, or increased vascularity on thyroid ultrasound (Figure 2), and clinically, he had no evidence of pain or enlargement to his thyroid gland, making traumatic injury to thyroid from his intubation or virally induced hyperthyroidism unlikely. A less common cause of acute transient hyperthyroidism is excess iodine administration in a phenomenon known as Jod-Basedow syndrome [5]. The time course of our patient's presentation shortly following administration of iodinated contrast supports iodine-induced hyperthyroidisim or Jod-Basedow syndrome as the most likely cause. At a dose of 78 ml of Omnipapague 300, our patient was exposed to approximately 23 grams organic iodine; many folds more than the International Council for the Control of Iodine Deficiency Disorders (ICCIDD) recommended a tolerable upper level of 1,100 μg per day in adults [1, 12] Significantly increased thyroglobulin levels well above the normal range, as were seen in our patient, support overactivity of the thyroid gland. Thyroglobulin levels are thought to correlate with iodine exposure and may be a potential biomarker of iodine overload [13, 14].

Although the diagnosis of Jod-Basedow Syndrome is not typically dependent on confirmed elevation in serum iodine levels, our patient's elevated iodine levels correlated directly with the change in thyroid functions, further supporting the diagnosis [1]. Although other case reports have noted even higher iodine levels, our initial serum measurement was obtained 10 days after contrast administration and 7 days following initial diagnosis of hyperthyroidism. Thus, the iodine levels were presumed to be higher at the onset of disease.

Jod-Basedow syndrome typically occurs in those who have underlying thyroid disease such as autoimmune thyroiditis, goiter formation, or in those with underlying kidney

Table 1: Thyroid function tests.

	12/28/ 17+	2/23/20 PCD 4	2/24/20 PCD 5*	2/27/20 PCD 8	2/28/20 PCD 9**	2/29/20 PCD 10	3/1/20 PCD11	3/6/20 PCD16***	3/11/20 PCD 21****
TSH (uIU/ml) 0.6–4.8	1.165	<0.0008	<0.0008	0.0009	0.008	0.009	0.008	0.011	0.822
Free T4 (ng/dL) 0.9–1.8 (ng/dL)	1.0	4.1	5.1	6.8	7.4	7.0	5.2	2.4	1.3
Total T4 (ug/dL) 4.5–10.9		15.0	16.5	26.9	26.3	24.7	21.5	8.1	6.4
Total T3 (ng/mL) 0.6–1.8		1.79	1.81	4.06	3.90	2.76	1.91	0.76	1.00
TSI (IU/L) <0.54IU/L			<0.10						
TPO ab (IU/ml) 0.0–9.0			<0.3						
Tg ag (IU/ml) 0.0–4.0			<0.9						

PCD: Post contrast day, +available as baseline from prior GI appointment for poor weight gain, *methimazole started, **hydrocortisone 100 mg q 8/ propranolol 40 mg q 8 hours started, ***methimazole stopped/Hydrocortisone stopped, ****propranolol stopped.

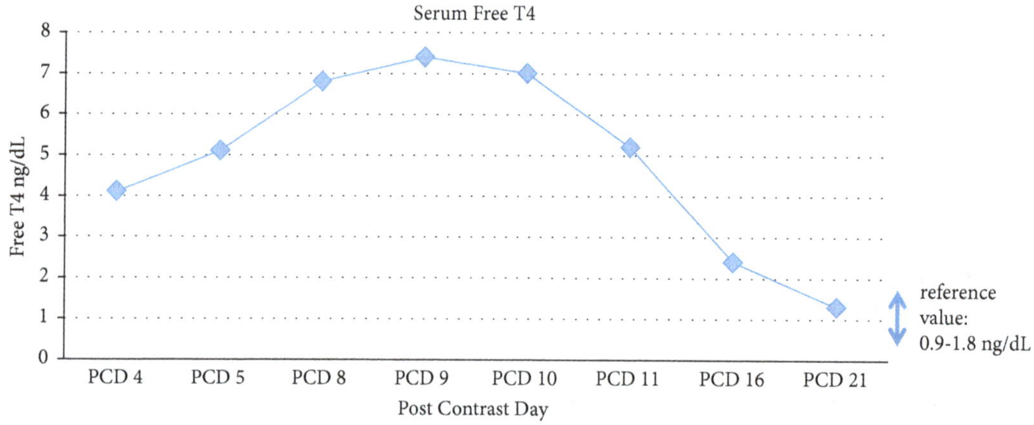

Figure 1: Serum Free T4 level in case study patient.

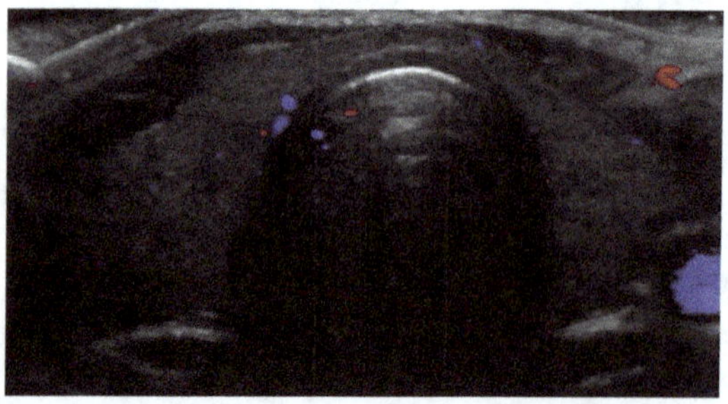

Figure 2: Thyroid ultrasound on post contrast day 7 reveals homogeneous and non enlarged thyroid gland measuring Isthmus: 0.2 cm, Right lobe: 2.3 × 4.3 × 0.9 cm Left lobe: 1.3 × 4.3 × 1.1 cm. Echogenicity is within normal limits with no increased vascularity.

disease as iodine is renally excreted. Our patient had previously documented routinely obtained thyroid function tests for an unrelated reason 2 years prior to this hospitalization (Table 1), decreasing our suspicion of prior underlying thyroid disease. Furthermore, the documented negative thyroid antibody status and normal renal function during the admission further excludes the typical underlying risk factors. We suspect that his underlying rhinovirus/enterovirus and EBV infections may have precipitated this thyroid response to iodinated contrast. The connection between viral infection and impaired thyroid function is well documented [15]. Specifically, EBV has been shown to have immunomodulatory effects and has been linked to autoimmune thyroid disease [16, 17]. In our patient, the exact mechanism of interaction between vial infection and response to iodine is not fully understood.

The reported timeline of contrast-induced hyperthyroidism in other case reports is variable, typically occurring from days to weeks following contrast administration [3, 14, 18]. However, there are reports of hyperthyroidism occurring as early as postcontrast day 1 [4]. While most cases of Jod-Basedow syndrome present as subclinical hyperthyroidism without clinical symptoms, our patient was overtly symptomatic with tremulousness and tachycardia. It not fully clear why the range of reactions to iodine exposure is so varied. Recent data point to a possible genetic predisposition [19]. Bronchospasm is not clearly associated with Jod-Baslow syndrome, and it remains unclear to date if this event in our patient was related to his thyroid disease or a reaction to his anesthesia [3, 4, 18].

This case also highlights the importance of managing side effects once medication is deemed necessary. Our patient developed both transmaminitis and hypertension. Transaminitis poses a clinical conundrum, as it has been described both as part of the natural history of hyperthyroidism [20] as well as a potential adverse effect of thionamides. In our case, the differential diagnosis additionally included EBV infection. Our decision to closely observe and continue methimazole therapy led to a successful outcome, but required a multidisciplinary effort involving other medical disciplines as well as the patient and patient's family. Steroid treatment was initiated in an effort to decrease peripheral conversion of T4 to T3 and to potentially avoid requiring increased Methimazole dosing. Thyroid function tests improved significantly once steroids were started, but our patient became significantly hypertensive at outpatient follow-up, and steroids were discontinued 6 days later. Given the uncertainty of the timeline and duration of our patient's hyperthyroidism, coupled with his significant clinical symptoms, we believe the steroid therapy was a valuable addition to the treatment regimen and was associated with significant clinical and biochemical improvement.

This case highlights the complexity of thyroid physiology and the importance of considering Jod-Basedow syndrome as a differential diagnosis even in previously healthy populations with no overt overlying risk factors. It also highlights the complexities involved in managing side effect profiles of treatment and the need for close follow-up. Although the majority of reported cases are in adults, it is important that pediatric providers are aware of the risk of this condition occurring in children as well.

Consent

Subjects have given their informed consent to publish their case.

Authors' Contributions

Apsan conceptualized the study (equal), wrote the original draft (lead), and reviewed and edited the manuscript (equal). Antal conceptualized the study and (equal) reviewed and edited the manuscript (equal).

References

[1] S. Y. Lee, C. M. Rhee, A. M. Leung, L. E. Braverman, G. A. Brent, and E. N. Pearce, "A review: radiographic iodinated contrast media-induced thyroid dysfunction," *The Journal of Clinical Endocrinology & Metabolism*, vol. 100, no. 2, pp. 376–383, 2015.

[2] H. Bürgi, "Iodine excess," *Best Practice & Research Clinical Endocrinology & Metabolism*, vol. 24, no. 1, pp. 107–115, 2010.

[3] A. J. van der Molen, H. S. Thomsen, and S. K. Morcos, "Contrast media safety committee, european society of urogenital radiology (ESUR). Effect of iodinated contrast media on thyroid function in adults," *European Radiology*, vol. 14, no. 5, pp. 902–907, 2004.

[4] C. M. Rhee, I. Bhan, E. K. Alexander, and S. M. Brunelli, "Association between iodinated contrast media exposure and incident hyperthyroidism and hypothyroidism," *Archives of Internal Medicine*, vol. 172, no. 2, pp. 153–159, 2012.

[5] H. R. Rose, "Jod Basedow syndrome," *in StatPearls, US National Library of Medicine*, Bethesda, MD, USA, 2021, https://www.ncbi.nlm.nih.gov/books/NBK544277/.

[6] K. Sarafoglou, *Pediatric Endocrinology and Inborn Error of Metabolism*, New YorkMcGraw Hill, New York, NY, USA, 2009.

[7] K. Markou, N. Georgopoulos, V. Kyriazopoulou, and A. G. Vagenakis, "Iodine-induced hypothyroidism," *Thyroid*, vol. 11, no. 5, pp. 501–510, 2001, PMID: 11396709.

[8] S. Melmed and R. H. Williams, *Williams Textbook of Endocrinology*, Elsevier/Saunders, Philadelphia, PA, USA, 12th edition, 2011.

[9] K. Lithgow and C. Symonds, "Severe thyrotoxicosis secondary to povidone-iodine from peritoneal dialysis," *Case Reports in Endocrinology*, vol. 2017, Article ID 2683120, 4 pages, 2017.

[10] L. Leuştean, C. Preda, M. C. Ungureanu et al., "Jod-basedow effect due to prolonged use of lugol solution-case report," *Revista Medico-Chirurgicala a Societatii de Medici si Naturalisti din Iasi*, vol. 118, no. 4, pp. 1013–1017, 2014, PMID: 25581962.

[11] E. Brotfain, L. Koyfman, A. Frenkel, A. Smolikov, A. Zlotnik, and M. Klein, "Iodine-induced hyperthyroidism-an old clinical entity that is still relevant to daily ICU practice: a case report," *Case Reports in Endocrinology*, vol. 2013, Article ID 792745, 4 pages, 2013.

[12] "Omnipaque™ (Iohexol) injection 140 180 240 300 350 140 350," 2021, https://www.accessdata.fda.gov/drugsatfda_docs/label/2017/018956s099lbl.pdf.

[13] A. M. Leung and L. E. Braverman, "Consequences of excess iodine," *Nature Reviews Endocrinology*, vol. 10, no. 3, pp. 136–142, 2014.

[14] A. M. El-Shirbiny, S. S. Stavrou, A. Dnistrian, M. Sonenberg, S. M. Larson, and C. R. Divgi, "Jod-basedow syndrome following oral iodine and radioiodinated-antibody administration," *Journal of Nuclear Medicine*, vol. 38, no. 11, pp. 1816-1817, 1997, Erratum in: Journal of Nuclear Medicine 1998 Mar;39(3):489.

[15] R. Desailloud and D. Hober, "Viruses and thyroiditis: an update," *Virology Journal*, vol. 6, no. 1, p. 5, 2009.

[16] A. Dittfeld, K. Gwizdek, M. Michalski, and R. Wojnicz, "A possible link between the epstein-barr virus infection and autoimmune thyroid disorders," *Central European Journal of Immunology*, vol. 41, no. 3, pp. 297–301, 2016.

[17] A. Janegova, P. Janega, B. Rychly, K. Kuracinova, and P. Babal, "The role of epstein-barr virus infection in the development of autoimmune thyroid diseases," *Endokrynologia Polska*, vol. 66, no. 2, pp. 132–136, 2015, PMID: 25931043.

[18] M. Higgs, E. Hull, and E. Lujan, "A case report of post-operative jöd-basedow phenomennon following oral and IV

iodine contrast administration," *Case Reports in Endocrinology*, vol. 2014, Article ID 980283, 3 pages, 2014.

[19] M. J. Cha, D. Y. Kang, W. Lee et al., "Hypersensitivity reactions to iodinated contrast media: a multicenter study of 196 081 patients," *Radiology*, vol. 293, no. 1, pp. 117–124, 2019, PMID: 31478801.

[20] S. Khemichian and T. L. Fong, "Hepatic dysfunction in hyperthyroidism," *Gastroenterology & Hepatology*, vol. 7, no. 5, pp. 337–9, 2011.

25

Weekly Intramuscular Injection of Levothyroxine following Myxoedema: A Practical Solution to an Old Crisis

Peter N. Taylor,[1,2] Arshiya Tabasum,[1] Gina Sanki,[3] David Burberry,[1] Brian P. Tennant,[3] James White,[4] Onyebuchi Okosieme,[1,2] Andrew Aldridge,[5] and Gautam Das[1]

[1] *Endocrinology and Diabetes Department, Prince Charles Hospital, Cwm Taf University Health Board, Merthyr Tydfil CF47 9DT, UK*
[2] *Thyroid Research Group, Institute of Molecular and Experimental Medicine, Cardiff University School of Medicine, Cardiff CF144XN, UK*
[3] *Biochemistry Department, Prince Charles Hospital, Cwm Taf University Health Board, Merthyr Tydfil CF47 9DT, UK*
[4] *Department of Medicine of the Elderly, Prince Charles Hospital, Cwm Taf University Health Board, Merthyr Tydfil CF47 9DT, UK*
[5] *Pharmacy, Prince Charles Hospital, Cwm Taf University Health Board, Merthyr Tydfil CF47 9DT, UK*

Correspondence should be addressed to Peter N. Taylor; taylorpn@cardiff.ac.uk

Academic Editor: Suat Simsek

An 82-year-old female with known hypothyroidism was admitted to hospital after being found on the floor. On examination, she was unkempt, confused, bradycardic, hypothermic, and barely arousable. Initial biochemistry revealed a thyroid stimulating hormone (TSH) of >100 mU/L and free thyroxine (FT_4) level of 1.5 pmol/L which supported a diagnosis of myxoedema coma. She was resuscitated and commenced on liothyronine, levothyroxine, and hydrocortisone and some improvement was made. It became apparent that she was hiding and spitting out her oral levothyroxine including levothyroxine elixir. Given the need for prompt alternative control, we sought advice from international experts where intramuscular levothyroxine was recommended. She was managed from day 50 onwards with intramuscular levothyroxine 200 mcg once a week, which was subsequently increased to 500 mcg. Thyroid function normalized and she made continual cognitive and physical progress and was discharged to a rehabilitation hospital. Her intramuscular levothyroxine was stopped and she was subsequently restarted on oral levothyroxine, with a plan for on-going close monitoring of her thyroid function. This report highlights the potential to use intramuscular levothyroxine in individuals with severe hypothyroidism arising from poor compliance with levothyroxine treatment or other potential causes such as impaired absorption.

1. Introduction

Myxoedema coma is a rare endocrine emergency with a high mortality rate of 25–70% [1]. It is uncommon nowadays due to widespread thyroid function testing and a low threshold for initiating levothyroxine therapy [2]. It has been reported that even after 5 years of levothyroxine therapy 21.5% of individuals persist in having a TSH level >5.0 mU/L [2] indicating widespread poor compliance or malabsorption. Myxoedema coma is more common in the winter months and in patients with poor compliance who are already known to have hypothyroidism [1]. Judicious use of levothyroxine, liothyronine, and hydrocortisone combined with supportive care is the mainstay of treatment for a favourable outcome.

In this paper we present an interesting case of myxoedema coma which was successfully managed with intramuscular levothyroxine as the compliance of the oral levothyroxine was poor. This is the first report which demonstrates the role of intramuscular levothyroxine in the management of myxoedema coma.

2. Case Report

An 82-year-old female was admitted in winter after being found unresponsive. She had a history of hypothyroidism and was prescribed levothyroxine 75 μg daily. Her sister reported that over the last few months she had been increasingly tired

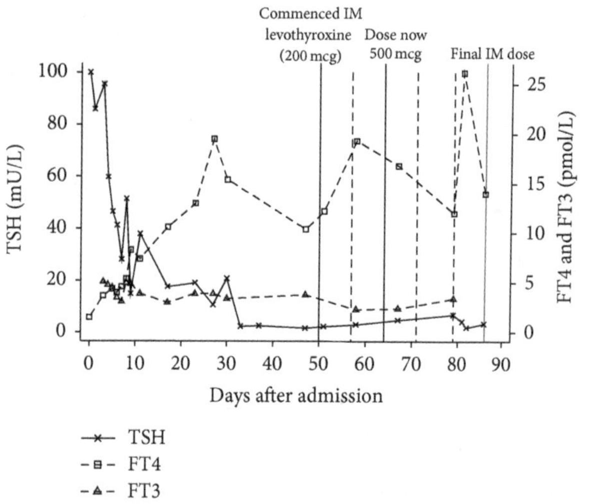

FIGURE 1: Thyroid function tests following admission. Intramuscular levothyroxine continued from day 50 until day 86 (end of graph) when converted to oral levothyroxine. Unbroken vertical lines refer to intramuscular levothyroxine initiation, dose change, and final IM dose. Dashed vertical lines refer to dates of other intramuscular levothyroxine injections.

and forgetful and was not compliant with her levothyroxine tablets.

On examination, her facies were consistent with myxedema and she was also found to be unkempt with evidence of self-neglect. She was bradycardic with a heart rate of 40 beats per minute and was profoundly hypothermic with a recorded temperature of 32.3 degrees Celsius and was barely arousable. Initial laboratory tests revealed a thyroid stimulating hormone (TSH) of >100 mU/L (0.27–4.2 mU/L) and free thyroxine (FT_4) of 1.5 pmol/L (11–25 pmol/L). She was resuscitated with warm fluids, oxygen, and a bear hugger and was given intravenous liothyronine and oral levothyroxine (initially via nasogastric tube) along with intravenous hydrocortisone in suspicion of a possibility of coexisting adrenal suppression.

Her clinical condition gradually improved over the next few days. Hypothermia resolved within 24 hours and her heart rate improved over a period of 48 hours. In due course her TSH began to normalize but her FT_4 levels remained inconsistent (Figure 1). She was therefore maintained on intravenous liothyronine for a longer period than that originally planned (up to day 38) as there were concerns regarding her compliance with oral tablets even within the hospital premises. It was highlighted by the ward nurses that she was regularly hiding her tablets underneath her pillow or spitting them out even if intake was tried with supervision. This was attributed to her poor cognitive state and ongoing impaired intellectual functioning. A further attempt was made with levothyroxine elixir, but unfortunately it was unsuccessful as well.

After significant deliberation and failed attempts to stabilize her TFTs on oral medications we embarked on trying her on a weekly intramuscular levothyroxine (200 mcg) regime. This resulted in more stable thyroid function (Figure 1). She did not report any side effects from intramuscular levothyroxine or symptoms of thyrotoxicosis. Her thyroid function stabilized over the next few weeks and she continued to make significant improvement with her physical and cognitive functions. Buoyed by her dramatic improvement we increased her dose to 500 mcg once a week on the 64th day and her TFTs were repeated on a weekly basis to monitor the change. One week later she was discharged to a community rehabilitation hospital, where she continued to make good progress. After almost 3 months of levothyroxine therapy, there was a modest improvement in her cognitive state to an extent which would sufficiently enable her to take her oral medication more reliably. As her TFTs and clinical state were progressing satisfactorily we stopped her intramuscular levothyroxine on day 86 and oral levothyroxine was recommenced. Our long term plan is to manage her with supervised once weekly oral dosing or consider her for once/twice weekly intramuscular levothyroxine therapy if her thyroid function becomes suboptimal again.

Poor compliance with medications which ought to be taken lifelong is a well-recognised problem [3]. Inadequate intake of levothyroxine which is usually designed for daily intake is reflected on TFTs with a persistently elevated TSH. One strategy in treating such cases hypothyroidism has been the use of once or twice weekly supervised oral therapy, although successful studies to date have been small [4, 5]. Previous case reports have successfully demonstrated the use of intramuscular levothyroxine therapy in patients with uncharacterized malabsorption [6], but use of parenteral levothyroxine therapy has not been studied rigorously to date and there are no well-established consensus guidelines at present [6].

Our strategy of a weekly intramuscular levothyroxine therapy did appear to stabilize our patient's thyroid status and allowed her clinical and cognitive state to improve continuously. It also provided us with a window of opportunity to ensure compliance when oral preparations were proving to be difficult. Moreover, whilst there was substantial variability in her thyroid function, we could reliably stabilize her TFTs without making her overtly hyperthyroid and further detrimental effects of ongoing hypothyroidism were suitably averted. To our knowledge this is the first time that the intramuscular route has been used to deliver levothyroxine in a patient with myxoedema coma. In individuals with such profound thyroid disturbance, poor circulation with impaired transport of intramuscular levothyroxine into the circulation might have been expected, but this did not appear to be the case in our patient.

In summary this case report crucially highlights that the intramuscular route for levothyroxine is a viable strategy even in profound hypothyroidism and would be useful in patients with either poor compliance or absorption. Although there was substantial variability in FT_4 levels on IM levothyroxine this may have been reduced by using twice weekly regime which we would consider if she requires IM levothyroxine again or when we encounter a similar patient.

3. Learning Point for Clinicians

This case report highlights the potential for severe harm that may arise due to poor compliance with thyroid hormone replacement. It also demonstrates that intramuscular levothyroxine is a viable treatment even in severe hypothyroidism and maybe particularly useful in individuals with poor compliance due to self-neglect and cognitive impairment or in patients with poor gastrointestinal absorption.

Acknowledgments

The authors acknowledge the support of Professor Colin Dayan from the Institute of Molecular and Experimental Medicine, Cardiff University School of Medicine, Cardiff, UK, and Professor John Geen from the Department of Biochemistry, Prince Charles Hospital, Cwm Taf University Health Board, Merthyr Tydfil, UK, for invaluable advice in managing this case.

References

[1] L. Wartofsky, "Myxedema coma," *Endocrinology and Metabolism Clinics of North America*, vol. 35, no. 4, pp. 687–698, 2006.

[2] P. N. Taylor, A. Iqbal, C. Minassian et al., "Falling threshold for treatment of borderline elevated thyrotropin levels-balancing benefits and risks: evidence from a large community-based study," *JAMA Internal Medicine*, vol. 174, no. 1, pp. 32–39, 2014.

[3] E. Vermeire, H. Hearnshaw, P. Van Royen, and J. Denekens, "Patient adherence to treatment: three decades of research. A comprehensive review," *Journal of Clinical Pharmacy and Therapeutics*, vol. 26, no. 5, pp. 331–342, 2001.

[4] J. Taylor, B. O. Williams, J. Frater, D. J. Stott, and J. Connell, "Twice-weekly dosing for thyroxine replacement in elderly patients with primary hypothyroidism," *The Journal of International Medical Research*, vol. 22, no. 5, pp. 273–277, 1994.

[5] S. Rangan, A. A. Tahrani, A. F. Macleod, and P. K. Moulik, "Once weekly thyroxine treatment as a strategy to treat non-compliance," *Postgraduate Medical Journal*, vol. 83, article e3, 2007.

[6] M. T. Hays, "Parenteral thyroxine administration," *Thyroid*, vol. 17, no. 2, pp. 127–129, 2007.

26

Therapeutic Challenges for Elderly Patients with Primary Hyperparathyroidism

Kenneth Sluis, Hyon Kim, Yuling He, Beatrice Wong, and Xiangbing Wang

Division of Endocrinology, Metabolism, and Nutrition, Department of Medicine, Rutgers University-Robert Wood Johnson Medical School, New Jersey, NJ 08903, USA

Correspondence should be addressed to Xiangbing Wang; wangx9@rwjms.rutgers.edu

Academic Editor: Mihail A. Boyanov

Primary hyperparathyroidism (PHPT) predominantly affects older adults, and parathyroidectomy can achieve definitive cure in symptomatic PHPT and asymptomatic meeting surgical criteria. As the population continues to age, the treatment of PHPT in octogenarians and nonagenarians presents a clinical conundrum. This case series presents the management of eight patients 85 years of age and older diagnosed with PHPT. A retrospective chart review of patients diagnosed with primary hyperparathyroidism were identified in a single institution. Those patients 85 years of age and older who were followed up for over one year were included in this case series. The literature on treatment options for this age group was also reviewed. Eight cases of PHPT patients aged 88 ± 2.5 years old with a follow-up average of 5.6 ± 4.4 years were reported in our case series. Six PHPT patients were medically managed and two PHPT patients underwent parathyroid resection. Most of the medically managed PHPT patients except for one had long-term stability of disease for over five years. The treatment of PHPT diagnosed in patients over 85 years of age presents a clinical challenge for which there is no clear consensus guideline. Our case series supports that medical therapy is a feasible option for PHPT patients over 85 years old.

1. Introduction

Primary Hyperparathyroidism (PHPT) is a common disease that increases in prevalence with advancing age. Prevalence peaks in women around 70–79 years of age (492 per 100,000) and in men over 80 years old (264 per 100,000) [1]. Most patients with PHPT initially present with asymptomatic hypercalcemia. Those that are symptomatic present with axial and extremity fractures, nephrolithiasis, and psychiatric disturbance [2]. Surgical resection of the involved glands is the standard of care for young or symptomatic patients with PHPT. Medical management is used as a bridge to surgery or in patients who refuse or cannot safely undergo surgery. Strategies include hydration with expectant management, stopping offending agents such as calcium supplementation and medications (thiazides, lithium) and using diuretics, bisphosphonates, selective estrogen receptor modulators, and cinacalcet [2]. Expectant management involves serial monitoring for worsening of symptoms without specific therapeutic intervention [3, 4].

Most of the literature on the treatment of PHPT is not age-specific. About 1.5% of patients over the age of 70 have PHPT [5]. As our population continues to age and as average life expectancy increases, the proportion of elderly patients with PHPT will also grow. Though the standard of care to manage PHPT is surgery to achieve cure, the role of surgery is less clear in the very elderly. The objective of our study is to report eight cases of PHPT patients over 85 years of age who were managed using medical or surgical treatment to elucidate differences in prognosis and outcomes.

2. Cases Presentation

We conducted a retrospective chart review of PHPT patients evaluated at Robert Wood Johnson University Hospital from January 2000 to September 2016. Our institution's IRB provided approval for our investigations. There were 556 patients diagnosed with PHPT during this time. The diagnostic criteria of PHPT included: (1) intact PTH > 65 pg/mL (normal range:

TABLE 1: Eight cases of PHPT in patients over age 85.

Case #	Clinical description
Case 1	An 86-year-old woman with a history of osteopenia, hyperlipidemia, and GERD was diagnosed with PHPT with a calcium level of 13 mg/dl, iPTH level of 66 pg/ml, 25OHD 34 ng/ml and creatinine 1.07 mg/dL. She underwent surgery and had successful removal of a right upper parathyroid gland. She achieved surgical cure with normalized calcium and iPTH levels. Her last calcium was 9.7 mg/dl, iPTH 12.4 pg/ml and 25OHD 54 ng/ml at her 2 year follow up visit.
Case 2	A 91-year-old woman with a history of hyperparathyroidism with parathyroidectomy of 3.5 glands 5 years ago, hypothyroidism, osteoporosis, and goiter presented with a calcium level of 11.6 and iPTH level of 500. She was diagnosed with relapse of PHPT, and was managed with cinacalcet, furosemide, and risendronate. Serum calcium was controlled for about 8 years, but creatinine started to rise. Ten years after the recurrence of PHPT, cinacalcet had to be lowered and her bisphosphonate had to be discontinued after a further increase in creatinine. She suffered a left hip fracture and a possible aspiration event during the subsequent hospitalization. She passed away from sepsis after 10 years' medical treatment of recurrence of PHPT.
Case 3	An 85-year-old woman with a history of a resected follicular Hurthle cell neoplasm presented with a calcium level of 11.5 mg/dl and iPTH of 279 pg/ml. She was diagnosed with PHPT and treated with cessation of hydrochlorothiazide, initiation of furosemide, and cinacalcet for 5 years. Cinacalcet dosage had to be increased after a year, but then subsequently discontinued due to worsening renal function (Cr 2.98–3.3 mg/dl). Five years after diagnosis her PTH level increased (483–511 pg/ml) but calcium was 10–11 mg/dL. She was hospitalized for cellulitis 6 years later and was discharged to hospice care for end-stage renal disease. She passed away at the age of 91.
Case 4	A 91-year-old man with a history of type 2 diabetes, hyperlipidemia, dementia, atrial fibrillation, and congestive heart failure was hospitalized for sepsis. He was found to have a calcium level of 11.1 mg/dl, iPTH 59 pg/ml, 24-hour calcium 203 mg, and 25OHD 26 ng/ml. He was diagnosed with PHPT. He was treated with calcitonin, oral hydration and furosemide. He was discharged to his long-term care facility. His calcium level remained normal up to 10.9 mg/dL with Cr 1.8 mg/dl at 1-year follow up.
Case 5	A 96-year-old woman with a history vitamin D deficiency, osteoporosis, and hypothyroidism was found to have a calcium level of 11.2 mg/dl, iPTH 165 pg/ml, and 24-hour urine calcium of 204 mg. A parathyroid scan showed a possible left lower pole adenoma. She refused surgery and was treated with zoledronic acid infusion for her osteoporosis. Calcium decreased to 10.2 mg/dL three years after diagnosis she was given a second zoledronic acid infusion. She was followed for 4 years and did well with serum calcium maintained from 10.2 to 10.7 md/dL and iPTH 147 pg/ml.
Case 6	An 86-year-old woman with a history of osteoporosis, hypertension and dementia was found to have a calcium level of 11.1 mg/dl, iPTH 100 pg/ml, and 25OHD 32 ng/mL. She did not tolerate bisphosphonate therapy and was treated with oral hydration, cessation of thiazide diuretic, and encouragement of physically activity. Two years after diagnosis, calcium levels were maintained in the high-normal range (10.2–10.5 mg/dl). Her dementia worsened and she suffered a left hip fracture 8 years after diagnosis. She passed away on hospice from a gangrenous wound after 8 years of expectant medical management of PHPT at age of 96.
Case 7	An 86-year-old woman with osteopenia treated with bisphosphonates and a selective estrogen receptor modulator, hypothyroidism, vitamin D deficiency and DVT was found to have a calcium level of 11.8 mg/dl, iPTH 128 pg/ml, 24-hour urine 142 mg, and 25OHD 31 ng/mL Sestamibi scan did not locate an adenoma. Expectant management with increased oral hydration, decreased milk intake, cessation of thiazides, and encouragement to increase activity was begun. Her calcium rose as high as 12.9 mg/dL but then settled to 11.2 mg/dL on subsequent measurement. She was followed without incident for 3 years.
Case 8	An 89-year-old woman with a history of hypothyroidism was found with a calcium level of 11.5 mg/dl, iPTH 95 pg/ml and 25OHD 24.6 ng/mL. She was asymptomatic and was managed expectantly with oral hydration and increased physical activity. Calcium was maintained from 10.2to 10.9 mg/dL and PTH 77–107 pg/ml. She was hospitalized for hypertensive urgency but otherwise had no sequelae for 6 years.

Note: PHPT = Primary hyperparathyroidism, iPTH = Intact parathyroid hormone, 25OHD = 25 hydroxyvitamin D.

10–65 pg/mL) or inappropriately normal levels in the presence of elevated serum calcium, (2) serum calcium > 10.6 mg/dL (normal range: 8.5–10.4 mg/dL), and (3) 24-hour urinary calcium > 100 mg/day (normal range: 100–250 mg/day). Eight PHPT patients aged 85 years and older with follow-up duration longer than one year were included for this study. Patient demographics, baseline characteristics, clinical presentation and overall clinical follow-up were examined.

Eight patients diagnosed with PHPT at the age of 85 years or older were included. The average age at diagnosis was 88 ± 2.5 years old. The average follow-up duration was 5.6 ± 4.4 years. The average calcium was 11.3 ± 0.78 mg/dL, iPTH was 166 ± 154 pg/mL and 24-hour urine calcium was 183 ± 35.5 mg at the time of diagnosis. All eight patients met guidelines [2, 5] for surgery by the serum calcium levels >1 mg/dl upper limit of normal, creatinine clearance <60 cc/min or T-score <2.5 (Table 1). Six PHPT patients were medically managed for one to eight years and two PHPT patients underwent parathyroid resection. The surgical group had a pre-operative serum calcium of 12.3 mg/dL while the medically managed group had an average of 10.9 mg/dL. For two patients treated surgically, one patient was cured with normal calcium and PTH levels but was only followed up for two years. One patient had recurrence of PHPT five years after surgery and required medical management with cinacalcet, loop diuretic, and bisphosphonate for ten years. Six patients were managed medically for an average of 5.2 years with minimal complications. Only one of the six patients experienced PHPT-related mortality. This patient had severe dementia, was on medical treatment for eight years, and passed away on hospice after a hip fracture. Of the other medically managed patients, three patients were managed with pharmaceutical therapy, one with bisphosphonate and two with cinacalcet. Two other patients were treated with nonpharmaceutical expectant management, which included oral hydration, discontinuation of HCTZ and maintaining physical activity. They had favorable outcomes after three to six years.

Patient vignettes are demonstrated in Table 1.

3. Discussion

The Endocrine Society consensus guidelines recommend parathyroidectomy for both symptomatic and asymptomatic PHPT. Surgery is readily offered for biochemical cure in younger, symptomatic or asymptomatic patients with PHPT meeting surgical criteria [2]. The benefits of parathyroidectomy include advantages in survival, increased bone density, reduced fatigue, and other subjective measures [6, 7].

Much of the current literature advocates for more aggressive surgical therapy for the elderly. However, the benefit of surgery at achieving cure for octogenarians and nonagenarians is less straightforward than for the young. There is increased risk for complications, prolonged operation time and increased length of stay in hospitals for patients over the age of 80 years [7, 8]. As our understanding of PHPT has evolved, different phenotypes of the disease have been recognized, the symptoms of which can be confounded by the aging process in this population [9]. Studies have shown that medically managed patients with PHPT could have stable disease for over ten years [9, 10]. Our expanded case series supports medical management as a reasonable option in the very elderly, especially those with comorbidities.

Literature in favor of medical management of the very old shows promise despite its smaller scope. Khan et al. [4] and Marcocci et al. [11] reviewed the rationale and evidence behind medical management and expectant monitoring. They found that medical management can be effective, and that patients' quality of life can be similar to those treated surgically. Jacobs et al. [3] described four patients with PHPT aged 79 to 87 years treated with medical management as a bridge to surgery or as sole therapy in poor surgical candidates or those refusing surgery. They employed saline hydration, pamidronate and cinacalcet. Medical therapy was a successful bridge to surgical cure with parathyroidectomy for two patients after two weeks to two months of treatment. Medical therapy was not tolerated for another and pursued indefinitely for the final patient. Wong reported two PHPT patients over the age of 90 treated with oral rehydration, bisphosphonate or cinacalcet. They experienced no PHPT related complications or fractures in a follow-up duration of seven months to four years [12].

The limitations of our study include small sample size and short duration of follow-up. One patient had baseline dementia, and 3 nonagenarian patients passed away after 6–10 years follow up, we did not have the data and therefore cannot compare quality of life, cognitive and muscle function before and after intervention.

In summary, our data suggest that medical therapy is a reasonable option for PHPT patients over 85 years old. As life expectancy increases and more patients are diagnosed with PHPT later in life, further consensus guidelines may need to specifically address treatment recommendations for patients over the age of 85 years. Studies with larger patient populations and randomized controlled trials are needed to support our findings.

References

[1] M. W. Yeh, P. H. Ituarte, H. C. Zhou et al., "Incidence and prevalence of primary hyperparathyroidism in a racially mixed population," *The Journal of Clinical Endocrinology & Metabolism*, vol. 98, no. 3, pp. 1122–1129, 2013.

[2] J. P. Bilezikian, M. L. Brandi, R. Eastell et al., "Guidelines for the management of asymptomatic primary hyperparathyroidism: summary statement from the fourth international workshop," *The Journal of Clinical Endocrinology & Metabolism*, vol. 99, no. 10, pp. 3561–3569, 2014.

[3] L. Jacobs, M. M. Samson, H. J. Verhaar, and H. L. Koek, "Therapeutic challenges in elderly patients with symptomatic hypercalcemia caused by primary hyperparathyroidism," *The Netherlands Journal of Medicine*, vol. 70, no. 1, pp. 35–38, 2012.

[4] A. Khan, A. Grey, and D. Shoback, "Medical management of asymptomatic primary hyperparathyroidism: proceedings of the third international workshop," *Journal of Clinical Endocrinology & Metabolism*, vol. 94, no. 2, pp. 373–381, 2009.

[5] H. Chen, S. Parkerson, and R. Udelsman, "Parathyroidectomy in the elderly: do the benefits outweigh the risks?" *World Journal of Surgery*, vol. 22, no. 6, pp. 531–536, 1998.

[6] J. Bollerslev, S. Jansson, C. L. Mollerup et al., "Medical observation, compared with parathyroidectomy, for asymptomatic primary hyperparathyroidism: a prospective, randomized trial," *The Journal of Clinical Endocrinology & Metabolism*, vol. 92, no. 5, pp. 1687–1692, 2007.

[7] G. B. Talpos, H. G. Bone3rd, M. Kleerekoper et al., "Randomized trial of parathyroidectomy in mild asymptomatic primary hyperparathyroidism: patient description and effects on the SF-36 health survey," *Surgery*, vol. 128, no. 6, pp. 1013–1021, 2000.

[8] D. C. Thomas, S. A. Roman, and J. A. Sosa, "Parathyroidectomy in the elderly: analysis of 7313 patients," *Journal of Surgical Research*, vol. 170, no. 2, pp. 240–246, 2011.

[9] J. P. Bilezikian, "Primary hyperparathyroidism," *The Journal of Clinical Endocrinology & Metabolism*, vol. 103, no. 11, pp. 3993–4004, 2018.

[10] M. R. Rubin, J. P. Bilezikian, D. J. McMahon et al., "The natural history of primary hyperparathyroidism with or without parathyroid surgery after 15 years," *The Journal of Clinical Endocrinology & Metabolism*, vol. 93, no. 9, pp. 3462–3470, 2008.

[11] C. Marcocci, J. Bollerslev, A. A. Khan, and D. M. Shoback, "Medical management of primary hyperparathyroidism: proceedings of the fourth international workshop on the management of asymptomatic primary hyperparathyroidism," *The Journal of Clinical Endocrinology & Metabolism*, vol. 99, no. 10, pp. 3607–3618, 2014.

[12] B. Wong and X. Wang, "Treatment of nonagenarians with primary hyperparathyroidism," *Journal of the American Geriatrics Society*, vol. 64, no. 10, pp. e112–e113, 2016.

27

Diabetes Mellitus, Extreme Insulin Resistance and Hypothalamic-Pituitary Langerhans Cells Histiocytosis

Mathilde Sollier,[1] Marine Halbron,[1] Jean Donadieu,[2] Ahmed Idbaih,[3] Fleur Cohen Aubart,[4] Corinne Vigouroux,[5] Martine Auclair,[5] Olivier Bourron,[1] Marie Bastin,[1] Géraldine Béra,[6] Philippe Touraine,[7,8] Jacques Young,[9] Héléna Mosbah,[1] Agnès Hartemann,[1] Fabrizio Andreelli,[1] and Chloé Amouyal[1]

[1] *Diabetology-Metabolism Dpt, Sorbonne Université, APHP, Institut Hospitalo–Universitaire de Cardiometabolisme et Nutrition (ICAN), Pitié-Salpêtrière-Charles Foix Hospital, 75013 Paris, France*
[2] *Hemato-Oncology Dpt, Trousseau Hospital, APHP, 75012 Paris, France*
[3] *Sorbonne Université, Inserm, CNRS, UMRS 1127, Institut du Cerveau et de la Moelle épinière, ICM, AP-HP, Hôpitaux Universitaires La Pitié Salpêtrière -Charles Foix, Service de Neurologie 2, Mazarin, 75013 Paris, France*
[4] *Department of Internal Medicine 2, Sorbonne Université, APHP, Institut Hospitalo–Universitaire de Cardiometabolisme et Nutrition (ICAN), Pitié Salpêtrière-Charles Foix Hospital, 75013 Paris, France*
[5] *Inserm UMRS 938, Centre de Recherche Saint–Antoine, Sorbonne Université, Reference Center for Rare Diseases of Insulin Secretion and Insulin Sensitivity, Institut Hospitalo–Universitaire de Cardiometabolisme et Nutrition (ICAN), Paris, APHP, Saint Antoine Hospital, Paris, France*
[6] *Nuclear Medicine Dpt, Sorbonne Université, APHP, Pitié-Salpêtrière-Charles Foix Hospital, 75013 Paris, France*
[7] *Department of Endocrinology and Reproductive Medicine, Pitié-Salpêtrière Hospital, APHP, Reference Center for Rare Endocrine Diseases of Growth, Reference Center for Rare Gynecological Pathologies, Institut Hospitalo–Universitaire de Cardiometabolisme et Nutrition (ICAN), Sorbonne University, 75013 Paris, France*
[8] *Pitié-Salpêtrière-Charles Foix Hospital, 75013 Paris, France*
[9] *Reproductive Endocrinology Department, Paris Sud University, APHP, Le Kremlin-Bicêtre, 94275, France*

Correspondence should be addressed to Fabrizio Andreelli; fabrizio.andreelli@aphp.fr

Academic Editor: Lucy Mastrandrea

Background. Langerhans Cell Histiocytosis (LCH) is a rare inflammatory neoplasm characterized by an infiltration of organs by Langerin + (CD207+) and CD1a+ histiocytes. Diabetes insipidus is a frequent manifestation of the disease, while diabetes mellitus is very rare. We report the first case of a 20-year-old man suffering from hypothalamopituitary histiocytosis and diabetes mellitus with serum anti-insulin receptor antibodies. *Case Presentation*. A 20-year-old patient was admitted for the evaluation of growth delay and hyperphagia. HbA1c level and fasting blood glucose were in the normal range. The diagnosis of hypothalamopituitary histiocytosis was based on histological features after biopsy of a large suprachiasmatic lesion identified on magnetic resonance imaging (MRI). Association of vinblastine and purinethol was started followed by a second-line therapy by cladribine. During the follow-up, the patient was admitted for recurrence of hyperglycemic states and extreme insulin resistance. The screening for serum anti-insulin receptor antibodies was positive. Each episode of hyperglycemia appeared to be correlated with tumoral activity and increase in serum anti-insulin receptor antibodies and appeared to be improved when the disease was controlled by chemotherapy. *Conclusion*. We report the first description of a hypothalamopituitary histiocytosis associated with serum anti-insulin receptor antibodies, extreme insulin resistance, and diabetes. Parallel evolution of glucose levels and serum anti-insulin receptor antibodies seemed to be the consequence of immune suppressive properties of cladribine.

1. Background

Langerhans Cell Histiocytosis (LCH) is a rare disease characterized by an infiltration of organs by Langerin+ (CD207+) and CD1a+ histiocytes [1, 2]. Although it can occur at any time of life with an incidence of 4.6 cases per million habitants, LCH is more frequent in children (with onset at a peak age of 1-3 years) [3]. The pathogenesis of LCH is not clear but is likely linked to an inflammatory neoplasm. The definitive diagnosis relies on histology with expression of CD1a antigen or CD207 antigen according to the revised criteria of the Histiocyte Society [1]. Multiple tissues can be concerned by LCH but the most frequent are bones, skin, and pituitary [4]. Indeed, a recent review of endocrine manifestations showed that pituitary deficiency associated with diabetes insipidus (DI) is one of the most frequent endocrine diseases observed at onset of LCH [5]. Endocrine pancreas is rarely concerned and to our knowledge only five cases of pancreatic infiltration by LCH cells have been reported in the literature [6–10]. In addition, association between LCH and diabetes mellitus with or without hypothalamopituitary involvement has been published [11–15]. We report for the first time the case of a 20-year-old man presenting a hypothalamopituitary histiocytosis and positive for serum anti-insulin receptor antibodies with a follow-up characterized by alternating periods of diabetes mellitus with extreme insulin resistance and periods of normoglycemia.

2. Case Presentation

The patient #1509232 is a young male with a history of polyuria and polydipsia since he was 11 years old. This symptom was neglected. The patient had a normal academic progression and medical work-up (at age of 14 years and 17 years) excluding several times the diagnosis of diabetes mellitus, as no hyperglycemia has been detected. At the age of 20 years and 5 months he became polyphagic and his weight increased from 60 to 90 kg without any other complaint. Finally, 5 months later, a brain MRI was performed and a large hypothalamus mass (20x20mm) with thickening of the pituitary stalk and compression of the third ventricle was observed. A strong contrast enhancement was observed after administration of gadolinium (Figures 1(a), 1(b), and 1(c)).

The patient was admitted in the department of endocrinology and the biological explorations concluded to a panhypopituitarism associated with diabetes insipidus. At the initial assessment, the following was also discovered: (i) the patient presented stage I obesity (BMI=26.6 kg/m2), (ii) delayed bone age relative to chronological age (resp., 16 years for a chronological age of 20), and (iii) a growth delay with a deceleration of linear growth at age of 15 years.

A stereotactic biopsy of the brain mass was performed at age of 21 years (Table 1, M1) and immunohistochemistry showed positive staining for CD1a and PS100, supporting the diagnosis of LCH. Presence of BRAF V600E mutation was explored because this mutation in LCH is associated with more severe disease than did those with wild-type BRAF and irreversible damage, such as neurologic and pituitary injuries [16]. In addition, presence of BRAF V600E mutation may offer the possibility of a targeted therapy by BRAF inhibitor (vemurafenib or PLX8394, a second-generation BRAF inhibitor) [17]. Unfortunately, the mutation was not observed and this has limited the possibility to use BRAF inhibitors). Disease work-up failed to find any extra pituitary-hypothalamic extension.

The patient was referred to the oncology department to start vinblastine (one infusion of 10mg per week) and purinethol (100mg per day) according to the French guidelines HL2010 protocol [18]. He did not receive corticosteroids. The patient signed an informed consent to be enrolled in the French LCH registry according to regulation [19].

One month after, the patient was admitted to the emergency room for altered consciousness (Table 1, M0). The blood tests showed hypernatremia at 164mmol/l and hyperglycemia at 25.8mmol/l without ketosis. Importantly, blood glucose levels were in the normal range 6 months before and at the time of the brain biopsy. After continuous administration of fluids and rapid acting insulin analogue (124UI/24hr), he was admitted to the diabetology department.

The search for type 1 diabetes (anti-GAD and anti-IA2 antibodies) was negative. C-peptide level was 9μg/l in the fasting state (normal range: 0.8-4.2 μg/l). The lipid profile showed hypertriglyceridemia at 5.7mmol/l (5,4g/l) and low HDL-cholesterol level at 0.41 mmol/l (0.16g/l). Blood pressure was normal at 125/68mmHg. The abdominal CT-scan found liver steatosis without any pancreatic abnormalities. The weight gain of 19kg during the last 3 months (body mass index: 32kg/m^2) was linked to eating disorder (especially binge-eating disorder). It was decided to continue the first-line therapy up to 6 infusions of vinblastine.

Intriguingly, soon after the diagnosis of diabetes mellitus, daily insulin needs grew up to 400UI per day (4.2UI/kg), indicating a significant insulin resistance state. We did not observe acanthosis nigricans or loss of subcutaneous tissue and we excluded hypersecretion of hyperglycemic hormones. We tested the hypothesis of antibodies against insulin receptors as a cause of insulin resistance. The screening for serum anti-insulin receptor antibodies was performed using a radioreceptor assay as described [20, 21]. In summary, Chinese Hamster Ovary cells overexpressing insulin receptor (CHO-IR) were incubated or not for 90 min at 22°C with control and patient's serum at different dilutions, washed, and then incubated for 90 min at 22°C with a tracer concentration of ^{125}I-insulin with or without unlabeled insulin.

The ability of patient's serum to inhibit binding of [^{125}I] insulin was expressed as a percent decrease of insulin binding at 1:3 dilution as compared to the reference value. At the diabetes diagnosis, insulin receptor antibodies were positive (42% decrease in insulin binding) (Table 1), allowing the diagnosis of type B insulin resistance, a disease often associated with autoimmune disorders or hematological diseases. We then excluded systemic lupus erythematous, multiple myeloma, and Hodgkin's disease. Interestingly, insulin receptor antibodies levels decreased when first-line therapy was achieved (19% decrease in insulin binding) in parallel to a spectacular decrease in daily insulin needs (Table 1).

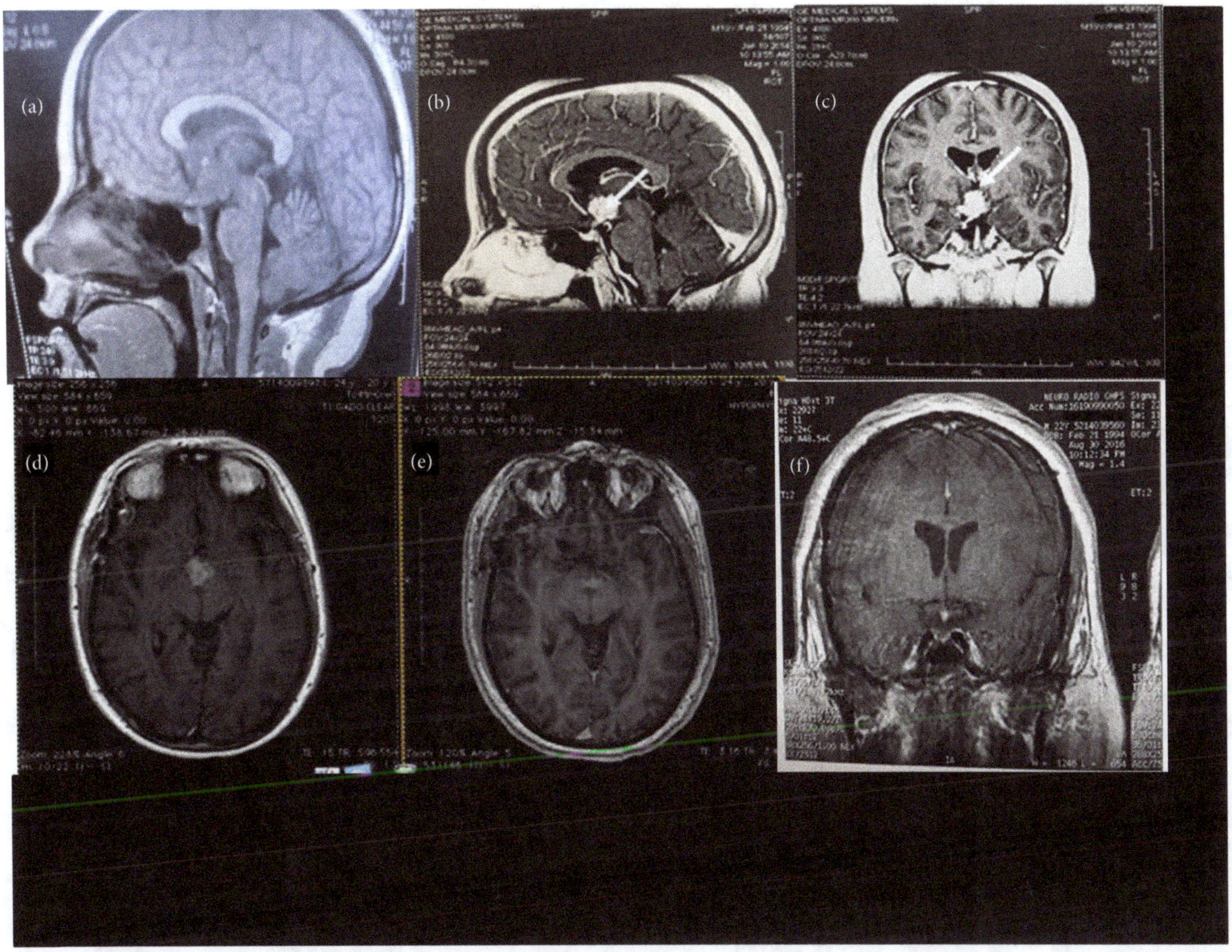

FIGURE 1: *Evolution of brain MRI during follow-up.* At diagnosis, the normal T1-weighted hyperintense signal of the posterior pituitary has disappeared (a). Contrast-enhanced hypothalamic mass after gadolinium infusion ((b) and (c)); compression of third ventricle and thickening of pituitary stalk (b). Comparison of brain MRI (T1 with gadolinium) at diagnosis (M0) (d) and at the end of the first-line therapy (e). MRI showed a significant decrease of the hypothalamic mass but the persistence of contrast enhancement after gadolinium. Brain MRI (T1 after gadolinium infusion) at M30 showing a hypothalamic lesion stable in size and with decreased hypersignal compared to previous MRI (f).

Insulin therapy could be discontinued and replaced by a monotherapy with metformin (850mg twice a day). HbA1c remained stable at 6.5% (48 mmol/mol) until M8. In contrast, no improvement of binge-eating disorder was observed and body mass index kept increasing significantly during this period (Table 1).

Seven months after initial diagnosis of diabetes mellitus, intensification of hypoglycemic therapy with sulfonylurea and liraglutide LAR added to metformin was needed because glucose levels increased. The change in glucose levels was observed at the same time as a further increase of serum insulin receptor autoantibodies at M8 and M10 (43 and 42 percent decrease of insulin binding to its receptor upon incubation of CHO-IR cells with patient's serum at 1:3 dilution, resp.) (Table 1). Although a significant decrease of the size of the brain mass was observed when compared to initial evaluation, persistence of contrast enhancement after gadolinium administration suggested an incomplete response to therapy (Figures 1(d) and 1(e)).

A second-line therapy was started, consisting in 6 cycles of cladribine (5mg/m2/24h, 5 days/week, each month) from month 12 to month 18 after the diagnosis. At M30, brain MRI showed a decrease of both tumor volume and contrast enhancement (Figure 1(f)). In addition, glucose levels were controlled with the association of metformin and liraglutide (HbA1c level decreased to 7.5% or 58mmol/mol). Diabetes improvement was associated with a decrease of insulin receptor antibodies levels until M31. Unfortunately, a new recurrence of uncontrolled diabetes (HbA1c: 11.2%, 99 mmol/mol) occurred at M32 needing insulin therapy. Insulin receptor antibodies were once again positive (36% inhibition of insulin binding by patient's serum at 1:3 dilution), while brain MRI did not reveal tumor recurrence.

It was decided to initiate new cycles of cladribine. The patient received a first cycle at M32 after diagnosis and a second one month later. During this period, insulin daily doses decreased from 300UI to 36UI at the end of cladribine cycles. Additionally, HbA1c level decreased from 11.2% to 8.6% (from

Table 1: *Evolution of blood glucose levels, BMI, and anti-insulin receptor antibodies in blood*. Evolution of fasting blood venous glycemia (measured at each administration of chemotherapy or at each assessment of anti-insulin receptor antibodies) and the ability of patient's serum to inhibit insulin binding to its receptor. The reduction of [^{125}I]insulin binding in the presence of patient's serum (used at 1:3 dilution) was measured on CHO cells overexpressing insulin receptor as described (18-20). Ins: insulin. Met: metformin.

	IMC (kg/m2)	Anti-insulin receptor antibodies	Blood glucose levels (mM)	Admissions	Therapy for diabetes	Therapy for histiocytosis
M-1	24		4,4	Stereotactic biopsy		
M0	31,5		25,8	Hyperosmolar hyperglycemic coma	Ins	Vinblastine + purinethol
M1	32		15		Ins + Met + sulfamides	Vinblastine + purinethol
M2	31	42	13		Ins + Met + sulfamides	Vinblastine + purinethol
M2	32,1	35	8,2		Ins + Met + sulfamides	Vinblastine + purinethol
M2	32,1	19	5,5		Met	Vinblastine + purinethol
M8	33,8	43	13,7	Relapse of hyperglycemia	Met + sulfamides + GLP-1 analog	Vinblastine + purinethol
M10	35,2	42	11		Met + sulfamides + GLP-1 analog	Cladribine
M20	35,2	49	11		Met + sulfamides + GLP-1 analog	Cladribine
M28	37,6	30	14,3		Met + sulfamides + GLP-1 analog	
M31	37,6	2	5,5		Met + GLP-1 analog	
M32	39	36	22	Relapse of hyperglycemia	Ins	Cladribine
M33	39	32	17		Ins	Cladribine

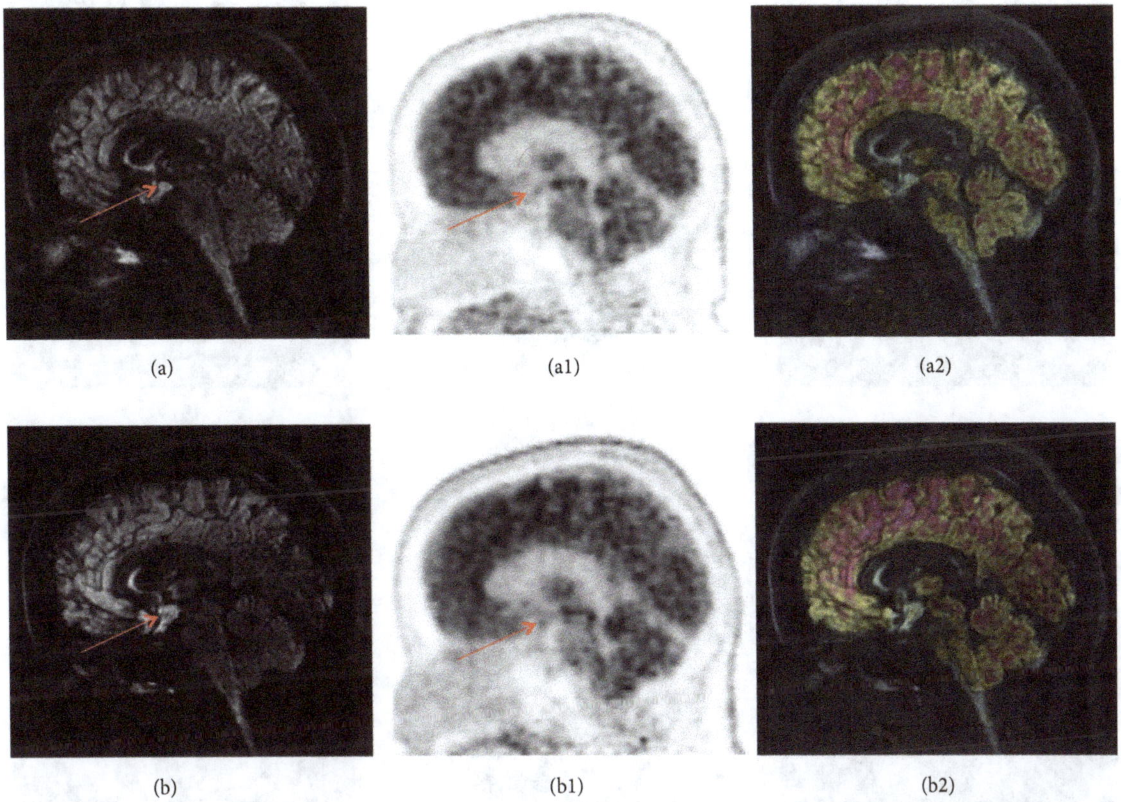

FIGURE 2: *Sagittal PET-MRI brain imaging.* Sagittal PET-MRI brain imaging with [18F]FDG at M32 (a, a1, a2) and at M35 (b, b1, b2) of follow-up. Nodular thickening of the floor of the third ventricle and pituitary infundibulum, in hyperintense FLAIR, without [18F]FDG-uptake, measuring 7 mm in height x 13 mm in the axial plane, without significant enhancement, globally unchanged from the previous MRI. Linear and fine enhancement of the pituitary infundibulum with stable appearance.

99 to 70 mmol/mol). The PET-MRI made during the relapse of diabetes at M32 showed a nodular thickening of the floor of the third ventricle and pituitary infundibulum with no [18F]-FDG-uptake (Figures 2 and 3). Control of diabetes was maintained until M35 and PET-MRI was unchanged at that time (Figures 2 and 3). The follow-up was marked by a very complex clinical disorder, with behavioural difficulties, polyphagy and agressivity; neurological difficulties, loss of memory; and very instable basal metabolic situation, hyperglycemia, and recurrent hypernatremia episodes. Four years after the diagnosis of LCH, the patients is actually frequently hospitalized in a psychiatric hospital.

3. Case Discussion

We reported a case of isolated hypothalamic-pituitary LCH and panhypopituitarism, with multiple episodes of extreme insulin resistance and diabetes mellitus. Each episode appeared to be associated with tumoral activity and appeared to be improved when brain tumor was controlled by chemotherapy.

Each period of hyperglycemia was characterized by important specificities. First, blood glucose levels were extremely high at each recurrence of diabetes and induced massive dehydration and hypernatremia in a context of diabetes insipidus. A second major characteristic was the insulin resistance state. Important doses of insulin (4UI/kg/D) were necessary to maintain glycemia around 11 mmol/l, regardless of how insulin was administered, intravenously or subcutaneously. The hyperglycemia periods alternated with periods of improvement of glucose homeostasis; oral hypoglycemic monotherapy with metformin was then sufficient to achieve the target of HbA1c (< 6.5% or 48 mmol/mol). Such fluctuations in glucose homeostasis and insulin resistance raise the question of the etiology of this diabetes. Low levels of ketone bodies and negativity of islet antibodies contributed to excluding the diagnosis of type 1 diabetes. The most frequent etiologies of insulin resistance (such as infectious disease, lipodystrophy, excessive secretion of hyperglycemic hormone, or corticosteroids therapy) were absent. In addition, the increase in body weight observed before onset of diabetes was not sufficient to explain by itself such an important level of insulin resistance at the discovery of diabetes.

Thus, we hypothesized that insulin resistance could be triggered by serum anti-insulin receptor antibodies. Indeed, in this condition (known as type B insulin resistance), such antibodies are known to reduce insulin (exogenous or endogenous) transduction signaling in insulin target

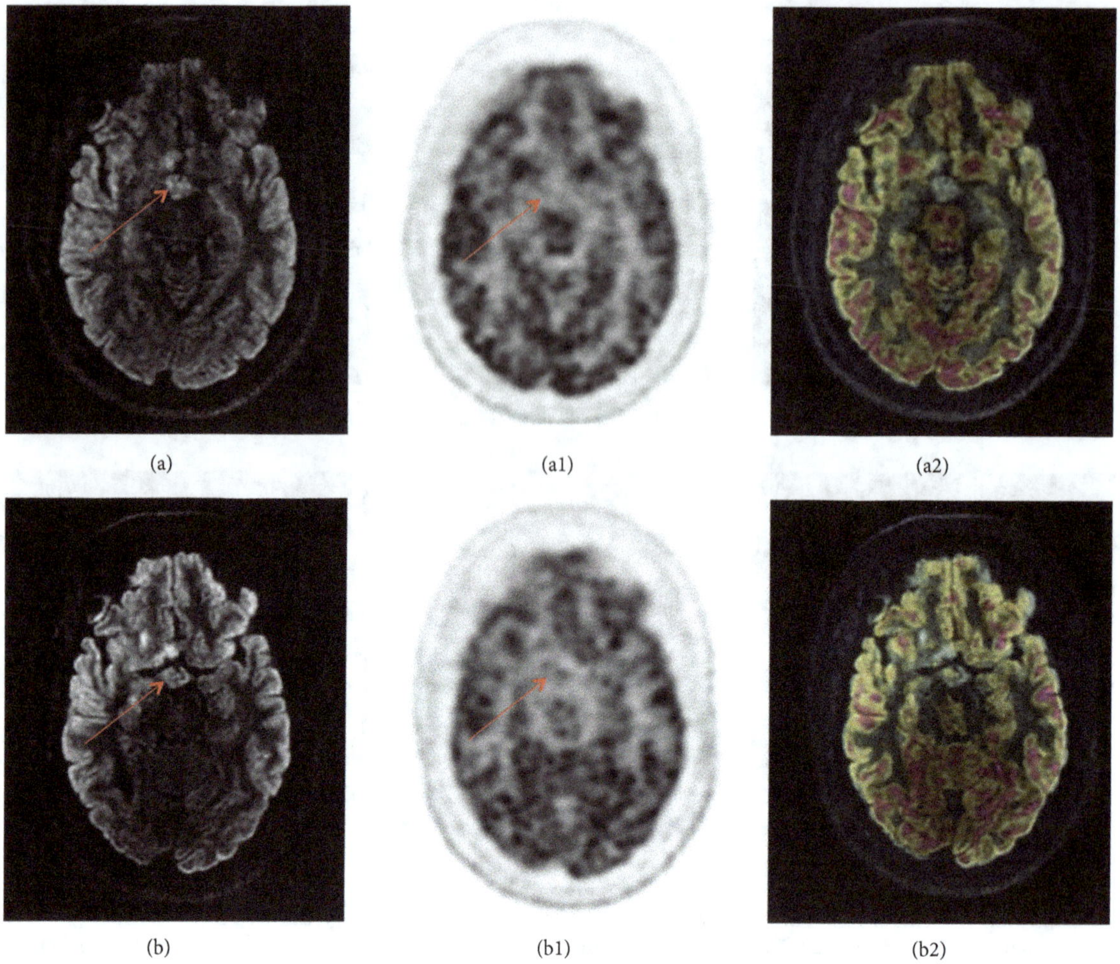

FIGURE 3: *Axial PET-MRI brain imaging.* Axial PET-MRI brain imaging with [18F]FDG at M32 (a, a1, a2) and at M35 (b, b1, b2) of follow-up.

tissues [22]. Arioglu et al. compared 24 patients with type B insulin resistance and admitted in their clinical center with representative case reports gathered from the literature [23]. Most type B insulin resistance was described in patients with systemic autoimmune diseases (especially systemic lupus erythematous) or associated with multiple myeloma and with Hodgkin's disease. All of these diseases were absent in our patient.

In our case, the positivity of anti-insulin receptor antibodies in blood and the observation of resistant hyperglycemic state despite intravenous or subcutaneous insulin therapy strongly suggested a possible causal link between these antibodies and the pathophysiology of diabetes. Accordingly, during the follow-up, we established a parallel evolution of serum insulin receptor antibodies and glucose homeostasis. In contrast, no correlation was found between serum insulin receptor antibodies (or control of diabetes) and body weight.

Whether positivity of insulin receptor antibodies and LCH is a direct relationship or a fortuitous association is not clear. Indeed, cases of diabetes mellitus associated with LCH are rare if we except a transient glycemic intolerance during corticoid steroid therapy. Among the 3200 cases in the national French LCH registry, which enrolled 56 cases of hypothalamic tumor, we failed to find any similar conditions [19, 24, 25]. In the literature, only nine cases with diabetes and LCH have been so far reported and summarized in Table 2.

As in our case, seven of these five observations have in common a diabetes insipidus as first symptom of LCH in the hypothalamic-pituitary region [7, 11–13, 15]. The onset of diabetes mellitus was described as a hyperglycemic hyperosmolar syndrome in three previously published observations [11, 12, 14]. As for our patient, hyperosmolarity was probably the consequence of massive glycosuria and polyuria, which leads to massive dehydration in a context of diabetes insipidus. In few observations, onset of diabetes was observed after a body weight gain in relation with hyperphagia when histiocytosis developed in the infundibulum as in our case [7, 11, 13, 15]. Only one publication reported massive insulin needs as observed in our case [12]. Lastly, localization of LCH in pancreas has been exceptionally observed in two cases without diabetes. Yu RC et al. reported the postmortem findings in an 18-month-old boy with infiltration of pancreas by cells with the characteristic features of LCH [9]. However, the islets of Langerhans were preserved. Muwakkit et al. published a case of disseminated LCH in a 4-week-old infant with a cystic lesion in the pancreas discovered at abdominal CT [10]. This lesion improved with systemic therapy of LCH.

TABLE 2: Characteristics and specific organ involvement of cases of diabetes mellitus associated with LCH.

Age at diagnosis of histiocytosis (years)	Sex	Diagnosis of histiocytosis	Diabetes insipidus	Delay between diagnosis of histiocytosis and diabetes	Pathophysiology of diabetes	Daily insulin needs	Reference
31	M	Bone biopsy	+	2 years	Central obesity, insulin resistance	NA	[11]
60	F	Autopsy (histiocytes cells in vertebral marrow, pituitary, lung	+	3 years	Central obesity, insulin resistance	3300 UI/day	[12]
26	M	Autopsy (histiocytes cells in pancreas)	+	2 years	Destruction of pancreatic islets by pancreas infiltration of histiocytosis	80UI/day	[7]
28	F	Lymph node biopsy	+	Few months	Central obesity, insulin resistance	NA	[13]
NA	M	Autopsy (histiocytes cells in skin, liver, bones)	-	6 months	NA	NA	[14]
54		Central nervous system, bones	+	NA	Glucocorticoids, overweight	NA	[15]
60	F	Central nervous system, bones	+	NA	Overweight	NA	[15]
54	M	Gengives	+	NA	Glucocorticoids, overweight	NA	[15]
45	F	Bones, lung, lymph nodes	-	NA	Obesity	NA	[15]

The first-line treatment used for LCH remains empirically derived chemotherapy [18], whereas cladribine has been proposed as a second-line therapy [26]. In contrast with the other cases published, we showed that therapy of LCH had beneficial effect on diabetes mellitus. The patient first received vinblastine and then cladribine as a second-line treatment because vinblastine cycles had only partial effect on brain mass volume. Cladribine therapy provided an excellent effect on brain mass volume. Improvement of glucose homeostasis (in parallel to decline of anti-insulin receptor antibodies in blood) was observed during first- and second-line therapy of LCH. Thus, it could be postulated that reduction of the brain mass volume and/or LCH activity will explain almost in part the improvement of glucose homeostasis. Nevertheless, it is difficult to determine if metabolic amelioration was a consequence of tumor shrinkage or an immune-suppressive effect but some arguments seemed to favor the latter. Indeed, recurrence of hyperglycemia exacerbation at M32 was not associated with changes of volume of the brain mass or its metabolic activity assessed by PET-MRI brain imaging with [18F]FDG. In contrast, this episode was closely correlated with the level of antibodies. Furthermore, at our knowledge, there is no publication about hypothalamic syndrome and anti-insulin receptor antibodies.

4. Conclusion

For the first time, we describe a case of LCH and diabetes and anti-insulin receptor antibodies. In this unique case, insulin resistance could be explained by presence of serum anti-insulin receptor antibodies with a direct link between anti-insulin receptor antibodies and LCH. We hypothesized that recurrent insulin resistant states can be assimilated to a paraneoplastic syndrome. We observed a positive effect of vinblastine and cladribine on glycemic control, probably explained by immune control independent of tumor size evolution.

Consent

Consent for publication has been obtained from the patient and a copy can be transferred to the editor upon request.

Authors' Contributions

Mathilde Sollier and Fabrizio Andreelli wrote the manuscript. Marine Halbron, Jean Donadieu, Ahmed Idbaih, Fleur Cohen Aubart, Marie Bastin, and Corinne Vigouroux provided critical revisions to the manuscript. Mathilde Sollier,

Marine Halbron, Jean Donadieu, Ahmed Idbaih, Fleur Cohen Aubart, Olivier Bourron, Philippe Touraine, Jacques Young, Héléna Mosbah, Agnès Hartemann, Fabrizio Andreelli, and Chloé Amouyal have been involved in the management of the patient. Jacques Young played a crucial role in the diagnosis of hypothalamic-pituitary Langerhans cells histiocytosis. Corinne Vigouroux and Martine Auclair carried out all determinations of serum anti-insulin receptor antibodies. Géraldine Béra performed PET-MRI brain imaging with [18F]FDG. All authors read and approved the final manuscript.

References

[1] J.-F. Emile, O. Abla, S. Fraitag et al., "Revised classification of histiocytoses and neoplasms of the macrophage-dendritic cell lineages," *Blood*, vol. 127, no. 22, pp. 2672–2681, 2016.

[2] J. Haroche, F. Cohen-Aubart, B. J. Rollins et al., "Histiocytoses: emerging neoplasia behind inflammation," *The Lancet Oncology*, vol. 18, no. 2, pp. e113–e125, 2017.

[3] A. Guyot-Goubin, J. Donadieu, M. Barkaoui, S. Bellec, C. Thomas, and J. Clavel, "Descriptive epidemiology of childhood Langerhans cell histiocytosis in France, 2000-2004," *Pediatric Blood & Cancer*, vol. 51, no. 1, pp. 71–75, 2008.

[4] The Writing Group of the Histiocyte Society, "Histiocytosis syndromes in children," *The Lancet*, vol. 329, no. 8526, pp. 208-209, 1987.

[5] P. Makras, K. I. Alexandraki, G. P. Chrousos, A. B. Grossman, and G. A. Kaltsas, "Endocrine manifestations in Langerhans cell histiocytosis," *Trends in Endocrinology & Metabolism*, vol. 18, no. 6, pp. 252–257, 2007.

[6] R. Goyal, A. Das, R. Nijhawan, D. Bansal, and R. K. Marwaha, "Langerhans cell histiocytosis infiltration into pancreas and kidney," *Pediatric Blood & Cancer*, vol. 49, no. 5, pp. 748–750, 2007.

[7] P. J. Hurley, G. C. Hitchcock, and J. D. Wilson, "Histiocytosis x and double diabetes," *Australasian Annals of Medicine*, vol. 16, no. 3, pp. 250–254, 1967.

[8] J. Sananes, F. Laurent, M. Joullie, B. Vergier, B. Damoo, and J. Drouillard, "Histiocytosis X revealed by pancreatic and pulmonary localisations," *European Radiology*, vol. 3, no. 5, pp. 468–470, 1993.

[9] R. C. Yu, A. Attra, C. M. Quinn, T. Krausz, and A. C. Chu, "Multisystem Langerhans' cell histiocytosis with pancreatic involvement.," *Gut*, vol. 34, no. 4, pp. 570–572, 1993.

[10] S. Muwakkit, A. Gharagozloo, A. K. Souid, and B. A. Spirt, "The sonographic appearance of lesions of the spleen and pancreas in an infant with Langerhans' cell histiocytosis," *Pediatric Radiology*, vol. 24, no. 3, pp. 222-223, 1994.

[11] I. Ben Ghorbel, M. Houman, S. B'chir, S. Chamakhi, and M. Miled, "Une forme disséminée d'histiocytose langerhansienne associant un diabète insipide et un diabète sucré," *La Revue de Médecine Interne*, vol. 22, no. 5, pp. 469–474, 2001.

[12] L. G. Rowntree and R. J. Poppiti, "Diabetes insipidus, diabetes mellitus, and insulin resistance with histiocytosis," *Journal of the American Medical Association*, vol. 156, no. 4, pp. 310–312, 1954.

[13] A. C. Thai, I. Sng, R. Suri, and J. S. Cheah, "Disseminated histiocytosis X with diabetes insipidus and diabetes mellitus in an adult female (histiocytosis with DI and DM)," *Annals, Academy of Medicine, Singapore*, vol. 17, no. 2, pp. 294–298, 1988.

[14] D. S. Trochtenberg and E. N. Dessypris, "Reversible hepatomegaly and diabetes mellitus in an adult with disseminated histiocytosis X," *The American Journal of the Medical Sciences*, vol. 299, no. 3, pp. 179–184, 1990.

[15] K. Alexandraki, P. Makras, A. Protogerou et al., "Cardiovascular risk factors in adult patients with multisystem Langerhans-cell histiocytosis: evidence of glucose metabolism abnormalities," *QJM: An International Journal of Medicine*, vol. 101, no. 1, pp. 31–40, 2007.

[16] S. Héritier, J. Emile, M. Barkaoui et al., "*BRAF* mutation correlates with high-risk langerhans cell histiocytosis and increased resistance to first-line therapy," *Journal of Clinical Oncology*, vol. 34, no. 25, pp. 3023–3030, 2016.

[17] S. Héritier, Z. Hélias-Rodzewicz, R. Chakraborty et al., "New somatic BRAF splicing mutation in Langerhans cell histiocytosis," *Molecular Cancer*, vol. 16, no. 1, p. 115, 2017.

[18] R. Haupt, M. Minkov, I. Astigarraga et al., "Langerhans cell histiocytosis (LCH): Guidelines for diagnosis, clinical work-up, and treatment for patients till the age of 18 years," *Pediatric Blood & Cancer*, vol. 60, no. 2, pp. 175–184, 2013.

[19] C. Rigaud, M. A. Barkaoui, C. Thomas et al., "Langerhans cell histiocytosis: therapeutic strategy and outcome in a 30-year nationwide cohort of 1478 patients under 18 years of age," *British Journal of Haematology*, vol. 174, no. 6, pp. 887–898, 2016.

[20] J. Maiza, M. Caron-Debarle, C. Vigouroux, and S. Schneebeli, "Anti-insulin receptor antibodies related to hypoglycemia in a previously diabetic patient," *Diabetes Care*, vol. 36, no. 6, p. e77, 2013.

[21] M. Auclair, C. Vigouroux, C. Desbois-Mouthon et al., "Anti-insulin receptor autoantibodies induce insulin receptors to constitutively associate with insulin receptor substrate-1 and -2 and cause severe cell resistance to both insulin and insulin-like growth factor I," *The Journal of Clinical Endocrinology & Metabolism*, vol. 84, no. 9, pp. 3197–3206, 1999.

[22] O. Bourron, M. Caron-Debarle, M. Hie et al., "Type B Insulin-resistance syndrome: a cause of reversible autoimmune hypoglycaemia," *The Lancet*, vol. 384, no. 9953, p. 1548, 2014.

[23] E. Arioglu, A. Andewelt, C. Diabo, M. Bell, S. I. Taylor, and P. Gorden, "Clinical course of the syndrome of autoantibodies to the insulin receptor (type b insulin resistance)," *Medicine*, vol. 81, no. 2, pp. 87–100, 2002.

[24] I. Marchand, M. A. Barkaoui, C. Garel, M. Polak, and J. Donadieu, "Central diabetes insipidus as the inaugural manifestation of langerhans cell histiocytosis: natural history and medical evaluation of 26 children and adolescents," *The Journal of Clinical Endocrinology & Metabolism*, vol. 96, no. 9, pp. E1352–E1360, 2011.

[25] S. Ng Wing Tin, N. Martin-Duverneuil, A. Idbaih et al., "Efficacy of vinblastine in central nervous system Langerhans cell histiocytosis: A nationwide retrospective study," *Orphanet Journal of Rare Diseases*, vol. 6, no. 1, p. 83, 2011.

[26] J. Donadieu, F. Bernard, M. Van Noesel et al., "Cladribine and cytarabine in refractory multisystem Langerhans cell histiocytosis: Results of an international phase 2 study," *Blood*, vol. 126, no. 12, pp. 1415–1423, 2015.

28

Horner Syndrome Secondary to Thyroid Surgery

Meliha Demiral,[1] Ciğdem Binay,[1] Enver Simsek,[1] and Hüseyin Ilhan[2]

[1] *Department of Pediatric Endocrinology, School of Medicine, Eskişehir Osmangazi University, Eskişehir, Turkey*
[2] *Department of Pediatric Surgery, School of Medicine, Eskişehir Osmangazi University, Eskişehir, Turkey*

Correspondence should be addressed to Meliha Demiral; drmelihad@hotmail.com

Academic Editor: Thomas Grüning

Horner syndrome (HS), caused by an interruption in the oculosympathetic pathway, is characterised by myosis, ipsilateral blepharoptosis, enophthalmos, facial anhydrosis, and vascular dilation of the lateral part of the face. HS is a rare complication of thyroidectomy. A 15-year-old female patient presented with solitary solid and large nodule in the right thyroid lobe. Ultrasound-guided fine-needle aspiration was performed and the cytological examination results were undefined. The patient underwent a total thyroidectomy. On postoperative day 2, she developed right-sided myosis and upper eyelid ptosis. HS was diagnosed. Interestingly, the patient exhibited an incomplete clinical syndrome with the absence of vasomotor symptoms. We herein report a case of HS in a 15-year-old female patient after total thyroidectomy. The possible causes of HS were ischaemia-induced nerve damage and stretching of the cervical sympathetic chain by the retractor during thyroidectomy. Clinicians should be aware of the possibility of this rare but important surgical complication.

1. Introduction

Horner syndrome (HS) was first described in 1869 by Johann Friedrich Horner [1]. The typical clinical features include myosis, ipsilateral blepharoptosis, enophthalmos, facial anhydrosis, and vascular dilation of the lateral part of the face. These conditions result from an interruption in the oculosympathetic pathway. The present literature review reveals that compression of the cervical sympathetic chain by large benign or malignant goitres may present as HS, and this has mostly been reported in adult patients [2–4]. However, HS has rarely been reported as a complication of thyroid surgery [5, 6]. We herein report a case of HS following total thyroidectomy in a 15-year-old girl.

2. Case Report

A 15-year-old female patient presented to the Pediatric Endocrinology Division at the Medical Faculty Hospital of Eskisehir Osmangazi University with a 2-month history of a noticeable neck mass. Physical examination revealed an enlarged thyroid gland with a palpable nodule in the right thyroid lobe. The patient had no other complaints related to thyroid disease. Her medical history was unremarkable. She had no history of previous radiation in her cervical region and no family history of thyroid disease. On physical examination, her weight was 64 kg (+1.16 standard deviation score), her height was 155 cm (−1.15 standard deviation score), her body mass index was 26.6 kg/m^2, and her blood pressure was 110/80 mmHg. A palpable nontender nodule measuring 35 mm × 20 mm completely covered the right thyroid lobe region. There was no evidence of cervical lymphadenopathy.

Thyroid function tests revealed thyroid stimulating hormone and free thyroxin levels of 1.0 mcIU/mL and 1.2 ng/dL, respectively. Thyroid peroxidase antibody and thyroglobulin antibody titres were negative. Thyroid ultrasonography showed markedly enlarged right and left lobes measuring 33 × 21 × 50 mm and 14 × 11 × 41 mm, respectively. A 31 × 19 × 38 mm solid nodule completely covered the right lobe with a hypoechoic halo. The patient underwent ultrasound-guided fine-needle aspiration, and the cytological examination results were undefined.

The patient then underwent a total thyroidectomy. On postoperative day 2, she developed right-sided myosis and upper eyelid ptosis (Figure 1). However, facial anhydrosis, enophthalmos, and a bitonal voice were not detected. Her

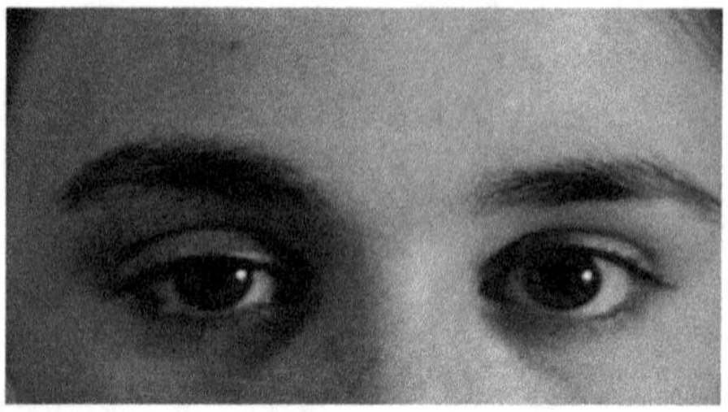

Figure 1: Myosis and eyelid ptosis were noted on the right side.

extraocular eye movements and visual acuity were normal. Brain magnetic resonance imaging, chest X-rays, neck computed tomography, and single-fibre electromyography showed no distinct pathology. No other complications such as bleeding, wound infection, vocal cord palsy, or findings of hypoparathyroidism were detected. Histological examination of the tissue obtained from the thyroidectomy revealed nodular thyroid hyperplasia. Euthyroidism was achieved by L-thyroxin replacement at a dose of 150 mcg/day. The patient has been followed up for 8 months. Six months after the thyroid surgery, physical examination findings were normal, and the patient exhibited no myosis or ptosis.

3. Discussion

The aetiologies of HS in childhood are classically divided into congenital and acquired causes. The major cause of acquired HS is postsurgical complications of the neck and thorax [7]. Noniatrogenic cases can be attributed to infection, trauma, vascular anomalies, and neoplasms such as sympathetic paraganglioma, neuroblastoma, schwannoma, and Ewing sarcoma [8–11].

Horner syndrome is a rare complication of thyroid disease. The majority of aetiologies involve compression of the cervical plexus. Thyroid carcinoma accounts for 21% of cases [12]. Of the reported cases, multinodular goitre, Riedel's and Hashimoto's thyroiditis, thyroid adenoma, and thyroid lymphoma have been associated with HS. Most of the reported cases occurred in an adult population [12, 13].

Horner syndrome following thyroid surgery is an extremely rare complication with an incidence of less than 0.2% to 0.3% among patients undergoing thyroidectomy [3]. Smith and Murley [14] reported 25 cases involving patients with iatrogenic injures following either partial or total thyroidectomy. Buhr et al. [15] also reported three cases of HS following modified radical neck dissection for medullary thyroid cancer. It has been postulated that HS might be caused not only by direct mechanical stress or compression of the stellate ganglion but also indirectly through anastomosis of the recurrent nerve, laryngeal superior nerve, and sympathetic nervous branches around the inferior thyroid artery [6]. The possible causes of HS after thyroid surgery have been attributed to the postoperative formation of a hematoma compressing the cervical sympathetic chain, ischaemia-induced damage caused by a lateral ligature on the inferior thyroid artery trunk, stretching of the cervical sympathetic chain by the tip of the retractor, and damage to communication between the cervical sympathetic chain and the recurrent laryngeal nerve during its identification [6].

In most cases, the HS is incomplete, exhibiting the absence of vasomotor symptoms, as in our case. The present case had some characteristics similar to those of previous cases, such as the onset of HS on postoperative day 2 and the lack of symptoms related to vascular or sweating dysfunction [16, 17].

The prognosis of HS has been proposed to be poor depending on the particular mechanism of injury. However, if the injury is related to hematoma formation, inflammation, or peripheral ligature of the inferior thyroid artery branches, the HS may spontaneously resolve. In the present case, postoperative hematoma and adherence were ruled out by neck ultrasonography and computed tomography. The nonrecurrent laryngeal nerve, which is rarely observed during thyroidectomy, is at high risk for damage [18]. The best way to avoid morbidity is routine identification of this nerve. About 70% of patients who develop HS after thyroidectomy have permanent damage or incomplete recovery, and the remaining 30% recover completely, but only after a much longer time (20 days to 15 months) [6]. The HS in our patient was reversible, and all findings of HS completely disappeared.

In conclusion, we have reported a case with HS resulting from thyroid surgery for benign pathology. While HS appears to be a very rare complication of thyroid surgery, clinicians should be aware of the possibility of this rare but important complication.

Disclosure

The English in this document has been checked by at least two professional editors, both native speakers of English.

Competing Interests

The authors declare that they have no competing interests.

References

[1] H. S. Amonoo-Kuofi, "Horner's syndrome revisited: with an update of the central pathway," *Clinical Anatomy*, vol. 12, no. 5, pp. 345–361, 1999.

[2] T. Yasmeen, S. Khan, S. G. Patel et al., "Clinical case seminar: Riedel's thyroiditis: report of a case complicated by spontaneous hypoparathyroidism, recurrent laryngeal nerve injury, and Horner's syndrome," *The Journal of Clinical Endocrinology & Metabolism*, vol. 87, no. 8, pp. 3543–3547, 2002.

[3] J. L. Harding, M. S. Sywak, S. Sidhu, and L. W. Delbridge, "Horner's syndrome in association with thyroid and parathyroid disease," *ANZ Journal of Surgery*, vol. 74, no. 6, pp. 442–445, 2004.

[4] I. Leuchter, M. Becker, R. Mickel, and P. Dulguerov, "Horner's syndrome and thyroid neoplasms," *Journal for Oto-Rhino-Laryngology and Its Related Specialties*, vol. 64, no. 1, pp. 49–52, 2002.

[5] E. Nordenström, M. Hallén, and J. Nordenström, "Horner syndrome is a serious complication in thyroid surgery. Dissection in nerve stimulation may be a risk factor, shown in three cases," *Lakartidningen*, vol. 108, pp. 2660–2661, 2011.

[6] L. Cozzaglio, M. Coladonato, R. Doci et al., "Horner's syndrome as a complication of thyroidectomy: report of a case," *Surgery Today*, vol. 38, no. 12, pp. 1114–1116, 2008.

[7] A. R. Jeffery, F. J. Ellis, M. X. Repka, and J. R. Buncic, "Pediatric Horner syndrome," *Journal of American Association for Pediatric Ophthalmology and Strabismus*, vol. 2, no. 3, pp. 159–167, 1998.

[8] N. R. Mahoney, G. T. Liu, S. J. Menacker, M. C. Wilson, M. D. Hogarty, and J. M. Maris, "Pediatric Horner syndrome: etiologies and roles of imaging and urine studies to detect neuroblastoma and other responsible mass lesions," *American Journal of Ophthalmology*, vol. 142, no. 4, pp. 651.e2–659.e2, 2006.

[9] A. Challapalli, L. Howell, M. Farrier, A. Kelsey, J. Birch, and T. Eden, "Cervical paraganglioma—a case report and review of all cases reported to the Manchester Children's Tumour Registry 1954–2004," *Pediatric Blood and Cancer*, vol. 48, no. 1, pp. 112–116, 2007.

[10] A. Kansal, A. Lahiri, and H. Nishikawa, "Sympathetic paraganglioma presenting with Horner's syndrome in a child," *Journal of Plastic, Reconstructive & Aesthetic Surgery*, vol. 59, no. 7, pp. 772–774, 2006.

[11] S. Bhagat, S. Varshney, S. S. Bist, and N. Gupta, "Pediatric cervical sympathetic chain schwannoma with Horner syndrome: a rare case presentation," *Ear, Nose and Throat Journal*, vol. 93, no. 3, pp. 1–3, 2014.

[12] D. Yip, R. Drachtman, L. Amorosa, and S. Trooskin, "Papillary thyroid cancer presenting as Horner syndrome," *Pediatric Blood and Cancer*, vol. 55, no. 4, pp. 739–741, 2010.

[13] J. N. Darvall, A. W. Morsi, and A. Penington, "Coexisting harlequin and Horner syndromes after paediatric neck dissection: a case report and a review of the literature," *Journal of Plastic, Reconstructive and Aesthetic Surgery*, vol. 61, no. 11, pp. 1382–1384, 2008.

[14] I. Smith and R. S. Murley, "Damage to the cervical sympathetic system during operations on the thyroid gland," *British Journal of Surgery*, vol. 52, no. 9, pp. 673–675, 1965.

[15] H. J. Buhr, T. Lehnert, and F. Raue, "New operative strategy in the treatment of metastasizing medullary carcinomas of the thyroid," *European Journal of Surgical Oncology*, vol. 16, no. 4, pp. 366–369, 1990.

[16] P. Solomon, J. Irish, and P. Gullane, "Horner's syndrome following a thyroidectomy," *Journal of Otolaryngology*, vol. 22, no. 6, pp. 454–456, 1993.

[17] M. El Hajjaji, C. Deflorenne, and B. Dachy, "Horner's syndrome associated with Guillain-Barre syndrome," *Revue Neurologique*, vol. 159, pp. 799–800, 2003.

[18] A. Toniato, R. Mazzarotto, A. Piotto, P. Bernante, C. Pagetta, and M. R. Pelizzo, "Identification of the nonrecurrent laryngeal nerve during thyroid surgery: 20-year experience," *World Journal of Surgery*, vol. 28, no. 7, pp. 659–661, 2004.

29

Complete Remission of Anaplastic Thyroid Carcinoma after Concomitant Treatment with Docetaxel and Radiotherapy

Ichiro Abe,[1,2] Satoko Karasaki,[1] Yayoi Matsuda,[1] Shohei Sakamoto,[1] Torahiko Nakashima,[3] Hidetaka Yamamoto,[4] Hisaya Kawate,[1] Keizo Ohnaka,[1] Hisashi Nakashima,[5] Kunihisa Kobayashi,[2] Yoshinao Oda,[4] Masatoshi Nomura,[1] and Ryoichi Takayanagi[1]

[1] *Department of Medicine and Bioregulatory Science, Graduate School of Medical Science, Kyushu University, Maidashi 3-1-1, Higashi Ward, Fukuoka 812-8582, Japan*

[2] *Department of Endocrinology and Diabetes Mellitus, Fukuoka University Chikushi Hospital, 1-1-1 Zokumyoin, Chikushino, Fukuoka 818-8502, Japan*

[3] *Department of Otorhinolaryngology, Graduate School of Medical Science, Kyushu University, Maidashi 3-1-1, Higashi Ward, Fukuoka 812-8582, Japan*

[4] *Department of Anatomic Pathology, Graduate School of Medical Science, Kyushu University, Maidashi 3-1-1, Higashi Ward, Fukuoka 812-8582, Japan*

[5] *Department of Internal Medicine, Haradoi Hospital, Aoba 6-40-8, Higashi Ward, Fukuoka 813-8588, Japan*

Correspondence should be addressed to Ichiro Abe; abe1ro@fukuoka-u.ac.jp

Academic Editor: Wayne V. Moore

Anaplastic thyroid carcinoma (ATC) although rare is the most lethal form of thyroid cancer. The mortality rate for ATC is very high, with a median survival time of only 5 months; the survival rate at 1 year after diagnosis is <20%. Management of ATC is extremely difficult and rife with uncertainties. Herein, we describe a 75-year-old woman who presented with ATC and was successfully treated using concomitant treatment with docetaxel and high-dose radiotherapy. This case appears to be the first to have been reported in the literature involving complete remission of ATC confirmed by autopsy, suggesting the therapeutic potential of this combination.

1. Introduction

Anaplastic thyroid carcinoma (ATC) is a rare carcinoma that accounts for 2% of all thyroid cancers [1] and has a slightly higher rate of occurrence in women; its incidence peaks in the sixth and seventh decades of life. ATC is one of the most aggressive cancers with patients having a median survival time of only 5 months; <20% of patients are alive at 1 year after diagnosis. The disease is locally advanced with infiltration of surrounding organs and blood vessels. Furthermore, 50% of patients have distant metastasis at diagnosis [2]. All patients are classified as stage IV, with the primary lesion restricted to the thyroid gland in stage IVA disease; locoregional lymph nodes may exist in stages IVA/IVB and stage IVC is defined by distant metastasis, according to the American Joint Commission on Cancer TNM staging system. It has long been thought that the most important factors associated with longer survival are completeness of surgical resection and high-dose external beam radiotherapy. Because progression of ATC is extremely rapid and no effective systemic chemotherapy has been established, its management is quite difficult and rife with uncertainties. The problems include the following: (1) should adjuvant radiotherapy and/or chemotherapy be used in the treatment of stage IVA disease; (2) which chemotherapy regimens should be recommended for stage IVB unresectable disease; (3) which systemic therapies should be considered for stage IVC patients; and (4) which clinical factors should be used to direct an appropriate therapeutic approach to the individual patient or help patients in their decision making regarding the pursuit of aggressive therapy or palliative/hospice care. All of these problems might be resolved when an effective treatment strategy including systemic chemotherapy has been established. Recently, high-dose radiotherapy plus combination chemotherapy has been shown to improve

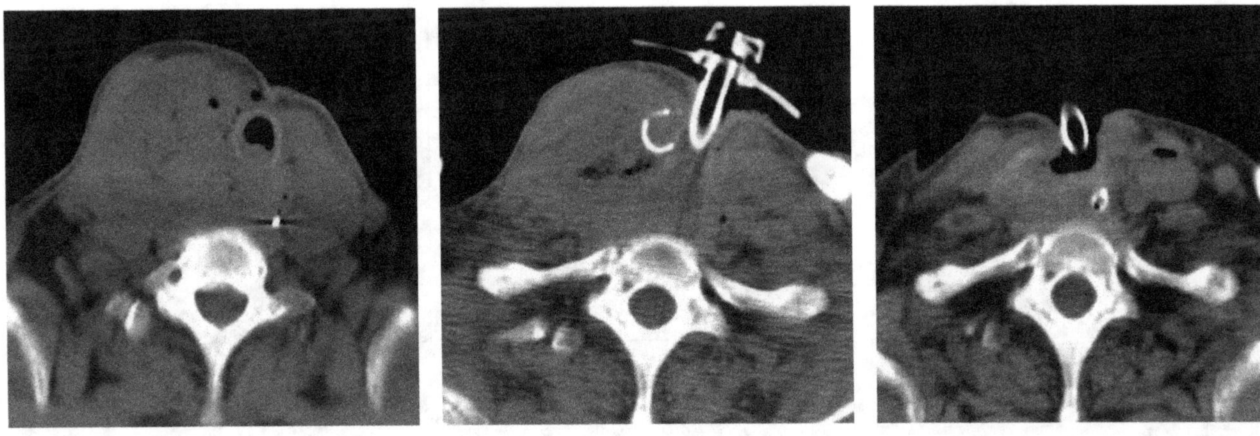

FIGURE 1: ATC in a 75-year-old woman. The cervical mass was inseparable from the strap muscles, tracheal wall, and carotid sheath. (a) Computed tomography scan showing a huge mass in the right thyroid robe on admission, (b) after surgical resection of a part of tumor and tracheotomy, and (c) after radiotherapy and seven cycles of chemotherapy.

long-term survival in ATC patients. In particular, the combination of radiotherapy and concomitant docetaxel has been reported to be highly effective [3]. Here, we report a case of complete remission of ATC at stage IVB after treatment using concomitant docetaxel and radiotherapy. In addition, complete remission was pathologically confirmed at autopsy, suggesting the therapeutic potential of this treatment combination.

2. Case Presentation

A 75-year-old woman presented at the nearby hospital with the complaints of neck swelling and respiratory discomfort. She had been diagnosed with type 2 diabetes mellitus 20 years previously and had been treated exclusively with diet therapy. The risk factors for ATC remain to be clarified [4]. She did not have any other past history such as thyroid tumor and special medical history. A right thyroid mass was detected using sonogram. Because a malignant tumor was suspected, the patient was referred to our hospital for further examination and treatment. A sonogram confirmed the presence of a very large tumor (46 × 44 × 78 mm) with homogenous appearance in the right thyroid lobe. The left thyroid lobe was dislocated to the opposite side. Abnormal cervical lymph nodes could not be detected by a sonogram. A diagnosis of undifferentiated carcinoma was made using fine needle aspiration cytology, and ATC was highly suspected. On physical examination, the patient presented with swelling of the neck and her peripheral capillary oxygen saturation (SPO_2) level was 93% (in room air). Her blood pressure was 124/78 mmHg and her body temperature was 37.1°C. The patient had a regular pulse rate, which was 100/min. Laboratory tests revealed an elevated white blood cell count of 12,110/mm^2 with 85.2% neutrophils and a C-reactive protein level of 13.98 mg/dL. The hemoglobin level was 10.0 g/dL and the platelet count was 541,000/μL. On biochemical investigation, the blood glucose level was found to be 276 mg/dL and the HgbA1c level was 10.0%. On thyroid function tests, TSH was 3.05 μU/mL (reference range: 0.30–4.30 μU/mL) and free T4 was 1.23 ng/dL (reference range: 0.90–1.70 ng/dL). However, she had elevated levels of anti-thyroid antibodies, an anti-thyroglobulin antibody: 407.6 U/mL (reference range: <28 U/mL), and an anti-microsomal antibody: 1,732 U/mL (reference range: <16 U/mL). Thyroglobulin was 4.0 ng/mL (reference range: <32.7 ng/mL). An irregularly shaped very large mass in the right thyroid together with tracheal compression was detected using a computed tomography (CT) scan as shown in Figure 1(a). A further examination using a whole-body CT revealed that the thyroid tumor was the only tumor present. To obtain an appropriate diagnosis of this thyroid tumor and to prevent asphyxiation, surgical resection of a part of tumor and tracheotomy were conducted (Figure 1(b)). Histological analysis of the tumor using hematoxylin and eosin staining revealed that the tumor was composed of polygonal cells, spindle cells, and multinucleated cells; necrosis was also present (Figures 2(a) and 2(a′)). Using immunohistochemistry, the tumor cells were negative for TTF1 (data not shown). An extremely high number of the cells were found to be positive for Ki-67, indicating a highly proliferative tumor (Figure 2(b)). Although the tumor cells were negative for p53 (Figure 2(c)), known to be positive for 60% of ATCs [5], based on these pathological findings and the clinical manifestation of the thyroid tumor, ATC at stage IVB was diagnosed.

After making a diagnosis of stage IVB ATC, combined therapy with docetaxel and radiation was started. The patient received external beam radiotherapy at a total dose of 46 Gy delivered in 2 Gy daily fractions. Docetaxel was administered intravenously at a dose of 40 mg/m^2 every 4 weeks; administration was initiated within the 1st week of radiotherapy. During the combined therapy, no severe adverse reactions developed, with the exception of mild radiation dermatitis. After the 3rd cycle of chemotherapy, a slight degree of tumor shrinkage of the thyroid tumor was observed on CT. The patient was discharged after the 4th cycle of chemotherapy.

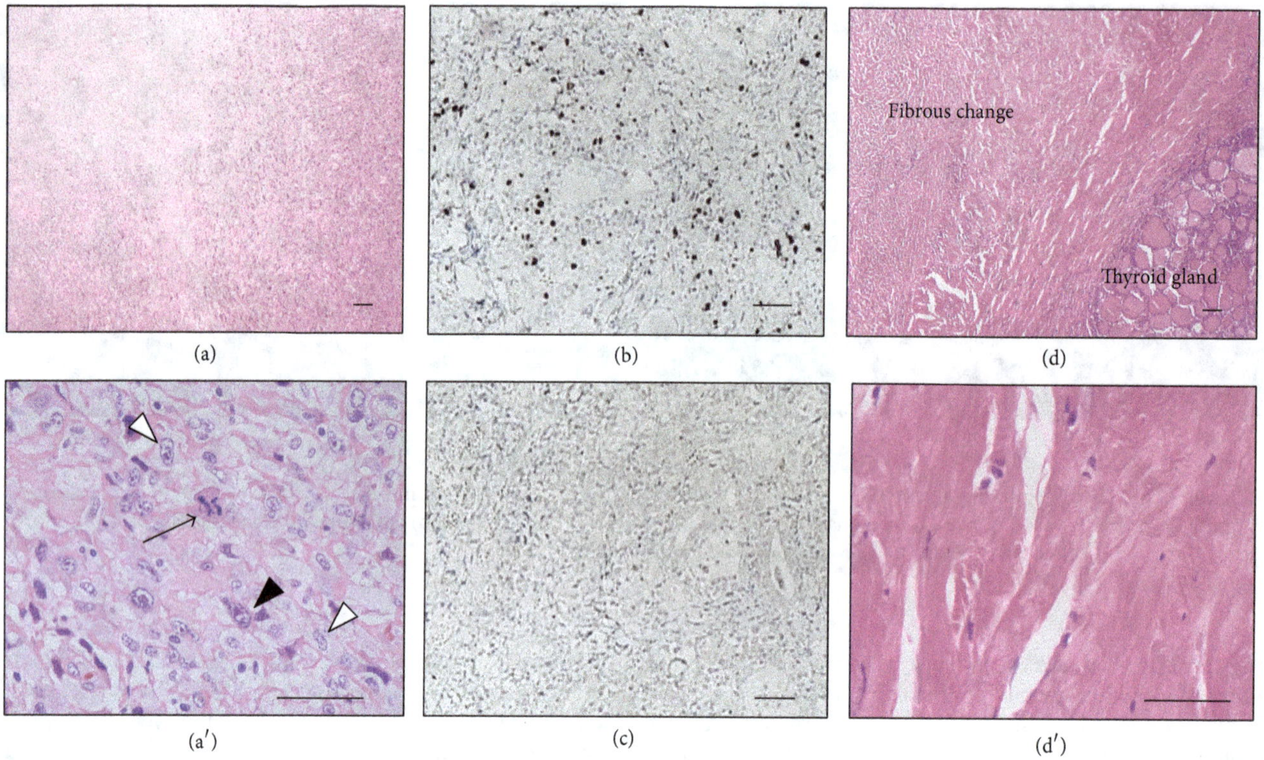

FIGURE 2: Pathological analysis of anaplastic thyroid cancer. (a, a′) Hematoxylin and eosin (HE) stained tumor section. High magnification is shown in the lower panel (a′). The tumor cells were composed of polygonal cells (closed arrowhead), spindle cells (open arrowheads), and multinucleated cells (arrow) with necrosis. (b) The Ki-67 labeling index was 50%. (c) The tumor cells were negative for p53. (d, d′) HE stained section of the thyroid gland after autopsy. It should be noted that the tumor is completely substituted by fibrotic tissue. Scale bars = 50 μm.

A whole-body PET-CT scan after 4th chemotherapy showed the right neck mass to be hypermetabolic with no metastasis. The patient continued chemotherapy with the same regimen every 8 weeks for >1 year (total 7 cycles) and further shrinkage of the thyroid tumor was observed; finally, the thyroid tumor could barely be detected on CT (Figure 1(c)). Unfortunately, the patient died suddenly 13 months after she referred to our hospital and 1 month after the seventh chemotherapy, with no worsening of the disease. Autopsy was carried out and the cause of death was identified as suffocation from sputum. Despite an extensive histopathological examination, there was no evidence of distance metastasis or malignant tissue in the thyroid gland; the tumor had been totally substituted with fibrotic tissue (Figures 2(d) and 2(d′)) indicating that the patient's ATC was in a complete remission.

3. Discussion

Because the progression of ATC is extremely rapid and aggressive, most patients initially present with a rapidly enlarging tumor in the neck, often causing progressive symptoms such as dyspnea. The disease is locally advanced with infiltration of the surrounding organs [2]. In the present case, the patient initially presented with a very large locally invasive tumor in the neck, which was diagnosed as stage IVB disease. Therefore, total resection of ATC could not be performed and systemic chemotherapy was concomitantly administered with radiotherapy to the localized lesion. An optimal treatment for ATC has not yet been established [6, 7]. American Thyroid Association guidelines for patients with stage IVA/IVB ATC recommended a multimodal approach including surgery, radiation, and systemic chemotherapy [8]. The ATC Research Consortium of Japan (ATCCJ) also reported that multimodal aggressive approach was effective to selected patients with ATC [9]. Cytotoxic drugs alone for advanced ATC are poorly effective. On the other hand, targeted biological agents including antiangiogenic agents and tyrosine kinase inhibitors might represent a viable therapeutic option. Axitinib [10], combretastatin A4 [11], sorafenib [12], and imatinib [13] have been tested in small clinical trials of ATC, with a promising disease control rate ranging from 33% to 75%. However, these findings have been derived from limited number of the patients. ATC is rare and thus it is difficult to advance evidence level of the diverse treatment of this deadly disease. Recently, Troch et al. reported that five ATC patients, who received radiotherapy at total doses of 50–60 Gy concomitantly with docetaxel administered intravenously at an absolute dose of 100 mg every 3 weeks, were alive after a median follow-up time of 21.5 months; four patients achieved complete remission of ATC that was confirmed by imaging analysis and clinical course [3]. Docetaxel arrests cell division by inhibiting microtubular depolymerization [14]. It has been reported that docetaxel increased the cell fraction in the G2/M phase of the cell cycle, considered to be the most radiosensitive phase, leading to radiation-sensitizing effects [15]. This may explain the mechanism underlying the synergistic effect of docetaxel and radiation. Taking these findings into account, we chose this combination therapy for the present case. Considering the age of the patient, the dosage of docetaxel was reduced and the dosing interval was extended. Although the dosage and the dosing interval of docetaxel were modified, ATC was well controlled during the whole clinical course. In addition, it should be noted that none of the severe adverse effects, with the exception of mild radiation dermatitis, was found at any time. Histopathological analysis during autopsy revealed complete remission of ATC. Our case appears to be the first reported in the literature involving complete remission of ATC after combination therapy, which could be pathologically confirmed. Our case report demonstrated the efficacy and a safety of combined therapy of radiotherapy with docetaxel to the aged patient with ATC. Although ATC is heterogeneous and it is difficult to standardize approach to treatment especially at an advanced stage, the best treatment involving a multimodal approach using a combination of radiotherapy and chemotherapy with docetaxel should be considered. Further analysis including the prospective randomized controlled study is required.

References

[1] F. D. Gilliland, W. C. Hunt, D. M. Morris, and C. R. Key, "Prognostic factors for thyroid carcinoma. A population-based study of 15,698 cases from the Surveillance, Epidemiology and End Results (SEER) program 1973–1991," *Cancer*, vol. 79, no. 3, pp. 564–573, 1997.

[2] E. Kebebew, F. S. Greenspan, O. H. Clark, K. A. Woeber, and A. McMillan, "Anaplastic thyroid carcinoma: treatment outcome and prognostic factors," *Cancer*, vol. 103, no. 7, pp. 1330–1335, 2005.

[3] M. Troch, O. Koperek, C. Scheuba et al., "High efficacy of concomitant treatment of undifferentiated (anaplastic) thyroid cancer with radiation and docetaxel," *Journal of Clinical Endocrinology and Metabolism*, vol. 95, no. 9, pp. E54–E57, 2010.

[4] V. Zivaljevic, K. Tausanovic, I. Paunovic et al., "Age as a prognostic factor in anaplastic thyroid cancer," *International Journal of Endocrinology*, vol. 2014, Article ID 240513, 5 pages, 2014.

[5] G. Gauchotte, C. Philippe, S. Lacomme et al., "BRAF, p53 and SOX2 in anaplastic thyroid carcinoma: evidence for multistep carcinogenesis," *Pathology*, vol. 43, no. 5, pp. 447–452, 2011.

[6] R. C. Smallridge and J. A. Copland, "Anaplastic thyroid carcinoma: pathogenesis and emerging therapies," *Clinical Oncology*, vol. 22, no. 6, pp. 486–497, 2010.

[7] R. Granata, L. Locati, and L. Licitra, "Therapeutic strategies in the management of patients with metastatic anaplastic thyroid cancer: review of the current literature," *Current Opinion in Oncology*, vol. 25, no. 3, pp. 224–228, 2013.

[8] R. C. Smallridge, K. B. Ain, S. L. Asa et al., "American Thyroid Association guidelines for management of patients with anaplastic thyroid cancer," *Thyroid*, vol. 22, no. 11, pp. 1104–1139, 2012.

[9] I. Sugitani, A. Miyauchi, K. Sugino, T. Okamoto, A. Yoshida, and S. Suzuki, "Prognostic factors and treatment outcomes for anaplastic thyroid carcinoma: ATC research consortium of Japan cohort study of 677 patients," *World Journal of Surgery*, vol. 36, no. 6, pp. 1247–1254, 2012.

[10] E. E. W. Cohen, L. S. Rosen, E. E. Vokes et al., "Axitinib is an active treatment for all histologic subtypes of advanced thyroid cancer: results from a phase II study," *Journal of Clinical Oncology*, vol. 26, no. 29, pp. 4708–4713, 2008.

[11] M. M. Cooney, P. Savvides, S. Agarwala et al., "Phase II study of combretastatin A4 phosphate (CA4P) in patients with advanced anaplastic thyroid carcinoma (ATC)," *Journal of Clinical Oncology*, vol. 24, no. 18S, p. A5580, 2006.

[12] G. Nagaiah, P. Fu, J. K. Wasman et al., "Phase II trial of sorafenib (bay 43-9006) in patients with advanced anaplastic carcinoma of the thyroid (ATC)," *Journal of Clinical Oncology*, vol. 27, no. 15S, p. A6058, 2009.

[13] H. T. Ha, J. S. Lee, S. Urba et al., "Phase II trial evaluating imatinib (I) in patients (pts) with anaplastic thyroid carcinoma (ATC)," *Journal of Clinical Oncology*, vol. 27, no. 15S, Article ID A6057, 2009.

[14] I. Ringel and S. B. Horwitiz, "Studies with RP 56976 (taxotere): a semisynthetic analogue of taxol," *Journal of the National Cancer Institute*, vol. 83, no. 4, pp. 288–291, 1991.

[15] L. H. Hartwell and T. A. Weinert, "Checkpoints: controls that ensure the order of cell cycle events," *Science*, vol. 246, no. 4930, pp. 629–634, 1989.

30

Locally Advanced Thyroglossal Duct Cyst Carcinoma Presenting as a Neck Mass

Niranjan Tachamo,[1] Brian Le,[2] Jeffrey Driben,[3] and Vasudev Magaji[4]

[1]*Department of Internal Medicine, Reading Health System, West Reading, PA 19611, USA*
[2]*Department of Pathology, Reading Health System, West Reading, PA 19611, USA*
[3]*ENT Head & Neck Specialists, Wyomissing, PA 19610, USA*
[4]*Department of Endocrinology, Reading Health System, West Reading, PA 19611, USA*

Correspondence should be addressed to Niranjan Tachamo; niranjantachamo@gmail.com

Academic Editor: Eli Hershkovitz

Thyroglossal duct cyst carcinoma is rare and occurs in just 1% of cases with thyroglossal duct cysts. It is not always possible to distinguish a thyroglossal cyst harboring malignancy from its benign counterparts unless biopsied, thus posing the dilemma. Currently there is no clear consensus on the optimal management of thyroglossal duct cyst carcinoma. Here we present the case of a 69-year-old female who presented with a midline neck mass and dysphagia and was found to have papillary thyroid cancer in the biopsy specimen of the neck mass. She underwent excision of the mass and the thyroglossal duct cyst along with total thyroidectomy; however, the thyroidectomy specimen showed no malignancy. Her lymph node mapping was negative and she is awaiting radioactive iodine treatment.

1. Introduction

Thyroglossal duct cyst is a developmental anomaly arising from the failure of thyroglossal duct to involute during embryological development [1]. It is the most common congenital anomaly of the neck [1, 2] and is present in approximately 7% of the general population [1, 3]. Uncommonly, thyroglossal duct cyst carcinoma (TDCC) may be found in 1% of cases, the majority being papillary carcinoma [2, 4]. It may be difficult to ascertain the presence of thyroid carcinoma originating exclusively from a thyroglossal duct cyst as there is no way to distinguish the carcinoma from a benign cyst preoperatively [3]. There is no consensus regarding the optimal management of TDCC.

2. Case Presentation

A 69-year-old female was seen in the office for a neck lump and dysphagia for 1 year. She denied any fever, night sweats, dysphonia, dysarthria, palpitations, or weight loss. There was no history of radiation to the head and neck. There was no family history of thyroid cancer. The neck mass was 4×5 cm, soft to palpation, freely mobile, and located in the midline at the level of the thyroid cartilage. She was evaluated with an ultrasonogram (US) of the neck which revealed a right mid to superior lobe hyperechoic nodule measuring $7 \times 3 \times 4$ mm, with mild increased vascularity, and a left inferior heterogeneous nodule measuring $1.5 \times 0.7 \times 0.7$ cm, along with submandibular lymph nodes, measuring $1.7 \times 0.9 \times 1.3$ cm on the right and measuring $2.1 \times 0.9 \times 1.1$ cm on the left. Computed tomography (CT) of the neck revealed a lobulated soft tissue mass at the level of the left side of the hyoid bone measuring 1.8×2.9 cm with no evidence of erosion of the hyoid bone or thyroid cartilage (Figures 1 and 2). Fine needle aspiration biopsy of the neck mass revealed papillary thyroid cancer. The patient underwent excision of the mass and thyroglossal duct cyst via a Sistrunk procedure with total thyroidectomy.

On histologic examination, within the central neck soft tissue there is a cystic structure, within which is a proliferation of papillary fronds (Figure 3). The cyst is lined by respiratory-type epithelium, consistent with thyroglossal

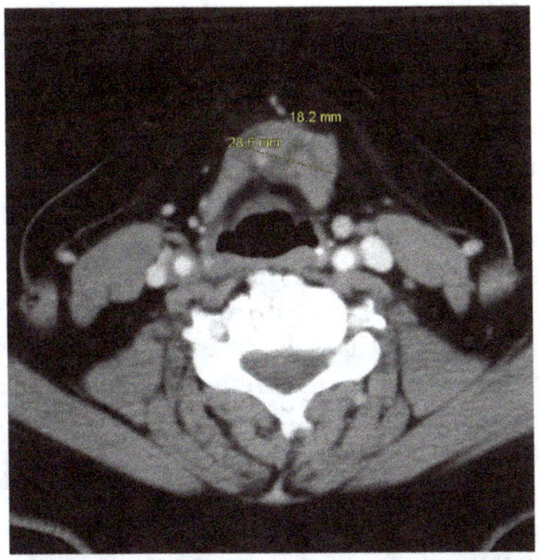

FIGURE 1: Transverse view of the CT neck that showed presence of a neck mass measuring 28.6 mm × 18.2 mm.

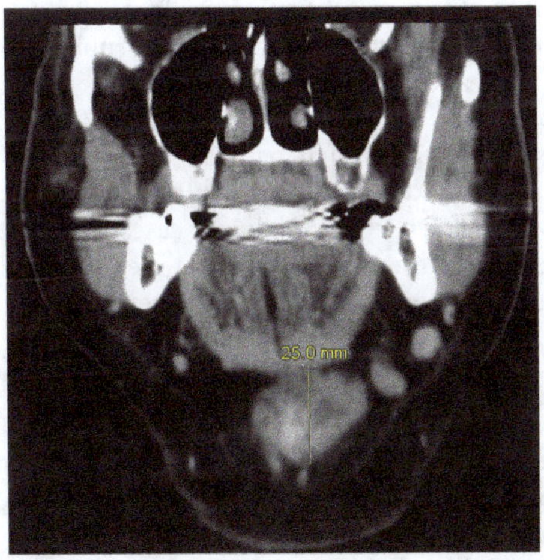

FIGURE 2: Axial view of the CT neck that showed presence of a neck mass measuring 25 mm in superior to inferior dimension.

duct cyst (Figure 4), while the intraluminal proliferation, which extends into adjacent soft tissue, demonstrates complex and arborizing fibrovascular cores lined by epithelioid cells (Figure 5). These cells are characterized by nuclear grooves with pseudoinclusions, peripheralization of nuclear chromatin, and some prominence of nucleoli (Figure 6). The morphologic features are diagnostic of papillary thyroid carcinoma. As there is no demonstrable tumor in the total thyroidectomy specimen concurrently reviewed, the tumor is deemed to have arisen from the thyroglossal duct cyst. Her lymph node mapping was negative and she is planned for treatment with radioactive iodine.

3. Discussion

The thyroid gland develops from the endodermal thickening at the base of the tongue and descends via the thyroglossal tract into its final position in the anterior neck inferior to the thyroid cartilage [2, 5, 6]. This thyroglossal tract usually disappears by 10th week of gestation [2, 5]. However, it fails to involute in 7% of cases [1, 4]. Cystic degeneration of this persistent duct forms a thyroglossal duct cyst, which is usually benign [5, 6]. So far, thyroglossal duct cyst is the most common congenital cause of neck swelling and accounts for more than 75% of midline neck swellings in childhood [6]. Between 1.5 and 45% of these cases show the presence of ectopic thyroid tissue [6].

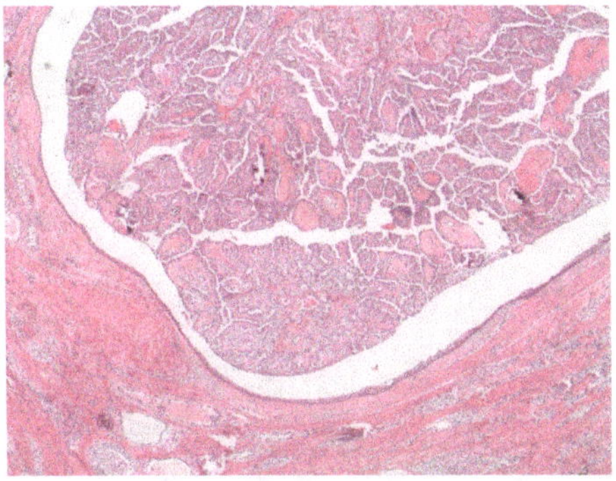

FIGURE 3: Central neck soft tissue demonstrating a cystic structure, within which is a proliferation of fibrovascular cores (H&E stain, 40x original magnification).

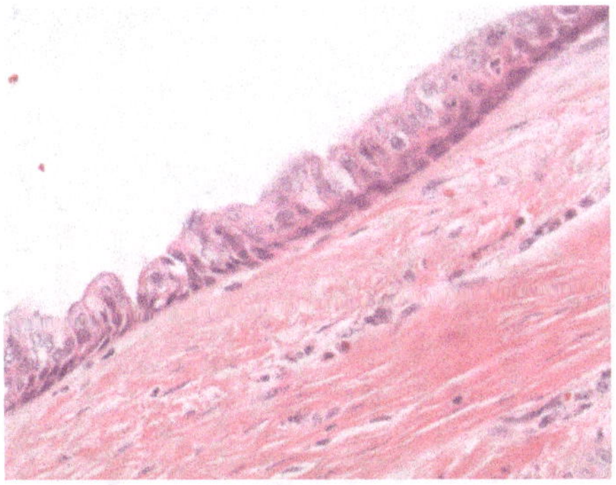

FIGURE 4: The cystic structure is lined by respiratory-type epithelium, consistent with thyroglossal duct cyst (H&E stain, 400x original magnification).

Thyroglossal duct cyst carcinoma (TDCC) is a rare phenomenon and occurs in just 1% of cases of thyroglossal duct cysts [2, 4]. TDCC is more common in females than in males. The mean age of presentation is 6 years in the pediatric population and 38 years in the adult population [4]. Well differentiated thyroid carcinomas account for 95% of TDCC, with papillary cancer being the most common. However, anaplastic thyroid carcinoma and squamous cell carcinoma arising from the cyst have been reported [1].

The origin of TDCC is not entirely clear, whether it arises de novo from the native thyroid tissue in the cyst wall or as a metastasis from the thyroid gland [1, 5]. Interestingly, medullary carcinoma in thyroglossal cyst has never been reported in literature, suggesting a de novo origin of TDCC [5]. In our case, the presence of papillary carcinoma in the thyroglossal duct cyst despite normal thyroid tissue on

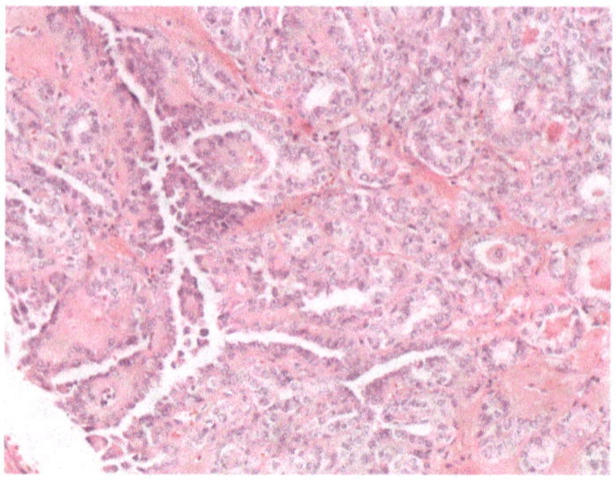

FIGURE 5: The proliferative tumor is characterized by complex and arborizing papillary fronds (H&E stain, 200x original magnification).

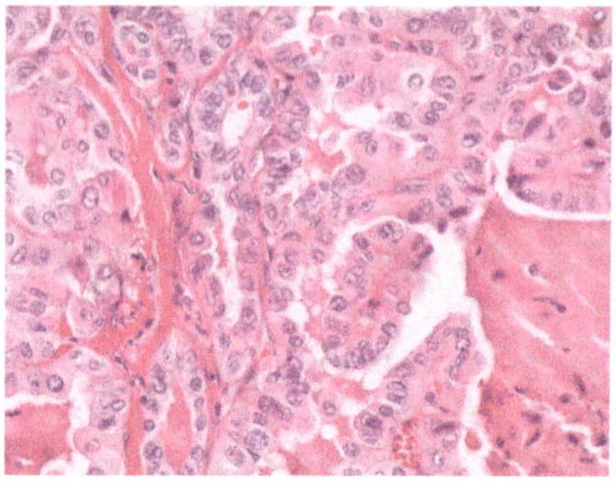

FIGURE 6: High-power view of the tumor, demonstrating cells with nuclear grooves, peripheralization of chromatin, and some prominence of nucleoli, diagnostic of papillary thyroid carcinoma (H&E stain, 400x original magnification).

surgical pathology supports the origin of the cancer from the thyroglossal duct remnant rather than metastasis. The most common papillary carcinomas have indolent growth and an excellent prognosis [1]. In one study, the 5- and 10-year survival rate were found to be 100% and 95.6%, respectively, with no disease-related deaths reported [7].

Most of the time, it is impossible to distinguish the thyroglossal duct cyst harboring malignancy from the benign counterparts [4–6]. Malignancy should be suspected if the thyroglossal duct cyst is hard, irregular, fixed, rapidly growing, and associated with palpable neck lymph nodes [2, 4]. Ultrasonogram (US) and fine needle aspiration cytology (FNAC) of the cyst may help diagnose TDCC preoperatively [5]. Calcifications within the cyst and/or regional calcifications suggest papillary carcinoma while a solid component suggests malignancy. However, TDCC may exist even with a normal US and FNAC [5].

The optimal management of TDCC is still controversial. In the study by de Tristan et al., TDCC was found to be present in just 1.4% (4 out of 352) of thyroglossal duct cysts, and all of them were papillary carcinoma. Three of the 4 patients underwent total thyroidectomy (TT) but none were found to have a second carcinoma in the thyroid suggesting that thyroidectomy was unnecessarily performed [8]. In this regard, some authors suggest tailoring the surgical strategy as per the risk group stratification [5].

Accordingly, it is recommended that the Sistrunk procedure (SP) alone be performed in low risk situations with a clinical and radiologically normal thyroid gland [4, 5]. The low risk situation is defined as age < 45 years, size < 4 cm, no prior radiation exposure, no soft tissue invasion, no distant or lymphatic metastasis, and no aggressive tumor histology [4, 5]. The addition of total thyroidectomy and radioactive iodine ablation (RAI) is done in high risk patients and in cases with positive surgical margins [5]. The rationale is that there was no significant overall survival benefit of TT and RAI in low risk patients. However, Bakkar et al. in their studies found a high rate (62.3%) of concomitant thyroid cancer and recommend routine addition of TT to SP [5]. Moreover, coexisting thyroid cancers may go undetected in US thyroid and the size of a TDCC may not be a reliable predictor of coexisting thyroid carcinoma. In this context, routine TT and RAI would eliminate the latent or residual disease and would positively impact the disease-free survival [5]. This treatment strategy would further facilitate the detection of persistent or recurrent disease based on serum thyroglobulin measurement and RAI scan [5]. However, prophylactic neck dissection is not recommended for papillary TDCC as occult node positivity is common in papillary carcinomas of the thyroid gland, and it does not prognosticate disease recurrence or disease-specific survival [5]. In our case, the patient was an elderly female with muscle invasion at the time of diagnosis, necessitating the need for extensive surgery.

4. Conclusion

TDCC is uncommon and is usually diagnosed postoperatively. The majority of the cases are papillary carcinoma and have a good prognosis with long-term survival. However, controversy still exists regarding the optimal management of TDCC. Whether total thyroidectomy with radioactive ablation and lymph node dissection should be performed even in low risk cases is still not clear, necessitating the need for more prospective studies.

References

[1] D. W. Jang, A. G. Sikora, and A. Leytin, "Thyroglossal duct cyst carcinoma: case report and review of the literature," *Ear, Nose & Throat Journal*, vol. 92, no. 9, pp. E12–E14, 2013.

[2] N. Maleki, M. Iranparvar Alamdari, I. Feizi, and Z. Tavosi, "Papillary carcinoma of the thyroglossal duct cyst: case report," *Iranian Journal of Public Health*, vol. 43, no. 4, pp. 529–531, 2014.

[3] A. K. Lira Medina, E. Fernandez Berdeal, E. Bernal Cisneros, R. Betancourt Galindo, and P. Frigerio, "Incidental papillary thyroid carcinoma in thyroglossal duct cyst case report," *International Journal of Surgery Case Reports*, vol. 29, pp. 4–7, 2016.

[4] R. Akram, J. J. Wiltshire, J. Wadsley, and S. P. Balasubramanian, "Adult thyroglossal duct carcinoma of thyroid epithelial origin: a retrospective observational study," *Indian Journal of Otolaryngology and Head & Neck Surgery*, vol. 68, no. 4, pp. 522–527, 2016.

[5] S. Bakkar, M. Biricotti, G. Stefanini, C. E. Ambrosini, G. Materazzi, and P. Miccoli, "The extent of surgery in thyroglossal cyst carcinoma," *Langenbeck's Archives of Surgery*, pp. 1–6, 2016.

[6] L. Gordini, F. Podda, F. Medas et al., "Tall cell carcinoma arising in a thyroglossal duct cyst: a case report," *Annals of Medicine and Surgery*, vol. 4, no. 2, pp. 129–132, 2015.

[7] S. G. Patel, M. Escrig, A. R. Shaha, B. Singh, and J. P. Shah, "Management of well-differentiated thyroid carcinoma presenting within a thyroglossal duct cyst," *Journal of Surgical Oncology*, vol. 79, no. 3, pp. 134–141, 2002.

[8] J. de Tristan, J. Zenk, J. Künzel, G. Psychogios, and H. Iro, "Thyroglossal duct cysts: 20 years' experience (1992–2011)," *European Archives of Oto-Rhino-Laryngology*, vol. 272, no. 9, pp. 2513–2519, 2014.

31

Case Report and Literature Review of Insulinoma in the Geriatric Population: An 86-Year-Old Female with Syncope of Unknown Origin

Gerry Samantha Eichelberger, [1] **Jordan Carbono**, [2] **Zachary Field**, [2] **KanwarAnoop Kainaur**, [3] **and Federico Montalvo** [1,2]

[1] *Florida State University College of Medicine, 1115 W. Call Street, Tallahassee, FL, USA 32304*
[2] *Department of Internal Medicine, Orlando Regional Healthcare, 21 W. Columbia St., Orlando, FL, USA 32806*
[3] *Department of Pathology, Orlando Regional Healthcare, 52 W. Underwood St., Orlando, FL, USA 32806*

Correspondence should be addressed to Gerry Samantha Eichelberger; gse12@my.fsu.edu

Academic Editor: Suat Simsek

Insulinomas are extremely rare pancreatic endocrine tumors. The tumor is characterized by endogenous hypersecretion of insulin and ensuing development of symptoms of neuroglycopenia and the catecholaminergic response. Symptoms may not always be present, particularly in patients compensating appropriately with increased appetites and caloric intake due to low glucose levels. Early localization of the disease is essential to prevent lethal hypoglycemia and timely treatment. This case report and literature review depict the case of a pancreatic insulinoma in an 86-year-old female, an exceptionally rare presentation based on age and absence of clinical symptoms for one or more years prior to hospitalization. Despite its rarity, similar presentations have been reported in the literature and are further outlined with characteristics and treatment plans. This case highlights a unique presentation of insulinoma and suggests the need for clinical vigilance and further study. It also discusses diagnosis, localization, and management of this uncommon disease in patients above the age of seventy-five.

1. Introduction

Pancreatic endocrine tumors are unusual findings. Among pancreatic endocrine tumors, the most common type is an insulinoma. Insulinomas are in fact quite rare with an annual incidence of four cases per million people in the general population [1]. Insulinomas occur more frequently in women than in men, with a 3 : 2 female-to-male ratio [2]. No racial predilection appears to exist. These tumors typically present in the fifth decade of life with a median age of diagnosis of 47 years of age, except in patients with a history of multiple endocrine neoplasia (MEN) type one syndrome, in whom the median age is typical during the second decade of life [3]. Insulinomas are typically sporadic, benign tumors, with a solitary small (<2 cm in diameter) mass [4]. However, 10% of insulinomas are multiple and occur as a part of MEN type one syndrome. The diagnosis is often delayed or missed due to the rarity of insulinomas and nonspecific symptoms.

Most symptomatic patients present with hypoglycemic episodes resulting from inappropriate intermittent insulin secretion by the tumor. Symptoms can include diaphoresis, tremor, palpitations, tachycardia, and neuroglycopenic symptoms such as personality changes, visual disturbances, weakness, confusion, syncope, seizures, and even coma. Diagnosis is achieved by satisfying the criteria of Whipple's triad—hypoglycemia (plasma glucose <50 mg/dL), neuroglycopenic symptoms, and prompt relief of symptoms following the administration of glucose. The gold standard for biochemical diagnosis includes measuring plasma glucose, insulin, C-peptide, and proinsulin during a 72-hour fast. This prolonged fasting test can detect up to 99% of insulinomas. Approximately 65% of patients will experience hypoglycemic episodes within the first 24 hours of fast [5].

Additionally, more than one imaging modality may be necessary for the localization of the tumor. Localization is performed using computed tomography (CT), magnetic resonance imaging (MRI), endoscopic ultrasonography (EUS), intra-arterial calcium stimulation test with hepatic venous sampling or angiography, and arterial stimulation venous sampling (ARVS). Because of their small size, localization is often difficult. Diagnosis of this pathology relies on a high index of suspicion based on clinical findings and symptomatology along with laboratory testing and imaging to aid in localization. Although medical therapy can be used in the initial treatment, surgical removal is often curative and is the standard of care to prevent permanent neurological deficits associated with prolonged hypoglycemia [6]. Nonetheless, surgery in the elderly population, particularly above the age of 75, can present with a greater risk of complications.

2. Case Presentation

An 86-year-old Caucasian female presents to the emergency room after a syncopal episode. She gives a history of multiple syncopal episodes in the past. Her most recent episode was three months ago and resulted in a fracture of her right femur, which was subsequently treated surgically. Detailed cardiac and neurological evaluations at that time were unable to establish a clear etiology for her syncope. The rest of her pertinent past medical history includes essential hypertension, hyperlipidemia, and breast cancer for which she underwent a bilateral mastectomy. Emergency responders found the patient unresponsive with a blood glucose of 38 mg/dL (70–99 mg/dL fasting). The patient received 50 mL of 50% dextrose in water and became responsive. Repeat glucose was 260 mg/dL. Upon further questioning, the patient admitted to skipping lunch to explain her low blood sugar. She also admitted to having multiple falls of unclear etiology during the past year.

At the time of her current admission, vital signs were notable for an elevated blood pressure of 151/70 mmHg. Physical examination, including complete neurological examination, was normal. Postural blood pressure readings did not show any orthostatic hypotension. Basic laboratory studies including a complete metabolic panel and complete blood count were normal except for the glucose level. Glucose was noted to be 125 mg/dL (70–99 mg/dL fasting). Her hemoglobin A_1C was noted to be 4.7% (4–5.6%); C-peptide was noted to be 2.16 ng/mL (0.78–5.19 ng/mL). Additional workup including TSH, electrocardiogram, troponins, and computerized tomography of the head were within normal limits.

Throughout the hospital course, the patient experienced recurrent hypoglycemic episodes. Fasting blood sugar was as low as 56 mg/dL on day three of her hospitalization requiring frequent doses of intravenous dextrose. Eventually, a continuous dextrose infusion was needed to maintain adequate blood glucose levels. The patient was tested for adrenal insufficiency with a morning cortisol level, which was found to be normal. Additionally, she was screened for exogenous hypoglycemic agents including sulfonylurea levels, which were negative.

Finally, the patient underwent a 72-hour fasting trial to assess for an insulinoma. The patient experienced symptomatic hypoglycemia within 48 hours, with a blood glucose of 32 mg/dL. Fasting trial was discontinued and insulin and C-peptide levels were 22.05 uIU/mL (1.90–23.00 uIU/mL) and 3.61 ng/mL (0.78–5.19 ng/mL), respectively, during the time of the hypoglycemic episode. High normal insulin and normal C-peptide levels in conjunction with very low plasma glucose levels strongly indicated the presence of an insulinoma.

Shown in Figure 1, the computerized tomography scans of the chest, abdomen, and pelvis demonstrated a well-defined enhancing pancreatic tail mass highly suggestive of insulinoma. The computerized tomography scans ruled out metastatic disease. The patient underwent elective laparoscopic-assisted pancreatic mass enucleation on day twelve of her hospitalization. Pathology results showed a low-grade well-differentiated noninvasive pancreatic neuroendocrine tumor, 1.5 cm diameter in size with no invasion present and negative margins as depicted in Figure 2.

Postoperatively, blood glucose levels normalized, without requiring any additional dextrose. The patient was discharged three days later. Two months after her hospitalization, the patient continued to show improvement in her clinical symptoms. She did not report any additional syncopal episodes or falls. Follow-up laboratory work demonstrated euglycemia. Repeat insulin and C-peptide levels were not obtained because of symptomatic improvement.

3. Discussion

Insulinomas have variable and nonspecific presentations particularly in the elderly population usually related to the hypoglycemic episodes. This can be attributable to the episodic and intermittent nature of the secretion of insulin from the tumor. Moreover, the pathogenesis of insulinomas remains unclear. In patients with insulinomas, there is continued secretion of insulin despite a low glucose level. Catecholaminergic and neuroglucopenic symptoms aid in reaching the diagnosis. However, due to the wide range of symptoms and severity, insulinomas can go undiagnosed for a substantial length of time. A broad differential diagnosis of syncope in the geriatric population further prevents prompt diagnosis of insulinoma. In fact, the median duration of symptoms before diagnosis remains variable and can be 12–18 months on average or even years in rarer circumstances from the onset of symptoms [7]. Delayed diagnosis and treatment of insulinomas represents a potentially dangerous condition. Early diagnosis prevents cognitive impairment as well as falls and improves the quality of life of elderly patients.

Insulinomas are defined by meeting Whipple's triad including hypoglycemia (plasma glucose <50 mg/dL),

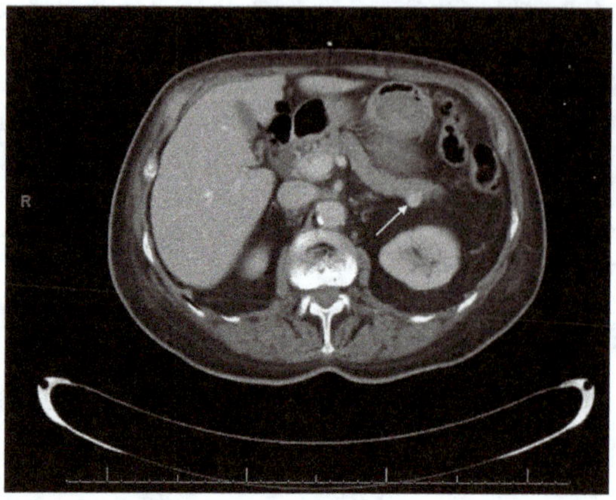

Figure 1: Computerized tomography of the abdomen and pelvis demonstrating enhanced pancreatic tail mass (1.5 cm) suggestive of insulinoma in the setting of unexplained hypoglycemia.

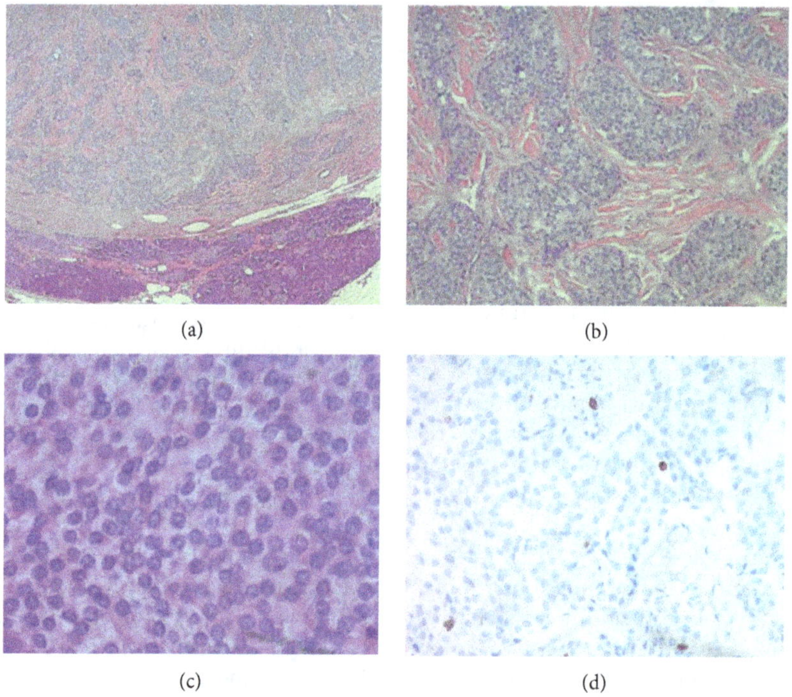

Figure 2: Low-grade pancreatic neuroendocrine tumor. (a) Low-power (20x) view shows a well-circumscribed nested pattern of the tumor cells within the eosinophilic stromal background with adjacent pancreatic parenchyma and (b) 100x view. (c) 400x exhibits uniform nuclei with "salt and pepper" chromatin. (d) 200x shows an immunohistochemical stain for Ki67, which demonstrated 1% reactivity, supporting a low-grade designation.

neuroglycopenic symptoms, and relief of symptoms following the administration of glucose. The 72-hour fasting test remains the gold standard for biochemical diagnosis with measurements of plasma glucose, insulin, C-peptide, and proinsulin levels during the onset of the hypoglycemic episodes. Various imaging modalities may be used to localize the tumor. Imaging type may be limited to what is available at each institution. However, studies have shown a higher sensitivity and preference for helical computerized tomography and endoscopic ultrasound, both of which have up to 94% sensitivity [8]. For most insulinomas, surgery can be curative. Alternatively, medical treatment with octreotide or streptozotocin may be used especially in those with contraindications to surgery or metastatic disease. In cases of malignant insulinomas, an aggressive medical approach is used for enhancing the quality of life by preventing hypoglycemic episodes and improving survival.

Exposure and recognition of an insulinoma case may be limited due to lack of clinical experience amongst healthcare providers. This is especially true in the event of an atypical presentation such as diagnosing insulinomas in the geriatric population. The importance of this case outlines the

TABLE 1: Outline of the literature with insulinoma cases including characteristics of patients, image modality of choice for diagnosis, location of tumor, and treatment plan.

Literature review of insulinomas in elderly patients (above 75 years of age)											
Name of study	Year	Age of presentation	Male vs. fatale	History of multiple endocrine neoplasia	Initial glucose level (mg/dL)	Glucose level within 72-hour fast trial	Imaging modality for diagnosis	Tumor size and location	Metastasis	Surgical management	Medical management
An elderly patient with an insulinoma who had prolonged dementia-like symptoms [12]	1998	77	Female	—	34 mg/dL	—	Abdominal ultrasound; mass not seen on CT or MRI; tumor localized via abdominal arteriography	1 cm tumor localized at the pancreatic tail	—	Pancreatectomy	—
Malignant insulinoma: spectrum of unusual clinical features [13]	2005	82	Female	No	26 mg/dL	—	Abdominal MRI	8.0 cm tumor localized at the dome of the liver	Yes	Percutaneous radiofrequency ablation	—
Successful treatment of insulinoma by a single daily dose of octreotide in two elderly female patients [14]	2006	76	Female	No	—	39 mg/dL after 6 hours	Abdominal angiography	1.5 cm tumor localized at the dome of the liver	No	Refused surgical management	Octreotide 50 μg subcutaneous once daily
Successful treatment of insulinoma by a single daily dose of octreotide in two elderly female patients [14]	2006	85	Female	No	61 mg/dL	37 mg/dL	Abdominal CT	1.5 cm tumor localized at the pancreatic uncus	No	Unsuitable for surgery due to obesity	Initial management was octreotide 100 μg subcutaneous once daily and subsequently reduced to octreotide 50 μg subcutaneous once daily
Pancreatic insulinoma coexisting with gastric GIST in the absence of neurofibromatosis 1 [15]	2009	76	Female	No	—	—	Abdominal CT	1.3 cm localized at the pancreatic tail	No	Pancreatectomy	Initial management with diazoxide

Table 1: Continued.

Literature review of insulinomas in elderly patients (above 75 years of age)											
Insulinoma in the elderly: a report of 3 cases and review literature [11]	2014	82	Female	Yes	—	—	Abdominal MRI	Unknown size; location initially pancreas with metastasis to liver	Yes	Pancreatectomy w/ partial hepatectomy (1993); radiofrequency (2004 and 2006); selective angiographic embolization (2010)	Metastasis in 2011: initial management with subcutaneous injection of octreotide 0.1 mg twice a day and switched to long-acting lanreotide 120 mg every four weeks upon discharge; further progression of metastasis in 2012; lanreotide was switched to diazoxide 100 mg three times a day w/ symptomatic improvement
Insulinoma in the elderly: a report of 3 cases and review literature [11]	2014	84	Male	No	—	—	Abdominal MRI	1 cm tumor localized at pancreatic tail that progressed to 2.2 cm in size	No	Refused surgery (2006); received unsuccessful selective embolization (2012)	Octreotide 0.2 mg three times a day
Insulinoma in the elderly: a report of 3 cases and review literature [11]	2014	85	Male	No	—	—	Abdominal MRI	4 cm tumor localized at the pancreatic head	No	Refused surgical management	Initial management with subcutaneous injection of octreotide 0.1 mg twice a day and switched to long-acting lanreotide 120 mg every four weeks upon discharge
Octreotide LAR was useful for avoiding hypoglycemia in an elderly patient with insulinoma [16]	2017	80	Female	No	—	—	—	—	No	Refused surgical management	Initial management with octreotide 50 mg subcutaneous injection every day; subsequently switched to lanreotide 120 mg every 4 weeks

Table 1: Continued.

Literature review of insulinomas in elderly patients (above 75 years of age)											
Insulinoma case report and literature review of insulinoma in 86-year-old female with late onset hypoglycemia of unknown origin	2020	86	Female	No	38 mg/dL	32 mg/dL	Abdominal CT	1.6 cm tumor localized at pancreatic tail	No	Pancreatectomy with enucleation	—

difficulty in diagnosing insulinomas in patients above the age of seventy-five. Syncopal episodes increase during aging with a prevalence of more than 20% in patients above the age of 75 [9]. Multiple etiologies of syncope exist including cardiovascular disease, arrhythmias, orthostatic hypotension, and neurological causes [10]. Risk factors for hypoglycemia in geriatric patients can include baseline dementia, polypharmacy, and inadequate diet, all of which are common characteristics of patients within this age group, making a diagnosis of an insulinoma more challenging [11]. Nonetheless, it is critical for healthcare providers to maintain insulinoma as a potential diagnosis in this patient population. Missing the diagnosis can lead to morbidity and mortality.

Despite the rarity of this disease, clinicians should be aware of the occurrence of insulinomas in the geriatric population, and how the clinical manifestations can widely vary. Table 1 depicts insulinoma cases in the geriatric population reported in the literature. Insulinomas are not restricted to a particular demographic or age group, as demonstrated by this case. While the classic demographic for insulinomas presents between 40 and 60 years of age, this patient presented at 86 years old, illustrating the wide demographic variance. Creating a proper differential diagnosis and having a high clinical index of suspicion will aid in making a diagnosis earlier. Healthcare providers that encounter syncope in the setting of hypoglycemic episodes should still consider the diagnosis of insulinoma in a geriatric patient. Ultimately, the best treatment is surgical removal or enucleation [11].Laparoscopic surgery can be performed; however, in approximately 44% of cases, open exploration was needed presenting greater possibility of complications [17]. Thus, in the geriatric population, particularly in those above the age of 75, the treatment plan can be medical or surgical. Due to the higher risks of surgical and postsurgical complications in this population, patients and physicians should engage in shared medical decision-making. However, with advancements in surgical techniques, more data are necessary to assess the relative risk and mortality from surgical management.

4. Conclusion

Insulinomas are a rare pancreatic endocrine tumor and disease, but can cause severe neurologic damage and complications resulting from repeated hypoglycemia in geriatric patients. Insulinomas are a difficult diagnosis to make and require a high index of clinical suspicion focusing on the significant recurrent hypoglycemic episodes. It is imperative for physicians to keep in mind insulinomas as a rare cause of syncope in patients above the age of 75 with hypoglycemic episodes, as missing the diagnosis can ultimately lead to morbidity and mortality. Patients and physicians should engage in shared medical decision-making of whether to opt for surgical or medical management, especially in the geriatric population who may be particularly vulnerable to complications.

Acknowledgments

The authors thank Dr. Vinayak Purandare, MD, from Florida State University College of Medicine for peer editing the case report.

References

[1] F. J. Service, M. M. McMahon, P. C. O'Brien, and D. J. Ballard, "Functioning insulinoma—incidence, recurrence, and long-term survival of patients: a 60-year study," *Mayo Clinic Proceedings*, vol. 66, no. 7, pp. 771–779, 1991.

[2] D. Andronesi, A. Andronesi, S. Andrei, A. Tonea, and I. Popescu, "Etiopathogeny of the insulinoma," *Annals of Fundeni Hospital*, vol. 13, no. 1-2, pp. 51–57, 2008.

[3] Z. A. Ali, "Insulinoma," 2013, https://emedicine.medscape.com/article/283039-overview.

[4] R. Sotoudehmanesh, A. Hedayat, N. Shirazian et al., "Endoscopic ultrasonography (EUS) in the localization of insulinoma," *Endocrine*, vol. 31, no. 3, pp. 238–241, 2007.

[5] F. J. Service and N. Natt, "The prolonged fast," *The Journal of Clinical Endocrinology & Metabolism*, vol. 85, no. 11, pp. 3973-3974, 2000.

[6] G. J. Abood, A. Go, D. Malhotra, and M. Shoup, "The surgical and systemic management of neuroendocrine tumors of the pancreas," *Surgical Clinics*, vol. 89, no. 1, pp. 249–266, 2016.

[7] K. Bouslama, H. Maghrebi, H. Bedioui, and K. Bouslama, "Pancreatic insulinoma: diagnostic approach and therapeutic modalities," *Journal Africain d'Hépato-Gastroentérologie*, vol. 8, no. 1, pp. 11–15, 2014.

[8] G. McAuley, H. Delaney, J. Colville et al., "Multimodality preoperative imaging of pancreastic insulinomas," *Clinical Radiology*, vol. 60, no. 10, pp. 1039–1050, 2005.

[9] E. S. Soteriades, J. C. Evans, M. G. Larson et al., "Incidence and prognosis of syncope," *New England Journal of Medicine*, vol. 347, no. 12, pp. 878–885, 2002.

[10] P. Goyal and M. S. Maurer, "Syncope in older adults," *Journal of Geriatric Cardiology*, vol. 13, no. 5, pp. 380–386, 2016.

[11] K. Bernaerts, L. Gers, A. Verhaegen, C. D. Block, and L. V. Gaal, "Insulinoma in the elderly: a report of three cases and review literature," *JSM Clinical Case Reports*, vol. 2, no. 1, p. 1020, 2014.

[12] H. Hattori, M. Matsumoto, H. Tsuchiya et al., "An elderly patient with an insulinoma who had prolonged dementia-like symptoms," *Nippon Ronen Igakkai Zasshi. Japanese Journal of Geriatrics*, vol. 35, no. 7, pp. 566–570, 1998.

[13] B. Hirshberg, C. Cochran, M. C. Skarulis et al., "Malignant insulinoma: spectrum of unusual clinical features," *Cancer*, vol. 104, no. 2, pp. 264–272, 2005.

[14] H. Kishikawa, Y. Okada, A. Hirose, T. Tanikawa, K. Kanda, and Y. Tanaka, "Successful treatment o finsulinoma by a single daily dose of octreotide in two elderly female patients," *Endocrine Journal*, vol. 53, no. 1, pp. 79–85, 2006.

[15] E. Alabraba, S. Bramhall, B. O'Sullivan, B. Mahon, and P. Taniere, "Pancreatic insulinoma co-existing with gastric GIST in the absence of neurofibromatosis-1," *World Journal of Surgical Oncology*, vol. 7, no. 1, p. 18, 2009.

[16] A. Kanno, K. Ide, K. Kurita, T. Terano, and K. Yamamoto, "Octreotide LAR was useful for avoiding hypoglycemia in an elderly patient with insulinoma," *Nihon Ronen Igakkai Zasshi. Japanese Journal of Geriatrics*, vol. 54, no. 2, pp. 172–178, 2017.

[17] D. E. Jaroszewski, R. T. Schlinkert, G. B. Thompson, and D. K. Schlinkert, "Laparoscopic localization and resection of insulinomas," *Archives of Surgery*, vol. 139, no. 3, pp. 270–274, 2004.

32

Treatment of Growth Hormone Deficiency via Daily Intravascular Injections in a Child with Bleeding Disorder

Emir Tas,[1] **Serife E. Uzun**,[2] **Vildan Tas**,[1] **and Juan D. Mejia-Otero**[1]

[1]*Department of Pediatrics, University of Arkansas for Medical Sciences, Little Rock, AR, USA*
[2]*College of Osteopathic Medicine, New York Institute of Technology, Glen Head, Long Island, NY, USA*

Correspondence should be addressed to Emir Tas; etas@uams.edu

Academic Editor: Wayne V. Moore

Objectives. The standard of treatment for pediatric growth hormone deficiency (GHD) is daily subcutaneous recombinant human growth hormone (rhGH) injections. The efficacy of rhGH treatment given as daily intravenous (IV) boluses is not known. *Case Presentation.* A female with protein C deficiency, a severe bleeding disorder characterized by thrombosis formation, was diagnosed with GHD at age four years. She has been receiving daily protein C infusion through a permanent port since the newborn period. GHD was treated with daily IV rhGH boluses given through the port following protein C infusion. She has reached a growth rate of 12 cm/year and had no side effects. Surprisingly, serum insulin-like growth factor-1 (IGF1) levels did not rise despite an excellent clinical response. *Conclusions.* IV administration may be an alternative route for GHD treatment in eligible patients with permanent vascular access. A rise in serum IGF1 levels may not be needed to achieve the growth-promoting effect of rhGH.

1. Introduction

Short stature is one of the most common referral reasons to pediatric endocrinology clinics. Among the various etiologies of short stature, growth hormone (GH) deficiency is the most common endocrine cause. Growth hormone deficiency (GHD) is estimated to have a prevalence of 1 in 4,000 to 10,000 and can be due to genetic defects, acquired causes, or idiopathic. Untreated GHD may have a profound impact on the overall health of the affected children with lasting consequences beyond childhood. Presenting symptoms and signs vary depending on the age of onset, but children with GHD usually come to medical attention with decelerated or stunted linear growth, delayed bone development, and delayed puberty. Screening tests for suspected GHD include measurement of serum growth factors, particularly insulin-like growth factor (IGF)-1, which is also used to assess adherence and monitor safety and as a guide to titrate GH dose during treatment. IGF1 is the primary mediator of GH-stimulated bone growth. Currently, the standard treatment of GHD involves daily subcutaneous injections of recombinant human growth hormone (rhGH). However, this administration route may be a source of stress in parents of children with severe underlying bleeding pathologies because of cutaneous bleeding risk. Although the likelihood of hitting a large vein in subcutaneous fat is practically zero, the parental anxiety associated with this may lead to nonadherence to GH treatment in such patients. There is a lack of knowledge regarding the efficacy and safety of daily intravenous (IV) administration of rhGH to treat GHD. We report the case of a patient with protein C deficiency who was diagnosed with GHD and successfully treated via daily IV rhGH boluses through an established port. To our knowledge, the IV route has not been previously used for long-term rhGH replacement therapy.

2. Case Presentation

A 2-year 5-month-old female was referred to for evaluation of short stature. She was born at term with a birth weight of 3845 grams and a length of 51 cm. Her history was notable for prolonged Neonatal Intensive-Care Unit (NICU) stay due to disseminated intravascular coagulation (DIC) characterized by multiple skin bruises and respiratory distress.

She required a chest tube and G-tube placement to treat chylothorax and feeding problems, respectively, and transfusion of multiple blood products to manage DIC. After an extensive workup, she was diagnosed with protein C deficiency and has begun daily IV protein C concentrate (Ceprotin®) treatment. She had no pulmonary or cardiac comorbidities upon discharge from the NICU around four months of age. The brain magnetic resonance imaging (MRI) showed nonspecific white matter injury with multiple small subdural bleeds with no known neurological sequela. She also developed right-sided blindness due to retinal detachment.

On presentation to the endocrinology clinic, she plotted below one percentile in the height-for-age and at the third percentile in the weight-for-age charts (Figure 1).

She was in no acute distress and had normal vital signs. She was developmentally at par for age. Physical examination was notable for the presence of a subcutaneous port-a-cath on the left upper chest for daily protein C concentrate infusion and well-healed small scar tissues on her chest and abdomen. She had no red reflex on the right eye and self-amputated toes on the left foot. There were no organomegaly or any other dysmorphic features. Laboratory showed undetectable insulin-like growth factor-1 (IGF-1) (<15 ng/mL) and low IGF-binding protein-3 (BP 3) (0.65 mg/L, reference range 0.8–3.9) levels, but normal thyroid studies (Table 1).

Over the next two years, she did not show catch-up growth despite improved nutritional status (Figure 1). She failed to demonstrate a normal response to the arginine-clonidine provocation test with a peak GH level of only 4.4 ng/mL and was diagnosed with GHD. Repeat brain MRI showed hypoplastic anterior pituitary without any evidence of residual white matter damage. Recombinant hGH therapy was recommended. Due to concerns of extensive bruising with daily rhGH subcutaneous injections, parents requested a trial of IV administration of rhGH therapy via her port-a-cath. They agreed to switch to subcutaneous administration if there were poor response. Parents were made aware of the off-label use of IV rhGH therapy and signed informed consent after obtaining clearance from the hematologist. The patient started standard rhGH therapy at a standard subcutaneous dose (0.3 mg/kg/week) at age 4 years and 9 months via daily IV boluses through her port-a-cath following daily protein C infusions. She had an excellent response with a growth velocity of 12 cm/year in the first year of treatment without any adverse effects. Surveillance tests for thyroid and glucose tolerance were normal. Linear growth was accompanied by a modest increase in serum IGF-1 levels a few months after starting rhGH therapy with a slight further rise in serum IGF-1 levels after 16 months of rhGH therapy (Table 1).

3. Discussion

Herein, we describe a child with congenital protein C deficiency who was later diagnosed with GHD. Congenital protein C deficiency is a rare and severe bleeding disorder, characterized by a hypercoagulable state as a result of homozygous or compound heterozygous mutation of the PROC gene [1]. Affected infants may present with purpura fulminans, disseminated intravascular coagulation (DIC), or intracranial hemorrhage due to venous thrombosis [2]. Prompt recognition of this condition is important as a delay in treatment initiation may result in irreversible consequences. Our patient presented with DIC in the newborn period with extensive skin bruising and has then suffered blindness, self-amputated toes, and white matter changes in the brain. She has had no further bleeding after protein C treatment has begun. However, she was found to have a small anterior pituitary gland while being worked up for GHD. Schmitt et al. described a case with suspected protein C deficiency who later developed hypothalamic failure manifesting with combined pituitary hormone deficiencies, including GHD [3]. Cerebrovascular occlusion due to protein C deficiency was hypothesized to be the etiology of panhypopituitarism. To our knowledge, isolated GHD has not been described previously in a patient with protein C deficiency.

Growth hormone has multiple effects on various tissues and organs in the body. Besides playing a crucial role in linear growth, it also has vital functions in metabolism and cardiovascular physiology [4]. GH regulates the endothelial function and hepatic synthesis of some coagulation factors. Studies in adults linked GHD and adverse cardiovascular outcomes, including increased thromboembolic events, but pediatric data are lacking [5]. Therefore, diagnosis and treatment of GHD in a child with an underlying bleeding disorder maybe even more important than simply focusing on the effect of GH on linear growth.

The somatomedin hypothesis suggests that GH mediates its functions, including bone growth, mainly through the induction of hepatic IGF1, which activates transmembranous receptors in chondrocytes [6]. However, Wu et al., in their animal studies, demonstrated that GH could independently promote linear bone growth even when the local IGF1 action is prevented [7]. Although the serum IGF1 level of our patient has fairly increased following over one year of GH replacement, it has remained below two standard deviations for age and sex. Our observation supports the notion that GH may promote linear growth independent of a significant increase in serum IGF1 levels even in humans.

The current standard approach for the treatment of GHD is daily subcutaneous injection of recombinant rhGH. However, this route of administration presented a challenge in our patient due to the risk of extensive bruising. Per parent's request and after clearance from her hematologist, we agreed to attempt a trial of intravenous administration of rhGH via her port-a-cath with an option to switch to subcutaneous administration if clinical responses were suboptimal. The half-life of exogenous rhGH is estimated to be around 10–15 minutes [8]. Jørgensen et al. showed that a single IV rhGH bolus in healthy adult men increased mRNA expression of IGF1 in adipose, but not in muscle tissue [9]. In a previous study conducted by the same group, the researchers compared the effects of three different IV rhGH administration schedules (two large boluses at 2000 and 0200 hours. vs. eight small boluses separated at 3-hour intervals vs. continuous infusion between 2000 and 0200

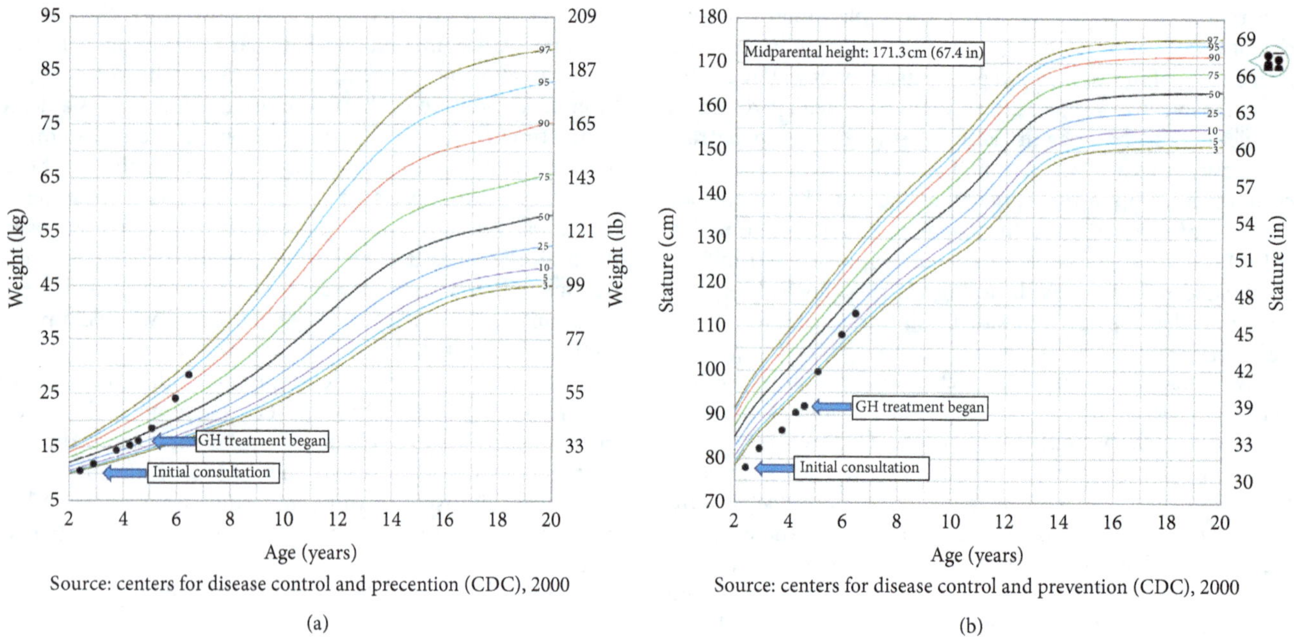

FIGURE 1: The weight (a) and height (b) data, at the time of initial consultation and when the growth hormone treatment has begun, indicated by arrows. GH, growth hormone.

TABLE 1: Laboratory results of selected biomarkers of the patient before and after growth hormone treatment.

Age (years, months)	$2^{5/12}$ years (before rhGH)	$3^{2/12}$ years (before rhGH)	$5^{2/12}$ years (5 months after rhGH)	$6^{1/12}$ years (16 months after rhGH)
IGF1 concentration (ng/mL)	<15	<15	29	41
IGF1 SDS score			−2.33	−2.17
IGFBP3 concentration (mg/L, RR: 0.8–3.9)	0.65	0.8	1.6	
TSH (mIU/L)	2.1		2.6	1.3
Free T4 (ng/dL)	1.1		0.9	0.9
Albumin (gr/dL)			4.3	
ALT (IU/L)			27	
AST (IU/L)			20	
HbA1c (%)			4.7	4.5
Protein C functional (%, RR: 40–92)	14	14	11	12

hours) on metabolic markers and IGF1 level. They found that the same amount of rhGH given as the two large boluses generated similar and significant metabolic responses on glucose and lipid markers than at baseline. All three schedules resulted in a considerable increase in IGF1 levels, but the two IV bolus groups had lower peaks in IGF1 and quicker return to baseline than the other two schedules [10]. The authors speculated that the serum GH level might need to be sustained above zero for prolonged periods to achieve its growth-promoting effects. In our patient, daily IV rhGH boluses markedly improved linear growth despite a modest increase of serum IGF1 levels.

Growth hormone stimulates hepatic IGF1 production via the activation of transmembranous receptors. Whether the expression of liver GH receptors is altered in patients with protein C deficiency or the administration of protein C concentrate immediately before the rhGH boluses had suppressed the normal hepatic response is not known. There is no standard dose for IV rhGH replacement. Moreover, we did not assess this treatment's direct effects on lipid metabolism, body composition, or cardiovascular markers. These would have provided direct evidence on the metabolic benefits of rhGH treatment on this patient.

4. Conclusions

IV administration may be an alternative route for treating GHD in eligible patients with permanent vascular access if there are challenges or potential side effects of subcutaneous administration. A significant rise in serum IGF1 levels may not be needed to achieve the growth-promoting effect of IV rhGH therapy.

Disclosure

The abstract of this manuscript was presented as a virtual poster at the annual Pediatric Endocrine Society meeting held online from April 30 to May 3, 2021.

References

[1] S. Ohga, A. Ishiguro, Y. Takahashi et al., "Protein C deficiency as the major cause of thrombophilias in childhood," *Pediatrics International*, vol. 55, no. 3, pp. 267–271, 2013.

[2] P. N. Knoebl, "Severe congenital protein C deficiency: the use of protein C concentrates (human) as replacement therapy for life-threatening blood-clotting complications," *Biologics: Targets & Therapy*, vol. 2, pp. 285–296, 2008.

[3] S. Schmitt, K. Auberger, T. Fendel, and W. Kiess, "Hypothalamic failure as a sequela of heterozygous protein C deficiency?" *European Journal of Pediatrics*, vol. 151, no. 6, pp. 428–431, 1992.

[4] J. Devesa, C. Almengló, and P. Devesa, "Multiple effects of growth hormone in the body: is it really the hormone for growth?" *Clinical Medicine Insights: Endocrinology and Diabetes*, vol. 9, Article ID CMED.S38201, 2016.

[5] C. Gazzaruso, M. Gola, I. Karamouzis, R. Giubbini, and A. Giustina, "Cardiovascular risk in adult patients with growth hormone (GH) deficiency and following substitution with GH—an update," *The Journal of Clinical Endocrinology & Metabolism*, vol. 99, no. 1, pp. 18–29, 2014.

[6] D. Le Roith, C. Bondy, S. Yakar, J.-L. Liu, and A. Butler, "The somatomedin hypothesis: 2001," *Endocrine Reviews*, vol. 22, no. 1, pp. 53–74, 2001.

[7] S. Wu, W. Yang, and F. De Luca, "Insulin-like growth factor-independent effects of growth hormone on growth plate chondrogenesis and longitudinal bone growth," *Endocrinology*, vol. 156, no. 7, pp. 2541–2551, 2015.

[8] P. C. Hindmarsh, D. R. Matthews, C. E. Brain et al., "The half-life of exogenous growth hormone after suppression of endogenous growth hormone secretion with somatostatin," *Clinical Endocrinology*, vol. 30, no. 4, pp. 443–450, 1989.

[9] J. O. L. Jørgensen, N. Jessen, S. B. Pedersen et al., "GH receptor signaling in skeletal muscle and adipose tissue in human subjects following exposure to an intravenous GH bolus," *American Journal of Physiology-Endocrinology and Metabolism*, vol. 291, no. 5, pp. E899–E905, 2006.

[10] J. O. L. Jørgensen, N. Møller, T. Lauritzen, and J. S. Christiansen, "Pulsatile versus continuous intravenous administration of growth hormone (GH) in GH-deficient patients: effects on circulating insulin-like growth factor-i and metabolic indices," *The Journal of Clinical Endocrinology & Metabolism*, vol. 70, no. 6, pp. 1616–1623, 1990.

33

An Interesting Cause of Hyperandrogenemic Hirsutism

Murat Atmaca,[1] İsmet Seven,[2] Rıfkı Üçler,[1] Murat Alay,[1] Veysi Barut,[2] Yaren Dirik,[2] and Yasin Sezgin[2]

[1]*Department of Endocrinology and Metabolism, Yuzuncu Yil University Faculty of Medicine, 65100 Van, Turkey*
[2]*Department of Internal Medicine, Yuzuncu Yil University Faculty of Medicine, 65100 Van, Turkey*

Correspondence should be addressed to Murat Atmaca; drmuratatmaca@hotmail.com

Academic Editor: Hidetoshi Ikeda

Mild clinical signs of hyperandrogenism such as hirsutism may appear during the menopausal transition as part of the normal aging process, but the development of frank virilization suggests a specific source of androgen excess. We report a case of a 68-year-old woman with signs of virilization that had started 6 months before. Clinical analyses revealed high levels of serum testosterone for a postmenopausal woman. Pelvic MRI and abdomen CT showed no evidence of ovarian and adrenal tumor. Postmenopausal hyperandrogenism can be the result of numerous etiologies ranging from normal physiologic changes to ovarian or rarely adrenal tumors. Our patient was found to have iatrogenic hyperandrogenism. This condition is rarely reported cause of virilization.

1. Introduction

The postmenopausal ovary remains hormonally active and secreting significant amounts of androgens and relatively less estrogens many years after menopause [1]. Although estrogen levels are reduced abruptly after menopause, androgen secretion declines gradually with aging and is maintained until later stages of life [2, 3]. Androgen secretion in pre- and postmenopausal ovaries depends on LH stimulation. The very high gonadotropin levels of menopause could maintain ovarian androgen production [2, 3]. This imbalance between estrogens and androgens after menopause is amplified further by the evolving decrease in sex hormone binding globulin (SHBG) concentrations and the subsequent increase of free androgen index [4]. As a result, menopause may be accompanied by the appearance of a few terminal hairs in the face and by a decrease in body and scalp hair that can be considered part of the normal menopausal process [5].

The development of true hirsutism (defined as the presence of excessive terminal hair in androgen-dependent areas), alopecia, or acne should not be considered normal in postmenopausal women. The main differential diagnosis of androgen excess in postmenopausal women is either tumoral causes, namely, androgen-secreting ovarian or adrenal tumors, or nontumoral causes, that is, polycystic ovarian syndrome, hyperthecosis, Cushing's syndrome, congenital adrenal hyperplasia, and iatrogenesis [6].

When hirsutism is accompanied by signs of virilization such as severe balding, deepening of the voice, or clitoromegaly, an underlying androgen-secreting tumor that may be malignant must be ruled out.

Here, a 68-year-old postmenopausal case with virilization is presented with a discussion referenced to the medical literature.

2. Case Report

A 68-year-old female was admitted in our clinic with complaints like gradually increased hirsutism and deepening of the voice. She was menopause at 52 years old and she has eight children. The medical history of the case showed that she was followed up due to hypertension for 5 years and had good tension control with telmisartan 80 mg daily. Also medical history of the case showed that she was diagnosed with osteoarthrosis and used some creams which contain probably nonsteroidal anti-inflammatory drugs but she does not remember the names of this drugs. She did not have any outstanding condition in family history. Her arterial blood pressure was measured as 140/90 mmHg, pulse was 84 beats/min, and body temperature was 36.9°C in

Table 1: Hormonal profiles of case.

	Normal range	Result
Follicle stimulating hormone	26,7–133,41 IU/L	30,09 IU/L
Luteinizing hormone	10,39–64,57 IU/L	13,04 IU/L
Estradiol	0–73,42 pmol/L	55,06 pmol/L
Total testosterone	0,38–1,97 nmol/L	25,40 nmol/L
Sex hormone binding globulin	19,8–155,2 nmol/L	43,1 nmol/L
Progesterone	0–636 pmol/L	318 pmol/L
17 OH progesterone	605–2723 pmol/L	302,57 pmol/L
Adrenocorticotropin hormone	0–10 pmol/L	3,3 pmol/L
Cortisol	100–535 nmol/L	330 nmol/L
1 mg dexamethasone suppression test	0–50 nmol/L	2,7 nmol/L
Dehydroepiandrosterone sulfate	270–540 nmol/L	508 nmol/L

her physical examination. Her face was plethoric and in her skin there was hirsutism especially in upper lip, chin, and upper abdomen areas. In these areas Ferriman-Gallwey score was 4. Abdomen and cardiovascular and respiratory system were also observed to be normal. There was no clitoromegaly or temporal baldness. In the hemogram of our case, polycythemia was observed (hemoglobin: 18 g/dL, hematocrit 54%). The electrolyte levels and biochemical levels were revealed to be normal. Testosterone was found to be 25,40 nmol/L in our case who was suspected to have hyperandrogenism due to the existent clinical pattern (testosterone normal range for women: 0,38–1,97 nmol/L). The other hormonal parameters were shown in Table 1. The case was hospitalized for differential diagnoses of hyperandrogenism including polycystic ovary syndrome (PCOS), congenital adrenal hyperplasia (CAH), Cushing's syndrome, and benign and malignant androgen-secreting ovarian and adrenal tumors. 17 OH progesterone level was detected 302,57 pmol/L and diagnosis of CAH was excluded. 1 mg dexamethasone suppression test was detected 2,7 nmol/L and Cushing's syndrome was excluded. Pelvic MRI and abdomen CT for androgen-secreting ovarian and adrenal tumors revealed that there was no adrenal and ovarian mass. In this imaging study right and left ovaries sizes, respectively, were 22 × 12 mm and 22 × 14 mm and adrenal configuration and size were normal. On the 4th day of her hospitalization, the control testosterone levels were detected 12 nmol/L. Testosterone levels were decreased every other day, respectively, 7,4 nmol/L, 4,3 nmol/L, and 2,1 nmol/L. This gradual decrease in testosterone levels was suggested to be due to exogenous androgen exposed. In our interview with the patient's husband it was showed that he has used transdermal testosterone gel since a year for impotence. Hyperandrogenism in our cases could be passed from her husband application region by skin contact. Our patient's husband has hidden his illness from patient and he said that he uses this gel for myalgia. Our patient has been using the husband's transdermal testosterone gel unconsciously for knee pain for 6 months.

3. Discussion

Mild hirsutism and alopecia in postmenopausal women can be considered part of the normal menopausal process [5]. The development of true hirsutism, alopecia, or acne should not be considered normal in postmenopausal women. The main differential diagnoses of androgen excess in postmenopausal women are polycystic ovary syndrome (PCOS), congenital adrenal hyperplasia (CAH), Cushing's syndrome, benign and malignant androgen-secreting ovarian and adrenal tumors, and iatrogenic causes [6].

PCOS is the most common cause of hyperandrogenism in women at reproductive age and diagnostic criteria are well defined in premenopausal women [7]. However, PCOS in postmenopausal women is not well defined, as no robust criteria are currently available and only recently age-based criteria for the definition of PCOS have been proposed [7–9]. In women with PCOS symptoms usually start in adolescence and gradually progress during reproductive years [10]. Our case's hirsutism occurred six months ago and deepening of the voice is concomitant with this symptom. Virilization symptoms and very high testosterone levels suggested excluding PCOS.

Congenital adrenal hyperplasia (CAH) is another cause of hyperandrogenism. Enzymatic deficiencies causing adrenal hyperplasia and excessive androgen production are mainly due to 21-hydroxylase and rarely to 3β-hydroxysteroid dehydrogenase and 11β-hydroxylase deficiencies [11–13]. Most of CAH cases are diagnosed and treated at a much younger age [14]. High testosterone levels such as our cases can be seen in simple virilizing or salt losing forms of CAH; however, these forms of CAH are associated with adrenal insufficiency and high ACTH, both of which the patient did not have.

Nonclassic adrenal hyperplasia (NCAH) arising from 21-hydroxylase deficiency is found in 1–10% of hyperandrogenic women depending on ethnicity and is associated with elevated 17-hydroxy-progesterone and adrenal androgen levels [11]. The prevalence of hirsutism in women with NCAH increases with age and the degree of hyperandrogenism may worsen in postmenopausal women [15]. In our case's medical history hirsutism occurred six months ago and before six months there was not any compliant of hirsutism. In reproductive her menscycles are regular along reproductive age. There was no adrenal hyperplasia or nodular lesion in abdomen CT and 17 OH progesterone levels were normal range. For these reasons NCAH was excluded.

Cushing's syndrome (CS) may also be diagnosed after menopause and cause symptoms or signs of androgen excess. Hirsutism can be found in approximately 50% of patients with CS mainly attributed to adrenal androgen excess; endogenous hypercortisolism also correlates positively with free androgen levels probably due to SHBG reduction [16]. In contrast to CS secondary to adrenal carcinomas, signs of hyperandrogenism are usually mild in women with the adrenocorticotropin-(ACTH-) dependent CS and are virtually absent in women with adrenal adenomas [17]. There was no adrenal mass in adrenal CT and 1 mg dexamethasone suppression test was detected 2,7 nmol/L and Cushing's syndrome was excluded.

When hirsutism is more severe and accompanied by symptoms or signs of virilization, ovarian hyperthecosis, adrenals, or the ovarian tumors should be excluded [6, 18].

The main nontumoral cause of postmenopausal ovarian biochemical hyperandrogenism seems to be ovarian hyperthecosis [19]. Hyperthecosis is a severe form of PCOS and results from an overproduction of androgens in the ovarian stromal cells [20]. Women typically present with slowly progressive acne and hirsutism (e.g., excessive male pattern hair growth), and they are likely to be virilized [21]. Although the exact aetiology is unclear, some authors claım that hyperthecosis ın postmenopausel women originate from elevated gonodotrophin productions. Patients with hyperthecosis typically have normal serum dehydroepiandrosterone sulfate (DHEA sulfate) concentrations [22, 23]. Ultrasonography in women with hyperthecosis usually shows a bilateral increase in ovarian stroma and the ovaries appear more solid [24]. Similarly MRI findings in ovarian hyperthecosis include symmetric bilateral ovarian enlargement [25]. Serious hyperandrogenemia, virilization symptoms, and normal DHEAS levels suggested hyperthecosis in our case but in pelvic MRI showed atrophic ovaries.

Tumorous hyperandrogenism is suspected when testosterone levels are greater than 3,5–5 nmol/L and is usually associated with abrupt onset and rapid evolution of symptoms or virilization [26]. Adrenal androgen-secreting tumors are rare but highly suggestive of malignancy. These tumors are easily identified on imaging techniques. Patients with adrenal androgen-secreting tumors typically have elevated serum dehydroepiandrosterone sulfate (DHEA sulfate) concentrations [27]. In our case DHEAS levels was normal and adrenal imaging did not detect any mass.

Androgen-producing ovarian tumors include lipoid, Leydig cell, granulosa-theca cell, and Sertoli-stromal cell tumors. These tumours are rare representing only 10% of all ovarian tumours [28, 29]. Ovarian androgen-secreting tumors are not easily identified in imaging techniques. Their ultrasonographic aspect depends on tumor type and ultrasonography studies for Sertoli-Leydig, steroid cell tumors, and thecomas have been reported negative in postmenopausal women [30–33]. Rapidly progressive virilization symptoms and very high testosterone levels suggested tumoral causes. Negativity of ovarian imaging does not exclude ovarian malignancy. Ovarian sampling, bilateral oophorectomy, or GnRH analogue treatment is suggested in these cases. Ovarian sampling is very difficult and invasive and, even at the best centers, sampling can accurately localize the ovarian tumor only 66% of the time [34].

We detected serious decrease in control testosterone levels. This condition, before further investigation, was suggested exogenous androgen exposed. Testosterone levels were decreased gradually every other day. Our patient has been using the husband's transdermal testosterone gel unconsciously for knee pain for 6 months. Iatrogenic or self-administration of androgenic drugs and supplements can induce symptoms and signs of hyperandrogenism via an increase in circulating androgen levels or an intrinsic androgenic activity of the drug. Drugs most commonly responsible include androgens, anabolic steroids, and antiepileptics [35]. Several case reports show that topical androgens may result in clinical syndromes of hyperandrogenism in exposed children and women [36].

In conclusion, iatrogenic causes of hyperandrogenemia should be kept in mind in differential diagnosis of hyperandrogenemia. Hospitalization to prevent from exposure and sequential testosterone level measurement can help in this condition's diagnosis.

References

[1] R. H. Fogle, F. Z. Stanczyk, X. Zhang, and R. J. Paulson, "Ovarian androgen production in postmenopausal women," *Journal of Clinical Endocrinology and Metabolism*, vol. 92, no. 8, pp. 3040–3043, 2007.

[2] A. V. Sluijmer, M. J. Heineman, F. H. de Jong, and J. L. H. Evers, "Endocrine activity of the postmenopausal ovary: the effects of pituitary down-regulation and oophorectomy," *The Journal of Clinical Endocrinology & Metabolism*, vol. 80, no. 7, pp. 2163–2167, 1995.

[3] E. Y. Adashi, "The climacteric ovary as a functional gonadotropin-driven androgen- producing gland," *Fertility and Sterility*, vol. 62, no. 1, pp. 20–27, 1994.

[4] S. Gershagen, A. Doeberl, S. Jeppsson, and G. Rannevik, "Decreasing serum levels of sex hormone-binding globulin around the menopause and temporary relation to changing levels of ovarian steroids, as demonstrated in a longitudinal study," *Fertility and Sterility*, vol. 51, no. 4, pp. 616–621, 1989.

[5] P. K. Thomas and D. G. Ferriman, "Variation in facial and public hair growth in white women," *American Journal of Physical Anthropolog*, vol. 15, no. 2, pp. 171–180, 1957.

[6] M. S. Rothman and M. E. Wierman, "How should postmenopausal androgen excess be evaluated?" *Clinical Endocrinology*, vol. 75, no. 2, pp. 160–164, 2011.

[7] R. S. Legro, S. A. Arslanian, D. A. Ehrmann et al., "Diagnosis and treatment of polycystic ovary syndrome: an endocrine society clinical practice guideline," *Journal of Clinical Endocrinology and Metabolism*, vol. 98, no. 12, pp. 4565–4592, 2013.

[8] D. Shah and S. Bansal, "Polycystic ovaries-beyond menopause," *Climacteric*, vol. 17, no. 2, pp. 109–115, 2014.

[9] S. Alsamarai, J. M. Adams, M. K. Murphy et al., "Criteria for polycystic ovarian morphology in polycystic ovary syndrome as a function of age," *The Journal of Clinical Endocrinology & Metabolism*, vol. 94, no. 12, pp. 4961–4970, 2009.

[10] R. Pasquali and A. Gambineri, "Polycystic ovary syndrome: a multifaceted disease from adolescence to adult age," *Annals of the New York Academy of Sciences*, vol. 1092, pp. 158–174, 2006.

[11] R. Azziz, L. A. Sanchez, E. S. Knochenhauer et al., "Androgen excess in women: experience with over 1000 consecutive patients," *Journal of Clinical Endocrinology and Metabolism*, vol. 89, no. 2, pp. 453–462, 2004.

[12] R. Azziz, E. L. Bradley Jr., H. D. Potter, and L. R. Boots, "3β-hydroxysteroid dehydrogenase deficiency in hyperandrogenism," *American Journal of Obstetrics & Gynecology*, vol. 168, no. 3 I, pp. 889–895, 1993.

[13] R. Azziz, L. R. Boots, C. R. Parker Jr., E. Bradley Jr., and H. A. Zacur, "11β-Hydroxylase deficiency in hyperandrogenism," *Fertility and Sterility*, vol. 55, no. 4, pp. 733–741, 1991.

[14] P. W. Speiser, R. Azziz, L. S. Baskin et al., "Congenital adrenal hyperplasia due to steroid 21-hydroxylase deficiency: an Endocrine Society clinical practice guideline," *Journal of Clinical Endocrinology and Metabolism*, vol. 95, no. 9, pp. 4133–4160, 2010.

[15] C. Moran, R. Azziz, E. Carmina et al., "21-hydroxylase-deficient nonclassic adrenal hyperplasia is a progressive disorder: a multicenter study," *American Journal of Obstetrics & Gynecology*, vol. 183, no. 6, pp. 1468–1474, 2000.

[16] G. A. Kaltsas, M. Korbonits, A. M. Isidori et al., "How common are polycystic ovaries and the polycystic ovarian syndrome in women with Cushing's syndrome?" *Clinical Endocrinology*, vol. 53, no. 4, pp. 493–500, 2000.

[17] C. Bertagna and D. N. Orth, "Clinical and laboratory findings and results of therapy in 58 patients with adrenocortical tumors admitted to a single medical center (1951 to 1978)," *American Journal of Medicine*, vol. 71, no. 5, pp. 855–875, 1981.

[18] M. Alpañés, J. M. González-Casbas, J. Sánchez, H. Pián, and H. F. Escobar-Morreale, "Management of postmenopausal virilization," *Journal of Clinical Endocrinology and Metabolism*, vol. 97, no. 8, pp. 2584–2588, 2012.

[19] S. Vaikkakara, E. Al-Ozairi, E. Lim et al., "The investigation and management of severe hyperandrogenism pre- and postmenopause: non-tumor disease is strongly associated with metabolic syndrome and typically responds to insulin-sensitization with metformin," *Gynecological Endocrinology*, vol. 24, no. 2, pp. 87–92, 2008.

[20] S. S. Braithwaite, B. Erkman-Balis, and T. D. Avila, "Postmenopausal virilization due to ovarian stromal hyperthecosis," *Journal of Clinical Endocrinology and Metabolism*, vol. 46, no. 2, pp. 295–300, 1978.

[21] S. H. Geist and J. A. Gaines, "Diffuse luteinization of the ovaries associated with the masculinization syndrome," *The American Journal of Obstetrics and Gynecology*, vol. 43, no. 6, pp. 975–983, 1942.

[22] R. Lindgren, C. Gunnarsson, A. Jakobsson, and M. Hammar, "Hypersecretion of ovarian androgens may be gonadotrophin dependent many years after menopause," *Maturitas*, vol. 34, no. 1, pp. 43–46, 2000.

[23] E. Krug and S. L. Berga, "Postmenopausal hyperthecosis: functional dysregulation of androgenesis in climacteric ovary," *Obstetrics & Gynecology*, vol. 99, no. 5, pp. 893–897, 2002.

[24] P. Rousset, A. Gompel, S. Christin-Maitre et al., "Ovarian hyperthecosis on grayscale and color Doppler ultrasound," *Ultrasound in Obstetrics and Gynecology*, vol. 32, no. 5, pp. 694–699, 2008.

[25] A. B. Rosenkrantz, D. Popiolek, G. L. Bennett, and E. M. Hecht, "Magnetic resonance imaging appearance of ovarian stromal hyperplasia and ovarian hyperthecosis," *Journal of Computer Assisted Tomography*, vol. 33, no. 6, pp. 912–916, 2009.

[26] C. I. Friedman, G. E. Schmidt, M. H. Kim, and J. Powell, "Serum testosterone concentrations in the evaluation of androgen-producing tumors," *The American Journal of Obstetrics and Gynecology*, vol. 153, no. 1, pp. 44–49, 1985.

[27] R. Libè, A. Fratticci, and J. Bertherat, "Adrenocortical cancer: pathophysiology and clinical management," *Endocrine-Related Cancer*, vol. 14, no. 1, pp. 13–28, 2007.

[28] K. Ireland and J. D. Woodruff, "Masculinizing ovarian tumors," *Obstetrical & Gynecological Survey*, vol. 31, no. 2, pp. 83–111, 1976.

[29] H. Fox, "Sex cord-stromal tumours of the ovary," *The Journal of Pathology*, vol. 145, no. 2, pp. 127–148, 1985.

[30] E. K. Outwater, B. Marchetto, and B. J. Wagner, "Virilizing tumors of the ovary: imaging features," *Ultrasound in Obstetrics and Gynecology*, vol. 15, no. 5, pp. 365–371, 2000.

[31] O. A. Sanz, P. R. Martinez, R. T. Guarch, M. J. I. Goñi, and J. L. Z. Alcazar, "Bilateral Leydig cell tumour of the ovary: a rare cause of virilization in postmenopausal patient," *Maturitas*, vol. 57, no. 2, pp. 214–216, 2007.

[32] D. Sanyal, W. G. Taylor, and M. I. Otter, "Bilateral thecomata in ovaries with normal ultrasonographic and radiological appearances, presenting with postmenopausal hirsutism and virilism," *Journal of Obstetrics & Gynaecology*, vol. 23, no. 4, pp. 457–458, 2003.

[33] E. Cserepes, N. Szücs, P. Patkós et al., "Ovarian steroid cell tumor and a contralateral ovarian thecoma in a postmenopausal woman with severe hyperandrogenism," *Gynecological Endocrinology*, vol. 16, no. 3, pp. 213–216, 2002.

[34] E. D. Levens, B. W. Whitcomb, J. M. Csokmay, and L. K. Nieman, "Selective venous sampling for androgen-producing ovarian pathology," *Clinical Endocrinology*, vol. 70, no. 4, pp. 606–614, 2009.

[35] K. A. Martin, R. J. Chang, D. A. Ehrmann et al., "Evaluation and treatment of hirsutism in premenopausal women: an endocrine society clinical practice guideline," *Journal of Clinical Endocrinology and Metabolism*, vol. 93, no. 4, pp. 1105–1120, 2008.

[36] C. Rolf, U. Knie, G. Lemmnitz, and E. Nieschlag, "Interpersonal testosterone transfer after topical application of a newly developed testosterone gel preparation," *Clinical Endocrinology*, vol. 56, no. 5, pp. 637–641, 2002.

34

Malignant Insulinoma with Multiple Liver Metastases and Hypercalcitoninemia in a Patient with Type 2 Diabetes Mellitus Presenting as Recurrent Episodes of Diaphoresis due to Severe Hypoglycemia

Marco Ciacciarelli,[1] **Gianluca Caruso**,[2] **Marco Rengo**,[3] **Piero Maceroni**,[3] **Carmen Misurale**,[1] **Eleonora D'Armiento**,[1] **Alessandro Polidoro**,[1] **Cristina Napoli**,[1] **Alberto Lombardini**,[1] **Umberto Ceratti**,[1] **Ruben Manuel Luciano Colunga Biancatelli**,[1] **Leonardo Calvosa**,[1] **Romina Milanese**,[1] **Sonia Ferri**,[1] **Teresa Massaro**,[1] **Andrea Lorusso**,[1] **Veronica Sorrentino**,[2] **Vincenzo Petrozza**,[2] **and Luigi Iuliano**[1]

[1]*Department of Medico-Surgical Sciences and Biotechnologies, Internal Medicine Unit, ICOT Hospital, "Sapienza" University of Rome, Via Franco Faggiana 1668, Latina 04100, Italy*
[2]*Department of Medico-Surgical Sciences and Biotechnologies, Pathology Unit, ICOT Hospital, "Sapienza" University of Rome, Via Franco Faggiana 1668, Latina 04100, Italy*
[3]*Department of Radiological Sciences, Oncology and Pathology, ICOT Hospital, "Sapienza" University of Rome, Via Franco Faggiana 1668, Latina 04100, Italy*

Correspondence should be addressed to Marco Ciacciarelli; marco.ciacciarelli@uniroma1.it

Academic Editor: Mihail A. Boyanov

Insulinoma is an insulin-producing pancreatic neuroendocrine tumor that can be malignant in about 10% of cases. Locoregional invasion, lymph node metastases, or remote metastases are the main criteria of malignant insulinoma. Its incidence in patients with pre-existing diabetes mellitus (DM) is exceptionally rare. In this report, we describe a 66-year-old man with long-standing type 2 DM who presented with recurrent episodes of diaphoresis due to severe hypoglycemia despite the withdrawal of insulin therapy, hypercalcitoninemia, and biochemical and radiological findings suggestive of metastatic malignant insulinoma. Unfortunately, after few days of diazoxide treatment, edema, hypotension, oliguria, and water retention were observed, patient's clinical status deteriorated rapidly, and he died in our department from acute renal failure.

1. Introduction

Insulinoma is an insulin-producing pancreatic neuroendocrine tumor (PNET) that can be malignant in about 10% of cases [1]. Locoregional invasion, lymph node metastases, or remote metastases are the main criteria of malignant insulinoma. The incidence of insulinoma, especially the malignant type, in patients with diabetes mellitus (DM) is extremely rare, and the diagnosis can be challenging due to concomitant glucose-lowering drugs, mistaken as the cause of hypoglycemia. Here, we report the case of a 66-year-old man with a medical history of long-standing type 2 DM diagnosed with malignant metastatic insulinoma, presented as recurrent episodes of diaphoresis. Furthermore, we discuss its relevance within the contest of PNETs and similar cases described in the literature, to aware physician of this, yet rare but dramatic and challenging disease that could affect the diabetic population.

2. Case

A 66-year-old man was admitted to our internal medicine department for recurrent episodes of severe hypoglycemia.

Type 2 DM was diagnosed when he was 31 years old and initially treated with oral antihyperglycemic agents. The patient discontinued oral antidiabetic agents and started insulin therapy 4 years before admission. At that time, he was treated with long-acting insulin glargine and insulin aspart. This insulin regimen was switched to insulin degludec/liraglutide 3 months before admission. While he was on insulin degludec/liraglutide, his home blood glucose monitoring ranged from 110 to 70 mg/dL. Five days before admission, while on insulin degludec/liraglutide in a dose of 18 IU daily, the patient started having recurrent episodes of diaphoresis. During those episodes, usually in the early morning before breakfast, his blood glucose levels were below 50 mg/dL. The patient suffered from several further episodes despite insulin dosage tapering and even after discontinuation. His past medical history was notable for heart failure with reduced ejection fraction, acute coronary syndrome, and osteomyelitis of the left foot. His family medical history included atrial fibrillation and DM. In addition to insulin, his therapy consisted in acetylsalicylic acid, bisoprolol, furosemide, ramipril, and atorvastatin. He denied oral antihyperglycemic agents. He had no known drug allergies, he was a former smoker, and he did not drink alcohol or use illicit drugs.

On admission, the patient's blood pressure was 130/80 mmHg, heart rate was 71 beats per minute, respiratory rate was 14 breaths per minute, and oxygen saturation was 98%, while he was breathing ambient air. The patient's body mass index was 26.7 kg/m^2 (height: 173 cm; weight: 80 kg), and the physical examination was unremarkable. Laboratory data on admission showed glucose 50 mg/dl, HbA1c 50 mmol/mol, normocytic anemia (hemoglobin 11.9 g/dL, hematocrit 34.8%, and mean corpuscular volume 85 fl), a normal white cell and platelet count, aspartate aminotransferase (AST) 87 IU/L (normal range: 17–59), alanine aminotransferase (ALT) 62 IU/l (normal range: 21–72), gamma glutamyl-transferase 545 IU/l (normal range: 15–73), alkaline phosphatase 177 IU/l (normal range: 38–126), total bilirubin 0.47 mg/dL (normal range: 0.20–1.30), lactate dehydrogenase 1021 IU/L (normal range: 313–618), albumin 3.5 g/dL (normal range: 3.6–5.5), INR 1.18, C-reactive protein 7.5 mg/dl (normal range: 0-1), erythrocyte sedimentation rate 90 mm/h (normal range: 0–15), fibrinogen 621 mg/dl (normal range: 170–410), iron 37 μg/dl (normal range: 49–181), and ferritin 776 ng/ml (normal range: 20–325). Viral markers for hepatitis B and C were negative.

Further blood tests were ordered to rule out endogenous hyperinsulinism: C-peptide was 4.2 ng/mL (normal range: 0.5–3), insulin 89 μIU/mL (normal range: 5–25), while the patient's glucose level was 40 mg/dL, and sulfonylurea screening test was negative, confirming endogenous hyperinsulinism. Markers of neuroendocrine tumors were severely increased: chromogranin A (CgA) was 1790 ng/ml (normal range: 0–100), and neuron-specific enolase (NSE) was 458 ng/ml (normal range: 0–11).

Given the high suspicion of insulinoma and the altered liver function tests on admission, a full-body CT scan was ordered. CT scan showed a 4.3 × 2.2 cm pancreatic tail mass containing calcifications with multiple regional lymphadenopathies (Figure 1). Multiple liver secondary lesions were found: the largest ones measuring 12 and 11 cm, respectively, in II-III and IVb-V segments. No lungs, bone, and brain metastases were detected. Additionally, a thyroid nodule of 2.6 cm was incidentally found. Hepatic metastases were highly suspected to be secondary to a malignant insulinoma, so ultrasound-guided percutaneous biopsies of the lesion in the II-III segments were performed (Figure 2). Histological findings of four core biopsies consisted of hepatocytes infiltrated by a poorly differentiated and focally necrotic proliferating tissue of medium-sized atypical epithelial cells with solid growth pattern (Figure 3). The cancer cells showed hyperchromatic nuclei with "salt and pepper" chromatin markedly Ki-67 positive, high mitotic index (10 figures × 10 HPF), and scant cytoplasm. Immunohistochemistry studies revealed the neuroendocrine nature and the partial insulin secreting activity of the lesion; CgA, synaptophysin, CD56, and CAM5.2 were diffusely positive; there was patchy (<5%) insulin expression. Ki-67 index was 40–50. These findings were consistent with the diagnosis of metastatic, poorly differentiated (G3), neuroendocrine carcinoma with morphology and immunophenotype favoring a pancreatic primary tumor. Thyroid ultrasound (Figure 4) showed a weakly hypoechoic solid nodule (2.8 × 3.2 × 1.3 cm) with a central cystic component and regular margins located in the isthmus and a markedly hypoechoic solid nodule (0.9 × 0.9 × 0.6 cm) adjacent to the lower pole of the left lobe. Calcifications and intranodular flow were absent in both nodules, and regional lymph nodes were not enlarged. The results of thyroid function tests were within normal limits (TSH 0.7 mUI/L, normal range: 0.46–4.68), as well as were parathormone (PTH) (80.1 pg/mL, normal range: 13.6–85.8), calcium (8.76 mg/dL, normal range: 8.4–10.2), and phosphorus (4.32 mg/dL, normal range: 2.5–4.5). Serum calcitonin was slightly raised (30 pg/mL, normal range: 0–6), but immunohistochemical staining of the liver lesions was negative for such markers.

The patient's hospital stay was characterized by different episodes of severe hypoglycemia (as low as 18 mg/dL) occurring especially at night and in the early morning, manifesting only with diaphoresis. During those episodes, the patient never lost consciousness or developed seizures and even never complained of confusion, amnesia, weakness, diplopia, blurred vision, palpitations, or hunger. In order to reduce the hypoglycemic events, we started a symptomatic treatment with diazoxide and IV infusion of 10% dextrose, while waiting for histopathological confirmation of the disease. Unfortunately, due to the severity of this malignancy, after 8 days of treatment edema, hypotension, oliguria, and weight gain of 10 kg were observed; the patient's clinical status deteriorated rapidly, and 3 days later, the patient died from acute renal failure. Postmortem examination was not carried out according to his family's request.

3. Discussion

PNETs are rare neuroendocrine malignancies that count only for the 2% of total pancreatic tumors. Their incidence is around 1 case per 100,000 people, and only about 10% of

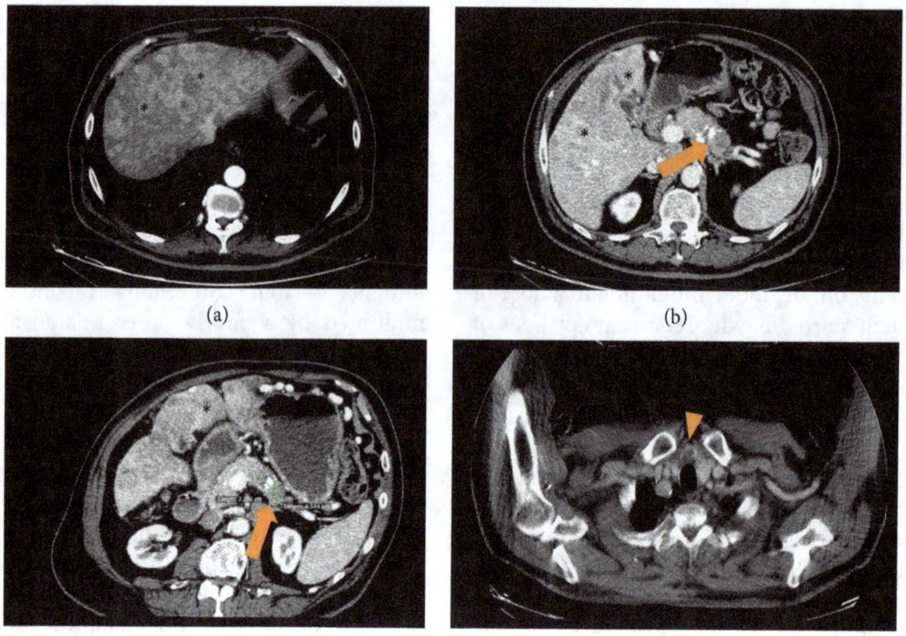

(c) (d)

FIGURE 1: CT images (a)–(c) show multiple hypervascular liver metastases (∗) and a focal solid lesion of the pancreatic tail (arrow). A thyroid nodule (arrow head) was also detected (d).

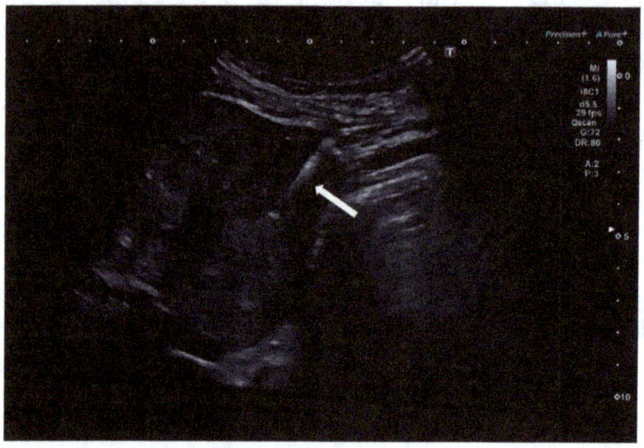

FIGURE 2: Ultrasound-guided percutaneous biopsies of the lesion located in the liver segments II-III. White arrow shows the needle penetrating in the subglissonian isoechoic/hypoechoic solid nodule with irregular margins (maximum diameter: 2.2 cm).

them are classified as functional, as they release hormones or peptides that cause specific symptoms and signs [2]. With an estimated incidence of 4 cases per 1 million person-years [3], insulinomas and insulin-producing tumors, are the most common functional PNETs, and unlike other PNETs, which are malignant in 50–100% of cases, they are malignant only in about 10% of cases [4].

Locoregional invasion, lymph node metastases, or remote metastases are the main criteria of malignant insulinoma. Most patients with malignant insulinoma have lymph node or liver metastases [5–7], and only rare metastases in other sites such as bones [8, 9], lungs [10], brain [11], ovaries [12, 13], and gallbladder [14]. Liver metastases at presentation count for almost 60% of the patients with PNETs [2].

In this report, we described a malignant insulinoma with multiple liver metastases in a 66-year-old man with longstanding type 2 DM. Although benign insulinoma occurs rarely in patients with pre-existing DM [15–17], malignant insulinoma in this population seems to be even rarer, and only sparse cases are described in the literature, in both type 2 [18–23] and type 1 DM [12, 24, 25]. However, despite the rare occurrence of insulinoma in diabetic population, clinicians should be aware of this possible differential diagnosis when managing diabetic patients with recurrent episodes of symptomatic hypoglycemia despite tapering and withdrawal of glucose-lowering drugs. We searched the PubMed database, and to the best of our knowledge, we collected the clinical, pathologic, and biochemical data of all previously reported cases of malignant insulinoma in patients with DM (Table 1). As reported by Yu et al. [26], short hypoglycemic symptoms duration before diagnosis of tumor seems to be common in patients with malignant insulinoma (median duration: 30 days). Furthermore, as shown in the same study, high proinsulin and CgA levels and a large proinsulin/insulin molar ratio should raise the suspicion of malignant insulinoma in patients with hyperinsulinemic hypoglycemia. In our case, similarly, hypoglycemic symptoms duration before diagnosis of malignant insulinoma was short (20 days), and CgA levels were markedly elevated (1790 ng/ml). Unfortunately, we could not measure proinsulin levels and calculate proinsulin/insulin molar ratio due to laboratory limitations.

Insulinoma is a pancreatic islet cell tumor which may be associated with multiple endocrine neoplasia type 1 (MEN-1). MEN-1 diagnosis was excluded because of age, a negative family medical history, and the absence of any clinical features of the most common endocrine and nonendocrine tumors associated with this rare syndrome. Primary

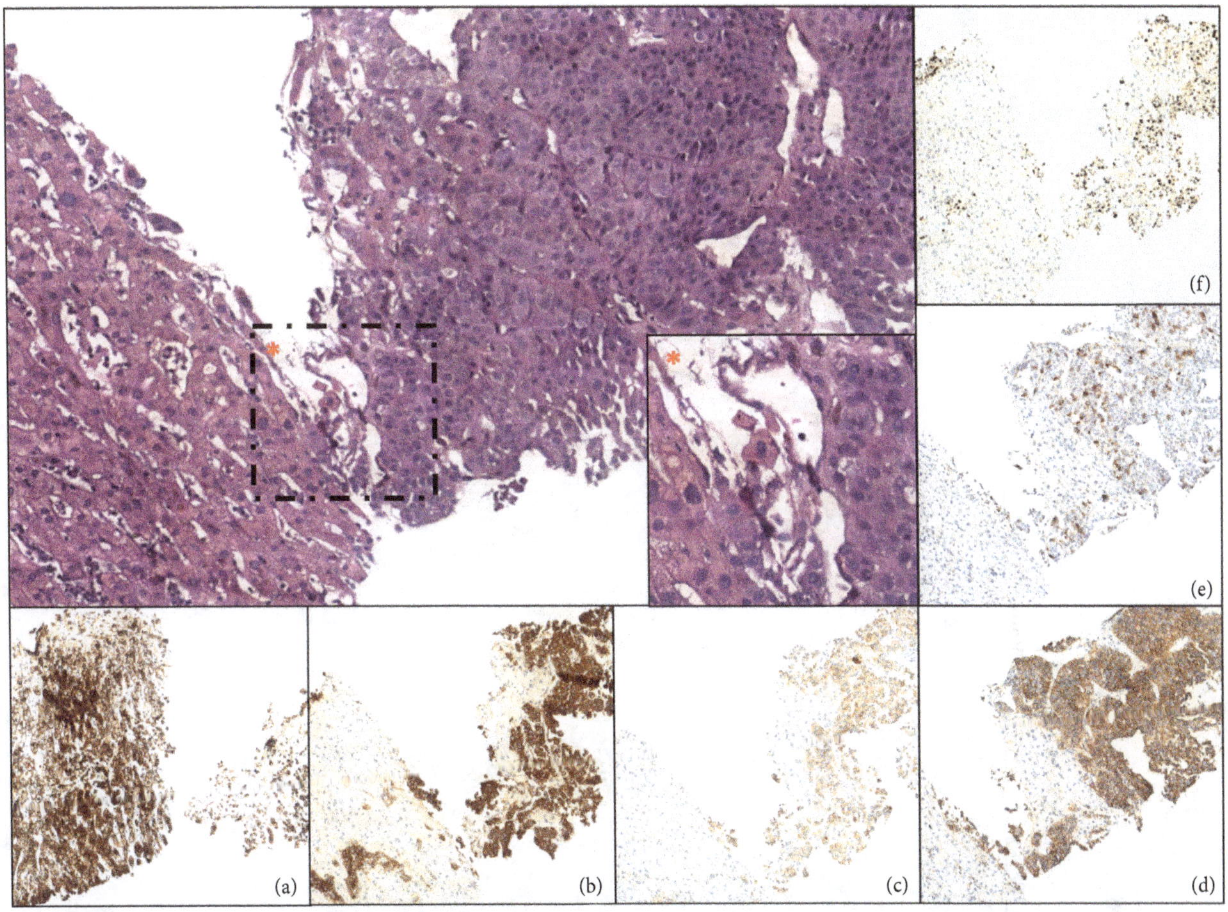

FIGURE 3: Poorly differentiated neuroendocrine carcinoma metastatic to the liver (H&E, magnification: 10x). The * box represents a detailed view of neoplasia (H&E, magnification: 40x). Immunohistochemical staining for CAM5.2 (a), synaptophysin (b), chromogranin A (c), CD56 (d), insulin (e), and Ki-67 proliferation index (f) (magnification: 10x).

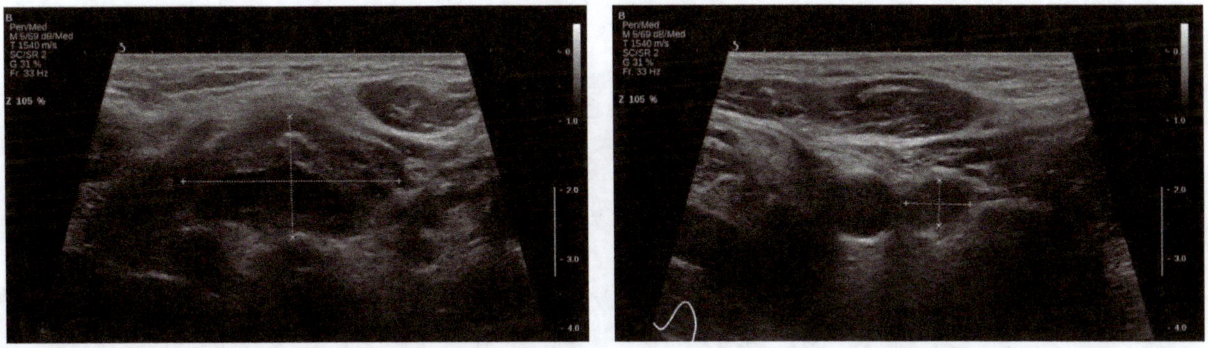

(a) (b)

FIGURE 4: Thyroid ultrasound. Weakly hypoechoic solid nodule ($2.8 \times 3.2 \times 1.3$ cm) with a central cystic component and regular margins located in the isthmus (a). Markedly hypoechoic solid nodule ($0.9 \times 0.9 \times 0.6$ cm) adjacent to the lower pole of the left lobe (b).

hyperparathyroidism is commonly associated with MEN-1, and at least 90% of patients develop it by the age of 50 years. The absence of history of osteoporosis or nephrolithiasis and normal serum calcium and PTH levels led us to rule out primary hyperparathyroidism. Since our patient had no symptoms or signs of a pituitary tumor, we did not order pituitary hormones (other than TSH) and pituitary MRI to rule out a pituitary tumor.

Metastatic insulinoma in our patient was extremely aggressive, and only progressively increased doses of diazoxide, up to 500 mg per day, were able to avoid severe hypoglycemic episodes. Unfortunately, as reported in other cases [19], our patient rapidly developed edema, hypotension, oliguria, and water retention secondary to diazoxide toxicity and died from acute renal failure. First-line chemotherapy regimen for poorly differentiated pancreatic

Table 1: Clinical, pathologic, and biochemical data of reported cases of malignant insulinoma in patients with diabetes mellitus.

Authors	Year	DM type	Age, sex	Site	Size (cm)	Metastases	Hypoglycemia symptoms	Insulin (μUI/ml)	C-peptide (ng/ml)	CgA (ng/ml)	Thyroid disease	Calcitonin (pg/ml)
Svartberg [12]	1996	1	33, F	Tail	Not reported	Liver Ovaries	Unconsciousness	86	8.4	Not reported	No	Not reported
Siraji [18]	2006	2	74, F	Tail, head	7.3 × 5.7 3 × 3 3.1 × 1.8	Liver	Diaphoresis Palpitations Confusion Seizures	39 (G: 28)	5.2	Not reported	No	Not reported
Schmitt [19]	2008	2	79, F	Body, tail	Not reported	Liver	Hunger Dizziness Tiredness	74 (G: 34)	9.7	↑ (404)	Hypothyroidism	Normal (<3)
FerrerGarcìa [20]	2011	2	78, M	Head	4.7 × 3	Liver	Not reported	23 (G: 35) (F)	4.6	↑ (834)	No	Not reported
Abbasakoor [21]	2011	2	67, F	Body	2.6 × 2 5-6	Liver Lymph nodes	Unconsciousness Anxiety Diaphoresis	91 (G: 19) (F)	8.2	Not reported	No	Not reported
Ademoglu [22]	2012	2	45, F	Head	0.8 × 0.7 0.9 × 1 0.7 × 0.7	Liver Lymph nodes	Confusion Diaphoresis	114 (G: 35) (F)	4.8	Not reported	No	Not reported
Lablanche [24]	2015	1	31, M	Head	6.3 × 5.6	Lymph nodes	Not reported	18 (G: 37) (F)	7.8	Not reported	Hashimoto thyroiditis	Not reported
Gjelberg [25]	2017	1	43, F	Tail	11 × 7	Liver Lymph nodes	Not reported	9 (G: 45) (F)	1.6	↑ (323)	Hypothyroidism	Normal
Our patient	2019	2	66, M	Tail	4.3 × 2.2	Liver	Diaphoresis	89 (G:40)	4.2	↑ (1790)	Thyroid nodules	↑ (30)

G: glucose (mg/dl); F: fasting.

neuroendocrine carcinoma consists with a combination of etoposide and either cisplatin or carboplatin. Unfortunately, when we obtained the report of histological analysis of liver biopsy, our patient was hemodynamically unstable and his renal function has worsened significantly, so we were not able to start chemotherapy with traditional regimen. Everolimus is an mTOR inhibitor with hyperglycemic and antitumoral effects indicated in treatment of malignant insulinoma. Given its toxicity, it is used as third-line treatment of recurrent episodes of hypoglycemia after failure of diazoxide and somatostatin analogs. The antitumoral effect of everolimus has been shown to improve progression-free survival of patients with well-differentiated PNETs. However, the antitumor efficacy of everolimus in poorly differentiated pancreatic neuroendocrine carcinoma remains to be determined.

Interestingly, our patient displayed increased serum calcitonin levels (30 pg/ml, normal range 0–6). Calcitonin is a peptide hormone secreted by C cells of the thyroid that acts as a physiologic antagonist to PTH, lowering blood calcium levels. Despite hypercalcitoninemia is a typical marker of medullary thyroid carcinoma (MTC), calcitonin can be found increased in several conditions: after exhausting physical activity, because of interfering drugs, in thyroid and non-thyroid diseases. These conditions should be always ruled out in cases with basal calcitonin values between 10 and 100 pg/mL [27], as observed in our patient.

He was sedentary, and at the time of blood sample analysis, he was not taking interfering drugs (e.g., omeprazole, glucocorticoids, or beta-blockers). In fact, bisoprolol was discontinued on admission in the attempt of increasing the adrenergic warning symptoms of hypoglycemia. Although glucagon-like peptide 1 analogs such as liraglutide are well known to cause slightly increases of calcitonin, we rejected this hypothesis because our patient discontinued liraglutide 22 days before calcitonin measurement.

Follicular and papillary thyroid carcinomas are thyroid diseases that may be associated to slightly raised calcitonin levels. Although the two thyroid nodules of our patient appeared benign and did not show any signs of malignancy (e.g., calcifications, intranodular flow, taller-than-wide shape, irregular margins, local invasion of surrounding structures, suspicious neck lymph nodes), we could not completely rule out any type of thyroid carcinoma, including MTC, as fine needle aspiration was not carried out due to severe worsening of the patient's clinical status. However, it is unlikely that ultrasound thyroid findings paired with thyroid malignancies and two different neuroendocrine tumors such as MTC and malignant insulinoma developed simultaneously.

Hypercalcitoninemia may also occur in nonthyroid diseases such as chronic renal failure, hyperparathyroidism-related hypercalcemia, and hypergastrinemia. Our patient had normal renal function, normal calcium levels, and no clinical features of conditions commonly associated with hypergastrinemia such as atrophic gastritis and gastrinoma; therefore, serum gastrin levels were not measured.

Hypercalcitoninemia due to ectopic calcitonin secretion by several types of PNETs, including insulinoma, has been described [28–33]; therefore, we measured calcitonin levels even if our patient had no family history of MTC or clinical and laboratory findings consistent with hyperparathyroidism or pheochromocytoma. Moreover, hypercalcitoninemia due to calcitonin-producing insulinoma has been documented in patients with benign thyroid nodules [31, 32].

Since a specific endocrine syndrome related to hypercalcitoninemia has not been identified yet, calcitonin-producing PNETs are currently classified as nonfunctional, unless they secrete "eutopic" biologically active hormones (insulin, glucagon, somatostatin, and pancreatic polypeptide). Interestingly, according to Uccella et al. [33], calcitonin expression is not related to either a more aggressive behavior or a worse prognosis, so it seems to not identify a separate subset of PNETs. The immunohistochemical detection of calcitonin in cells from pancreatic mass and the normalization of its value after tumor resection are important findings in confirming the diagnosis of calcitonin-producing insulinoma [29, 31, 32]. Due to the history of heart failure with reduced ejection fraction and the high suspicion of liver metastases, we performed a less-invasive diagnostic procedure such as liver biopsy rather than endoscopic ultrasound-guided biopsies of the pancreatic mass, as successfully reported in similar cases [5–7]. To the best of our knowledge, the few cases of calcitonin-producing insulinoma reported in the literature were not associated to metastases in liver or in other sites. In our case, immunohistochemistry of the liver lesion was negative for calcitonin; however, it should be noted that immunostaining of hepatic lesions secondary to calcitonin-producing PNETs may be negative for calcitonin probably because metastases can dedifferentiate and lose their secretory activity [34].

Despite the diagnosis of malignant insulinoma in our patient was made with biopsy of liver metastasis rather than biopsy of the pancreatic mass, in the absence of other apparent causes of hypercalcitoninemia, we hypothesized that cells of the pancreatic malignancy were able to produce calcitonin with following elevation of this serum marker.

4. Conclusion

In conclusion, although very rare, malignant insulinoma can occur in patients with both type 2 and type 1 DM. Most patients with malignant insulinoma have lymph node or liver metastases at presentation. Malignant insulinoma with liver metastases should always be considered as a cause of recurrent episodes of symptomatic hypoglycemia in diabetic patients with altered liver function tests, especially when severe hypoglycemia persists after withdrawal of glucose-lowering agents.

Furthermore, this case underlines that hypercalcitoninemia in patients with thyroid nodules is not necessarily due to MTC. Several physiologic and pathologic conditions other than MTC have been associated with increased calcitonin levels, including calcitonin-producing PNETs. Since the majority of PNETs are malignant, nonfunctional and hence represent a diagnostic challenge for physicians, all patients with raised calcitonin levels and thyroid nodules not clearly suggestive of MTC should be submitted to a careful investigation in order to rule out a calcitonin-producing PNET, a rare but recognized cause of hypercalcitoninemia.

References

[1] B. Hirshberg, C. Cochran, M. C. Skarulis et al., "Malignant insulinoma," *Cancer*, vol. 104, no. 2, pp. 264–272, 2005.

[2] A. Lewis, D. Li, J. Williams, and G. Singh, "Pancreatic neuroendocrine tumors: state-of-the-art diagnosis and management," *Oncology (Williston Park, NY)*, vol. 31, no. 10, pp. el–12, 2017.

[3] F. J. Service, M. M. McMahon, P. C. O'brien, and D. J. Ballard, "Functioning insulinoma-incidence, recurrence, and long-term survival of patients: a 60-year study," *Mayo Clinic Proceedings*, vol. 66, no. 7, pp. 711–719, 1991.

[4] D. W. Lee, M. K. Kim, and H. G. Kim, "Diagnosis of pancreatic neuroendocrine tumors," *Clinical Endoscopy*, vol. 50, no. 6, pp. 537–545, 2017.

[5] C. Toyoda, K. Hosokawa, Y. Atsumi et al., "Malignant insulinoma with extensive liver metastases presenting as disturbance of consciousness," *Internal Medicine*, vol. 37, no. 5, pp. 476–479, 1998.

[6] R. Baldelli, G. Ettorre, G. Vennarecci et al., "Malignant insulinoma presenting as metastatic liver tumor. Case report and review of the literature," *Journal of Experimental & Clinical Cancer Research: CR*, vol. 26, no. 4, pp. 603–607, 2007.

[7] A. Barnabei, E. Askin, F. Kose et al., "Erratum to: rapidly progressing malignant insulinoma presented with multiple liver metastases: a case report," *Journal of Gastrointestinal Cancer*, vol. 41, no. 4, pp. 272–274, 2010.

[8] C. S. Hesdorffer, M. Stoopler, and J. Javitch, "Aggressive insulinoma with bone metastases," *American Journal of Clinical Oncology*, vol. 12, no. 6, pp. 498–501, 1989.

[9] A. Naganuma, H. Mayahara, C. Morizane et al., "Successful control of intractable hypoglycemia using radiopharmaceutical therapy with strontium-89 in a case with malignant insulinoma and bone metastases," *Japanese Journal of Clinical Oncology*, vol. 42, no. 7, pp. 640–645, 2012.

[10] A. Albu, A. Zirnea, O. Georgescu, D. Terzea, D. Jinga, and S. Fica, "Malignant insulinoma with hepatic and pulmonary metastases associated with primary hyperparathyroidism. Case report and review of the literature," *Journal of Medicine and Life*, vol. 1, no. 2, pp. 210–217, 2008.

[11] J. L. Frazier and J. D. Weingart, "Metastatic insulinoma to the brain," *Endocrinologist*, vol. 19, no. 1, p. 5, 2009.

[12] J. Svartberg, M. Stridsberg, E. Wilander, D. E. H. Andersson, and B. Eriksson, "Tumour-induced hypoglycaemia in a patient with insulin-dependent diabetes mellitus," *Journal of Internal Medicine*, vol. 239, no. 2, pp. 181–185, 1996.

[13] O. Bélissant Benesty, T. Cassou-Mounat, C. Vatier, J.-N. Talbot, and F. Montravers, "Tumor heterogeneity detected by 68Ga DOTATOC and 18F-FDG PET/CTs in one malignant insulinoma with involvement of the portal splenic confluence and ovarian metastases," *Clinical Nuclear Medicine*, vol. 41, no. 11, pp. 874–876, 2016.

[14] M. Imamura, E. Miyashita, K. Miyagawa, S. Matsuno, and T. Sato, "Malignant insulinoma with metastasis to gallbladder and bone, accompanied by past history of peptic ulcer and hyperthyroidism," *Digestive Diseases and Sciences*, vol. 32, no. 11, pp. 1319–1324, 1987.

[15] L. A. Kane, C. S. Grant, T. B. Nippoldt, and F. J. Service, "Insulinoma in a patient with NIDDM," *Diabetes Care*, vol. 16, no. 9, pp. 1298–1300, 1993.

[16] H. Ishii, T. Ito, S. Moriya, Y. Horie, and M. Tsuchiya, "Insulinoma—a statistical review of 443 cases in Japan," *Nippon Rinsho*, vol. 51, no. Suppl, pp. 199–206, 1993.

[17] W.-Y. Lei, T.-E. Wang, T.-L. Chen, W.-H. Chang, T.-L. Yang, and C.-Y. Wang, "Insulinoma causing hypoglycemia in a patient with type 2 diabetes," *Journal of the Formosan Medical Association*, vol. 106, no. 5, pp. 392–396, 2007.

[18] E. S. Siraj, G. Samuel, S. Saber, S. Samuel, A. H. Hamrahian, and S. S. K. Reddy, "Metastatic malignant insulinoma in a patient with type 2 diabetes mellitus: case presentation and literature review," *Endocrine Practice*, vol. 12, no. 4, pp. 411–416, 2006.

[19] J. Schmitt, S. Boullu-Sanchis, F. Moreau et al., "Association of malignant insulinoma and type 2 diabetes mellitus: a case report," *Annales d'Endocrinologie*, vol. 69, no. 1, pp. 69–72, 2008.

[20] J. Ferrer-García, M. Tolosa-Torréns, C. Hernando-Meliá, L. Arribas-Palomar, and C. Sánchez-Juan, "Everolimus resolving hypoglycemia, producing hyperglycemia, and necessitating insulin use in a patient with diabetes and nonresectable malignant insulinoma," *Endocrine Practice*, vol. 17, no. 2, pp. e17–e20, 2011.

[21] N. O. Abbasakoor, M. L. Healy, D. O'Shea et al., "Metastatic insulinoma in a patient with type 2 diabetes mellitus: case report and review of the literature," *International Journal of Endocrinology*, vol. 2011, Article ID 124078, 5 pages, 2011.

[22] E. Ademoğlu, U. Unlütürk, K. Ağbaht, A. Karabork, and D. Corapçioğlu, "Type 2 diabetes mellitus in a patient with malignant insulinoma manifesting following surgery," *Diabetic Medicine*, vol. 29, no. 7, pp. e133–137, 2012.

[23] V. I. Podzolkov, N. A. Dragomiretskaia, T. V. Koroleva, N. N. Kavtaradze, H. H. Iakovleva, and A. V. Podzolkov, "A rare case of hypoglycemia in an elderly patient with type 2 diabetes mellitus: malignant metastasizing insulinoma," *Klin Med (Mosk)*.vol. 92, no. 2, pp. 65–70, 2014.

[24] S. Lablanche, M. Chobert-Bakouline, O. Risse, M.-H. Laverrière, O. Chabre, and P.-Y. Benhamou, "Malignant insulinoma may arise during the course of type 1 diabetes mellitus: a case report," *Diabetes & Metabolism*, vol. 41, no. 3, pp. 258–261, 2015.

[25] H. K. Gjelberg, D. Hoem, C. S. Verbeke, J. Eide, J. G. Cooper, and A. Molven, "Hypoglycemia and decreased insulin requirement caused by malignant insulinoma in a type 1 diabetic patient: when the hoof beats are from a zebra, not a horse," *Clinical Case Reports*, vol. 5, no. 6, pp. 761–768, 2017.

[26] R. Yu, N. N. Nissen, A. Hendifar et al., "A clinicopathological study of malignant insulinoma in a contemporary series," *Pancreas*, vol. 46, no. 1, pp. 48–56, 2017.

[27] S. P. Fan, D. M. Lourenço, M. A. Santos, M. R. Tavares, R. A. Toledo, and J. E. de Menezes Correia-Deur, "Hypercalcitoninemia is not pathognomonic of medullary thyroid carcinoma," *Clinics (Sao Paulo)*.vol. 64, no. 7, pp. 699–706, 2009.

[28] A. Ooi, I. Nakanishi, T. Kameya, Y. Funaki, and K. Kobayashi, "Calcitonin-producing insulinoma: an immunohistochemical and electron microscopic study," *Pathology International*, vol. 36, no. 12, pp. 1897–1903, 1986.

[29] D. E. Price, S. R. Absalom, K. Davidson, A. Bolia, P. R. F. Bell, and T. A. Howlett, "A case of multiple endocrine neoplasia:

hyperparathyroidism, insulinoma, GRF-OMA, hypercalcitoninaemia and intractable peptic ulceration," *Clinical Endocrinology*, vol. 37, no. 2, pp. 187-188, 1992.

[30] A. Gaulier, J. Cahen, J. L. Buisson, G. Périé, G. Vacher, and B. Poulet, "Pancreatic insulinoma, adenomatosis of the Wirsung's duct and chronic pancreatitis. Apropos of a case," *Archives d'anatomie et de cytologie pathologiques*, vol. 41, no. 5-6, pp. 245–250, 1993.

[31] M. J. G. M. Bugalho, L. Roque, L. G. Sobrinho et al., "Calcitonin-producing insulinoma: clinical, immunocytochemical and cytogenetical study," *Clinical Endocrinology*, vol. 41, no. 2, pp. 257–260, 1994.

[32] P. Pusztai, B. Sármán, G. Illyés et al., "Hypercalcitoninemia in a patient with a recurrent goitre and insulinoma: a case report," *Experimental and Clinical Endocrinology & Diabetes*, vol. 114, no. 05, pp. 217–221, 2006.

[33] S. Uccella, A. Blank, R. Maragliano, F. Sessa, A. Perren, and S. La Rosa, "Calcitonin-producing neuroendocrine neoplasms of the pancreas: clinicopathological study of 25 cases and review of the literature," *Endocrine Pathology*, vol. 28, no. 4, pp. 351–361, 2017.

[34] E. Giannetta, D. Gianfrilli, C. Pozza et al., "Extrathyroidal calcitonin secreting tumors," *Medicine*, vol. 95, no. 3, p. e2419, 2016.

35

Dramatic Response to First Line Single Agent Pembrolizumab in Anaplastic Thyroid Carcinoma

Valérie Spalart,[1] Barbara Legius,[2] Kurt Segers,[3] Johan Coolen,[4] Brigitte Maes,[5] and Lynn Decoster[2]

[1]*AZ Turnhout, Department of Internal Medicine, Turnhout, Belgium*
[2]*AZ Turnhout, Department of Pulmonology/Respiratory Oncology, Turnhout, Belgium*
[3]*AZ Turnhout, Department of Pathology, Turnhout, Belgium*
[4]*University Hospitals Leuven, Department of Radiology, Leuven, Belgium*
[5]*Jessa Hospital Hasselt, Laboratory for Molecular Diagnostics, Department of Clinical Biology, Hasselt, Belgium*

Correspondence should be addressed to Lynn Decoster; lynn.decoster@azturnhout.be

Academic Editor: Lucy Mastrandrea

Anaplastic thyroid carcinoma (ATC) is a deadly disease with very limited therapeutic options. There is an urgent need for new and efficacious drugs. Unfortunately accrual in clinical trials is problematic because of the rarity of the disease and often poor performance status at diagnosis. Recently some data have emerged suggesting a role for immunotherapy in the treatment of ATC. We describe the case of a 75-year-old patient with poor performance status and compromised airway and oesophagus at diagnosis, showing a rapid and dramatic response to first line single agent pembrolizumab. Disease progression in the brain occurred 16 months after initial diagnosis. At that time there was ongoing extracranial disease control.

1. Introduction

Anaplastic thyroid carcinoma (ATC) is a rare and aggressive disease representing 1-2% of all thyroid cancers but accounting for 50% of annual thyroid cancer related mortality. Approximately 50% of patients present with metastatic disease and treatment options are limited except for a subset of patients with BRAF-mutated tumors. Recent data suggest a potential role for immunotherapy in this disease desperate for new therapies. We describe a patient with poor performance status at presentation showing a rapid and dramatic response to first line single agent pembrolizumab.

2. Case Presentation

A 75-year-old female never smoker presented to the ear, nose and throat specialist with hoarseness, dry cough, difficulty swallowing and a 3 kg weight loss since 1 month.

5 years earlier she was treated with radioactive iodine for a toxic multinodular goiter. She also had a past medical history of a stage *Ic* well-differentiated serous papillary ovarian carcinoma treated with surgery and adjuvant chemotherapy.

On clinical examination, a multinodular and enlarged thyroid gland was palpated. A computed tomography (CT) scan of the neck and chest revealed a large mass (8 × 9 cm) in the anterior mediastinum involving the right thyroid lobe and causing deviation of both trachea and oesophagus. There were multiple pathologically enlarged cervical, supraclavicular and mediastinal lymph nodes as well as multiple bilateral lung metastases (Figure 1). Further staging revealed a bone metastasis in the right iliac crest. During bronchoscopy paralysis of the right vocal cord was noticed as well as invasion of the trachea with reduction of tracheal diameter estimated at 25%. No intracranial metastases were present on baseline brain CT imaging. A biopsy of a cervical lymph node was performed showing diffuse infiltration by an abnormal epithelial cell proliferation. The abnormal cells were large with large and hyperchromatic nuclei. Multiple mitotic figures were present as well as necrosis and several infiltrating lymphocytes. Immunohistochemical studies on the neoplastic cells were negative for thyroid transcription factor-1 (TTF-1), PAX-8,

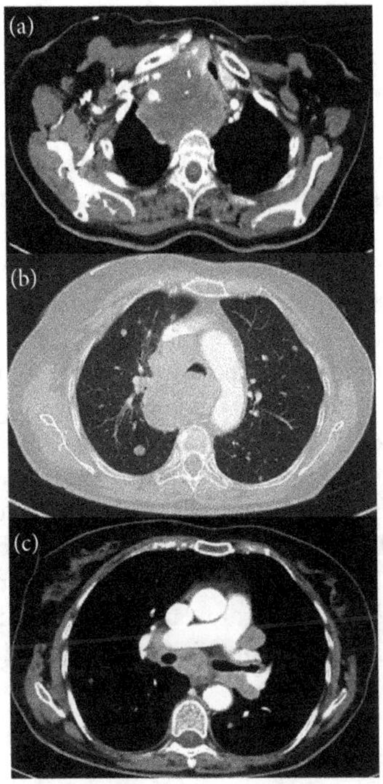

FIGURE 1: Baseline chest CT showing a large mass originating from the right thyroid lobe (a), with lung metastases (b), and hilar and mediastinal lymph nodes (c). (a), (c) images in mediastinal window. (b) image in lung window.

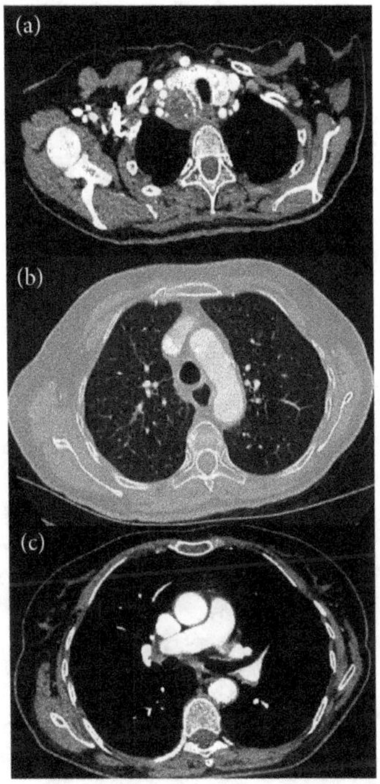

FIGURE 2: Chest CT after 3 cycles of pembrolizumab showing marked regression of primary tumor (a), lung metastases and (b), lymph nodes (c).

thyroglobulin, cytokeratin AE1/AE3, cytokeratin 7, CD 45, CD 34 and S-100. The pathological findings were compatible with an anaplastic large cell malignancy.

The case was discussed at the multidisciplinary tumor board and based on clinical presentation, imaging and pathology a diagnosis of primary anaplastic thyroid cancer was made. Next generation sequencing (NGS, TRUSEQ, MISEQ, ILLUMINA) was negative for molecular drivers. PDL1-staining was positive with a high expression (60% of tumor cells). At that point the clinical condition of the patient was rapidly deteriorating due to dysphagia with impaired food intake. The possibility of palliative stenting of the oesophagus was discussed with the gastroenterologist but was considered technically impossible. The patient was unfit for a clinical trial. Based on occasional case reports describing exceptional response to immunotherapy in patients with anaplastic thyroid cancer, the patient was offered the possibility of treatment with pembrolizumab. After only 2 cycles, the patient noticed a marked improvement of dysphagia and after 3 cycles, a near complete response was seen on CT (Figure 2). Thyroid function was thoroughly monitored during treatment and remained normal at all times.

After 8 cycles however, the patient developed a severe grade 4 colitis (bloody stools, severe dehydration with hypotension) requiring aggressive fluid resuscitation and treatment with systemic steroids. Due to further clinical deterioration infliximab was administered, after which gradual improvement occurred. 3 months after the last administration of pembrolizumab, there were no signs of tumor progression. As most guidelines recommend permanent discontinuation of immunotherapy after grade 4 gastro-intestinal toxicity, a watchful waiting approach was proposed with follow-up CT of the chest and neck every 3 months.

6 months later (16 months after diagnosis), the patient presented to the emergency department with gait difficulties, falling tendency to the left, left-sided facial palsy and hypoesthesia of the left upper arm. Magnetic resonance imaging (MRI) of the brain revealed a 19 × 18 × 19 mm lesion in the right thalamus. Stereotactic biopsy of this lesion was compatible with metastasis of known anaplastic large cell carcinoma. There were no signs of extra-cranial tumor progression (Figure 3). Stereotactic radiotherapy to the brain lesion was performed. However her neurological condition did not improve. Because of poor performance status, previous grade 4 gastro-intestinal toxicity and mainly intracranial treatment failure, a re-challenge with pembrolizumab was not considered nor was second line chemotherapy. The patient was referred for hospice care. She died 18 months after initial diagnosis.

3. Discussion

Anaplastic thyroid carcinoma (ATC) is a rare and aggressive disease with a median overall survival of less than 6 months and a 1-year survival of only 20%. In metastatic disease particularly, treatment options are limited [1]. The evidence for conventional chemotherapy is scarce as large randomized trials are lacking. Taxanes, doxorubicin and platin have shown some activity either as single agent or in combination, with response rates between 15% and 25% [2].

Lately promising results were reported with targeted therapies. In a single-arm, open-label study 17 ATC-patients

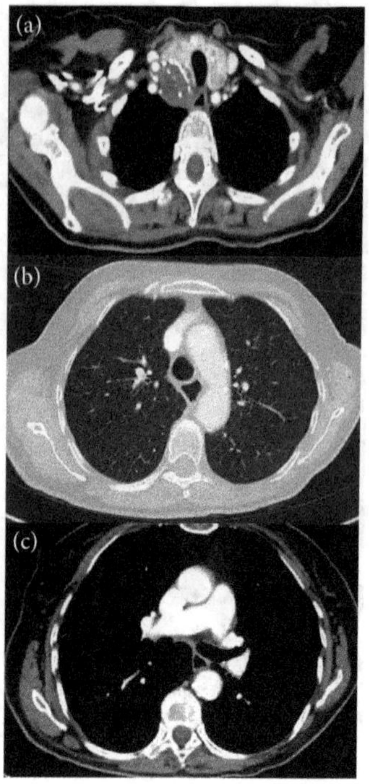

FIGURE 3: Chest CT 6 months after start of pembrolizumab showing ongoing response.

were treated with the multikinase-inhibitor lenvatinib. The objective response rate was 24%, the median progression-free survival (PFS) was 7.4 months and the median overall survival (OS) 10.6 months [3]. More importantly, in BRAF-mutated tumors, the combination of the selective kinase inhibitors (dabrafenib and trametinib) achieved a response rate of 69% and a 1-year survival of 80% [4]. Unfortunately resistance to these targeted therapies inevitably occurs.

The role of immunotherapy in ATC remains to be elucidated. Kolllipara et al. described an exceptional response with immunotherapy (nivolumab) in a patient with BRAF positive ATC who showed a mixed response to the BRAF-inhibitor vemurafenib [5]. In a small retrospective series of salvage pembrolizumab added to a kinase inhibitor at time of progression, partial response rate was 42% with a median OS from the start of pembrolizumab of 6.9 months [6]. Little is known about the role of single agent immunotherapy. In 30 ATC patients treated with the PD1-inhibitor spartalizumab, partial response was observed in less than 20% [7]. On the contrary, Khan et al. reported 2 out of 4 partial responses in ATC patients treated with pembrolizumab [8]. Currently 2 clinical trials are examining the role of immunotherapy-only in ATC patients (pembrolizumab in NCT02688608; nivolumab plus ipilimumab in NCT03246958).

In most ATC-trials however, accrual is hampered by the rarity of the disease and the often poor performance status at initial diagnosis. In a review article on diagnosis and management of ATC, Chintakuntlawar et al. state that it might therefore be reasonable to consider PD-1 inhibitors in these patients [1]. Occasional case reports might further build the evidence for the use of immunotherapy in a disease desperate for new treatment options.

We hereby describe a case of metastatic ATC treated with single agent pembrolizumab as first line therapy. Our case illustrates that a rapid and clinically meaningful response can be obtained even in a very sick patient with compromised airway and oesophagus. Clinical benefit occurred after only 2 cycles of pembrolizumab and near complete response was obtained after 3 cycles. Unfortunately, Pembrolizumab had to be discontinued because of grade 4 colitis and relapse occurred in the brain 14 months after initial diagnosis. At that moment there was ongoing extra-cranial disease control. As the initial impressive response to immunotherapy in our patient is intriguing we retrospectively assessed tumor infiltrating lymphocytes (TILs) on H&E slides from a metastatic lymph node. Stromal TILs (sTILs) could not be scored as no stroma was present in the biopsies. The percentage of intratumoral infiltrating lymphocytes (iTILS) was 30%. Whether PD-L1 or H&E based assessment of TILs (and at which cut-off) are predictive biomarkers in anaplastic thyroid cancer is a question that hopefully can be answered by ongoing or future clinical trials.

Author's Contributions

LD had the idea for the manuscript. VS and LD drafted the manuscript. LD and BL took part in the clinical management of the patient. JC was responsible for radiographic diagnosis. KS was responsible for pathological diagnosis. BM was responsible for molecular diagnosis. All authors contributed to and approved the final version of the manuscript.

References

[1] A. V. Chintakuntlawar, R. L. Foote, J. L. Kasperbauer, and K. C. Bible, "Diagnosis and management of anaplastic thyroid cancer," *Endocrinology and Metabolism Clinics of North America*, vol. 48, no. 1, pp. 269–284, 2019.

[2] M. E. Cabanillas, M. Zafereo, G. B. Gunn, and R. Ferrarotto, "Anaplastic thyroid carcinoma: treatment in the age of molecular targeted therapy," *Journal of Oncology Practice*, vol. 12, no. 6, pp. 511–518, 2016.

[3] M. Tahara, N. Kiyota, T. Yamazaki et al., "Lenvatinib for anaplastic thyroid cancer," *Frontiers in Oncology*, vol. 7, 2017.

[4] V. Subbiah, R. J. Kreitman, Z. A. Wainberg et al., "Dabrafenib and trametinib treatment in patients with locally advanced or metastatic BRAF V600-mutant anaplastic thyroid cancer," *Journal of Clinical Oncology*, vol. 36, no. 1, pp. 7–13, 2018.

[5] R. Kollipara, B. Schneider, M. Radovich, S. Babu, and P. J. Kiel, "Exceptional response with immunotherapy in a patient with anaplastic thyroid cancer," *The Oncologist*, vol. 22, no. 10, pp. 1149–1151, 2017.

[6] P. C. Iyer, R. Dadu, M. Gule-Monroe et al., "Salvage pembrolizulmab added to kinase inhibitor therapy for the treatment of anaplastic thyroid carcinoma," *Journal for Immunotherapy of Cancer*, vol. 6, no. 1, p. 68, 2018.

[7] L. J. Wirth, E. Eigendorff, J. Capdevila et al., "Phase I/II study of spartalizumab (PDR001), an anti-PD1 mAb, in patients with anaplastic thyroid cancer," *Journal of Clinical Oncology*, vol. 36, no. 15, pp. 6024–6024, 2018.

[8] S. A. Khan, P. Kurian, B. Mobley et al., "Relationship of anaplastic thyroid cancer high tumor mutation burden and MSI-H status with response to anti-PD1 monotherapy," *Journal of Clinical Oncology*, vol. 36, no. 15, pp. e18114–e18114, 2018.

36

Psychiatric Symptoms due to Thyroid Disease in a Female Adolescent

Nelly Capetillo-Ventura[1] **and Inmaculada Baeza**[2]

[1] *Department of Psychiatry, "Dr. José Eleuterio González" University Hospital, UANL, Avenida Francisco I. Madero and Avenida Gonzalitos, Mitras Centro, 64460 Monterrey, NL, Mexico*
[2] *Department of Child and Adolescent Psychiatry and Psychology, Institut Clínic de Neurociencies, Hospital Clínic, IDIBAPS, CIBERSAM, Barcelona, Spain*

Correspondence should be addressed to Nelly Capetillo-Ventura; dranellycv@hotmail.com

Academic Editor: Masashi Demura

The hypothalamic-pituitary-thyroid axis is involved in the production of thyroid hormone which is needed to maintain the normal functioning of various organs and systems, including the central nervous system. This study reports a case of hypothyroidism in a fifteen-year-old female adolescent who was attended for psychiatric symptoms. This case reveals the importance of evaluating thyroid function in children and adolescents with neuropsychiatric symptoms.

1. Background

The hypothalamic-pituitary-thyroid axis is involved in the production of thyroid hormone which is needed to maintain the normal functioning of various organs and systems, including the central nervous system [1]. Both hypothyroidism and hyperthyroidism can cause symptoms attributable to psychiatric illness. The lack of pathognomonic symptoms to differentiate thyroid disease from psychiatric disorders makes it difficult to distinguish between the two conditions in some cases [2].

Hypothyroidism is the most common abnormality of thyroid function in children and adolescents [3]. The prevalence of thyroid dysfunction between 11 and 18 years is 1% and the most common cause of acquired hypothyroidism is chronic lymphocytic thyroiditis (Hashimoto's thyroiditis), with a 2 : 1 female predominance, and, secondly, endemic goiter due to iodine deficiency. Hypothyroidism in children can be classified as primary or secondary (central) and can be congenital or acquired and transient or permanent [4].

Most adults with Hashimoto's thyroiditis are asymptomatic [5]. There are few published articles about this issue in children and adolescents. This paper reports a case of hypothyroidism in a female adolescent who was attended for psychiatric symptoms.

2. Case Report

A fifteen-year-old female adolescent was admitted to the child and adolescent acute psychiatric unit of our hospital for the first time after remaining isolated in her home for four months. She had initiated treatment in the outpatient clinic of her district in June 2013, attending only one visit and refusing all psychiatric treatment thereafter.

There was a family history of schizophrenia in second degree relative on her mother's side. The patient's medical history, according to her family, included recurrent acute bronchitis until 10 years of age. No history of alcohol or tobacco consumption or psychoactive substance use was reported. The patient was very selective and restrictive in her meals since her childhood. She only ate biscuits, ham croquettes, bread, and omelettes.

Regarding school, she described acceptable performance until the previous academic year when she presented some difficulties, and her teachers decided to change her to another classroom with a lower academic level.

Her premorbid personality was described as quiet and shy, with some difficulty in social relationships, but with a group of friends at the beginning of the episode. She lived with her parents and an 18-year-old sister in a mid-size city (with a population of about 216,000 inhabitants).

The patient reported that during the previous academic year she had been separated from her friends due to the change of classroom and at the same time she had begun to suffer digestive cramps and headaches, and as a result she stopped going to school. She stayed at home, with no interest in leaving the house, playing computer games and surfing the internet all day from April 2013 until her admission in our department 6 months later. The family explained that she had also become withdrawn from them, showing little interest in conversation, giving only monosyllabic answers, and gesturing in response to her parents' questions. She showed neglect in her personal hygiene and apathy regarding her physical appearance.

At the time of her admission, the mental status examination showed she was conscious and oriented in time, place, and person, though unkempt and exhibiting psychomotor retardation, poor eye contact, and limited language, answering questions with monosyllables or gestures. She also displayed emotional lability when discussing sensitive issues like friends and school and showed hypothymia, poorly reactive mood, apathy, weakness, and anhedonia and was only interested in computer usage. She did not exhibit impaired sensory perception, self-referentiality, or psychotic behavior, though she was sleeping from 4:00 am to noon. Her food intake was very selective, limited to certain specific foods, but there was no loss of appetite. The patient denied having suicidal ideation.

In the first interview, apathy and depressive moods were observed when she spoke about life events related to her friends at school and how this situation interfered with her functioning. Physical examination revealed a weight of 83.1 kg, height of 1.63 m, body mass index of 31.3, body mass index standard deviation score of 2.689, and blood pleasure of 120/80 mmHg. She denied muscular pain and no goiter or myxedema.

Soon after admission, a blood test and electrocardiogram (EKG) were performed. EKG, liver function tests, electrolytes, and whole blood count were within normal limits. Due to her isolation at home and selective food intake, levels of some vitamins were analyzed; vitamin D3 and folic acid levels were insufficient (vitamin D3: 20.9 ng/mL insufficient with levels above 30 ng/mL and folic acid: 2.3 ng/mL insufficient with levels above 3 ng/mL). The thyroid function test showed thyroid-stimulating hormone (TSH) levels of 24.159 mIU/L (reference range: 0.400–4.00), free thyroxine (FT4) 0.93 ng/dL (reference range: 0.80–2.00), and triiodothyronine (T3) 1.08 ng/mL (reference range: 0.70–1.90), with antithyroid peroxidase antibodies >1300 IU/mL (reference range: <35).

We requested interconsultation with the endocrinology department where hypothyroidism secondary to Hashimoto's thyroiditis was diagnosed, and treatment with levothyroxine 50 micrograms/day was recommended. We began folic acid (5 mg/day) and vitamin D (0.266 mg/alternate days) supplementation too.

During her hospital stay, the patient adapted well to the rules of the unit, was sociable with peers, and showed no behavioural disturbances at any time.

After 8 days in our acute unit, the patient showed significant improvement in mood and social interaction and was discharged. Monitoring continued in the outpatient clinic, while the patient maintained the same pharmacological treatment. At six weeks, the patient was asymptomatic; she had returned to school showing acceptable performance and socialization with family and classmates. The new thyroid function test showed TSH 9.096 mIU/L and FT4 1.21 ng/dL. Six-months after discharge, the improvement persisted, and thyroid function was TSH 6.935 mIU/L and FT4 1.35 ng/dL and antithyroid peroxidase antibodies decreased, with 75 micrograms/day of levothyroxine.

3. Discussion

This paper reports a case of hypothyroidism in a female adolescent who was attended for psychiatric symptoms. The literature highlights the importance of measuring thyroid function in patients with refractory mood disorders, rapid cycling, mixed episodes, and treatment with mood stabilizers (especially lithium) and in whom there is no improvement after treatment is initiated. In our department, thyroid function tests are routinely requested for adolescent patients with affective symptoms from the initial assessment whenever there are clinical manifestations of hypothyroidism such as decreased school performance, fatigue and sluggishness, emotional lability, and depressed or altered mood. This behavior may simulate other disorders of adolescence [4, 6]. The abnormalities found on physical examination include short stature, apparent excess weight (more fluid retention than obesity), having a puffy face with a dull, placid expression, bradycardia, pseudohypertrophy of the muscles, and delayed deep tendon reflexes. The thyroid gland may be normal in size, not palpable, or diffusely enlarged [7]. As for the laboratory analysis, determining the levels of TSH and FT4 is usually sufficient to make a diagnosis. Primary hypothyroidism presents high TSH and low free T4. Secondary hypothyroidism presents with low or normal TSH and decreased FT4. Autoimmune thyroiditis is confirmed by positive antithyroid antibodies (anti-TPO 85–90% higher) but its positivity does not imply hypothyroidism. [6]. In the National Health and Nutrition Examination Survey (NHANES III) from 1988 and 1994, 6.3 percent of adolescents (12 to 19 years of age) had positive antithyroglobulin antibodies (Tg Ab) and 4.8 percent had positive antithyroid peroxidase antibodies (TPO Ab) [8].

In paediatrics, the most common age of presentation of autoimmune thyroiditis is adolescence, though the disease may occur at any time even, in rare cases, in children under one year of age [9]. The initial presence of goiter and elevated thyroglobulin antibodies, the presence of celiac disease, and a progressive increase in thyroperoxidase antibodies and TSH value predict a progression toward overt hypothyroidism [10].

Thyroid hormones exert their influence on the central nervous system through a variety of mechanisms: modulation of gene expression of several groups of proteins, some of them with known physiopathological implications in mood disorders and the influence on serotonin and noradrenergic neurotransmission, known to be one of the modes of action of antidepressants [11].

T4 is the treatment of choice in children and adolescents with hypothyroidism. The goals of treatment are to restore normal growth and development, including pubertal development [7]. In patients who present with severe, longstanding hypothyroidism, slow correction with FT4 is advisable in order to minimize the potential development of unwanted side effects (deterioration in school performance, short attention span, hyperactivity, insomnia, and behavioral difficulties). In such patients, the replacement dose should be increased slowly over several weeks to months [12]. McClelland et al. recommended a period of closer observation before making any adjustments in the dose of thyroxine in order to detect noncompliance [13]. Several reports indicate that in hypothyroid patients the thyroid hormone replacement alleviates depressive symptoms, and thyroid supplements are accepted as an effective treatment option for affective disorders. The cumulative dose of levothyroxine over preceding weeks is best reflected in the serum TSH, and noncompliant patients require careful education as to the rationale for treatment [14]. In the patient we present, the TSH levels diminished after six weeks of treatment, which means there was adequate therapeutic compliance and hence clinical improvement.

The natural course of juvenile autoimmune thyroiditis is quite variable, and thyroid functions should be monitored periodically to detect hypothyroidism in all children and adolescents including those who are initially euthyroid or have subclinical hypothyroidism. Patients who are not receiving treatment at the time of presentation may require treatment subsequently. Levothyroxine therapy may have beneficial effects on the clinical course of the disease and on antibody titers [15].

Diagnosis of hypothyroidism is particularly important in adolescence because this condition retards growth in height and development of secondary sexual characteristics; delayed onset of puberty can also occur and diagnosing autoimmune thyroiditis (AT) at an early stage offers the opportunity for a timely intervention. Its potential association with papillary thyroid carcinoma is an additional reason for a careful follow-up of patients with AT [16].

4. Conclusions

Our case is an example of how neuropsychiatric symptoms in children and adolescents may have their etiology in an alteration of the functioning of the hypothalamic-pituitary-thyroid axis. After a proper diagnosis is made, treatment can focus on controlling the signs and symptoms presented, thus avoiding overmedication and preventing future complications in other body systems. Evaluation of thyroid functioning may be prudent in children and adolescents with neuropsychiatric symptoms, and we recommended including TSH and T4 blood levels in the complementary tests for differential diagnoses.

Abbreviations

EKG: Electrocardiogram
TSH: Thyroid-stimulating hormone
FT4: Thyroxine
T3: Triiodothyronine.

Consent

Written informed consent was obtained from the patient and her parents for publication of this case study.

Authors' Contribution

Nelly Capetillo-Ventura conceptualized and drafted the initial paper. Inmaculada Baeza reviewed and revised the paper and approved the final paper submitted. Nelly Capetillo-Ventura and Inmaculada Baeza approved the final paper submitted and agree to be accountable for all aspects of the work.

References

[1] P. M. Yen, "Physiological and molecular basis of Thyroid hormone action," *Physiological Reviews*, vol. 81, no. 3, pp. 1097–1142, 2001.

[2] F. Bello and S. G. Kojchen, "Función tiroidea y patología psiquiátrica," *Boletín de la Escuela de Medicina*, vol. 29, no. 3, 2000.

[3] M. L. Rallison, B. M. Dobyns, F. R. Keating, J. E. Rall, and F. H. Tyler, "Occurrence and natural history of chronic lymphocytic thyroiditis in childhood," *The Journal of Pediatrics*, vol. 86, no. 5, pp. 675–682, 1975.

[4] M. Bettendorf, "Thyroid disorders in children from birth to adolescence," *European Journal of Nuclear Medicine*, vol. 29, no. 2, pp. S439–S446, 2002.

[5] E. Sarı, A. Karaoglu, and E. Yeşilkaya, "Hashimoto's thyroiditis in children and adolescents," in *Autoimmune Disorders: Current Concepts and Advances from Bedside to Mechanistic Insights*, F.-P. Huang, Ed., InTech, 2011.

[6] C. Aguilá, "Hipotiroidismo en adolescentes," *Adolescere*, vol. 12, no. 1, pp. 24–31, 2013.

[7] S. La Franchi, *Acquired Hypothyroidism in Childhood and Adolescence*, UpToDate, 2007.

[8] J. G. Hollowell, N. W. Staehling, W. Dana Flanders et al., "Serum TSH, T4, and thyroid antibodies in the United States population (1988 to 1994): National Health and Nutrition Examination Survey (NHANES III)," *Journal of Clinical Endocrinology and Metabolism*, vol. 87, no. 2, pp. 489–499, 2002.

[9] T. P. Foley Jr., V. Abbassi, K. C. Copeland, and M. B. Draznin, "Brief report: hypothyroidism caused by chronic autoimmune thyroiditis in very young infants," *The New England Journal of Medicine*, vol. 330, no. 7, pp. 466–468, 1994.

[10] A. Monzani, F. Prodam, A. Rapa et al., "Endocrine disorders in childhood and adolescence. Natural history of subclinical hypothyroidism in children and adolescents and potential effects of replacement therapy: a review," *European Journal of Endocrinology*, vol. 168, no. 1, pp. R1–R11, 2013.

[11] S. Gloger, C. Fardella, R. Santis, and J. Bitran, "Relevancia del estudio tiroideo en pacientes con trastornos psiquiátricos," *Revista Médica de Chile*, vol. 125, pp. 1351–1356, 1997.

[12] R. Brown, "Autoimmune thyroiditis in childhood," *Journal of Clinical Research in Pediatric Endocrinology*, vol. 5, no. 1, pp. 45–49, 2013.

[13] P. McClelland, A. Stott, and W. Howel-Evans, "Hyperthyrotrophinaemia during thyroxine replacement therapy," *Postgraduate Medical Journal*, vol. 65, no. 762, pp. 205–207, 1989.

[14] A. Sevinc and H. Savli, "Hypothyroidism masquerading as depression: the role of noncompliance," *Journal of the National Medical Association*, vol. 96, no. 3, pp. 379–382, 2004.

[15] S. Özen, Ö. Berk, D. G. Şimşek, and Ş. Darcan, "Clinical course of Hashimoto's thyroiditis and effects of levothyroxine therapy on the clinical course of the disease in children and adolescents," *JCRPE Journal of Clinical Research in Pediatric Endocrinology*, vol. 3, no. 4, pp. 192–197, 2011.

[16] V. Skarpa, E. Kousta, A. Tertipi et al., "Epidemiological characteristics of children with autoimmune thyroid disease," *Hormones*, vol. 10, no. 3, pp. 207–214, 2011.

Isolated Adrenocorticotropin Deficiency Associated with Delirium and Takotsubo Cardiomyopathy

Masanori Murakami,[1] Noriko Matsushita,[2] Rie Arai,[3] Naohiro Takahashi,[1] Ryuki Kawamura,[2] Sayaka Suzuki,[1] Sachio Takekawa,[1] Fumiko Iwashima,[1] Takashi Shibui,[2] Akihiro Hata,[2] Yoshihiro Ogawa,[4] and Toshiyuki Horiuchi[1]

[1] *Department of Endocrinology and Metabolism, Tokyo Metropolitan Health Medical Treatment Corporation Toshima Hospital, 33-1 Sakae-cho, Itabashi-ku, Tokyo 173-0015, Japan*
[2] *Department of Cardiology, Tokyo Metropolitan Health Medical Treatment Corporation Toshima Hospital, 33-1 Sakae-cho, Itabashi-ku, Tokyo 173-0015, Japan*
[3] *Department of Psychiatry, Tokyo Metropolitan Health Medical Treatment Corporation Toshima Hospital, 33-1 Sakae-cho, Itabashi-ku, Tokyo 173-0015, Japan*
[4] *Department of Molecular Endocrinology and Metabolism, Graduate School of Medical and Dental Sciences, Tokyo Medical and Dental University, 1-5-45 Yushima, Bunkyo-ku, Tokyo 113-8510, Japan*

Correspondence should be addressed to Toshiyuki Horiuchi, endocrine@toshima-hp.jp

Academic Editors: T. Kita, W. V. Moore, and Y. Moriwaki

We report a 65-year-old woman with isolated adrenocorticotropic hormone (ACTH) deficiency. The patient was transported to the emergency outpatient department by ambulance complaining of malaise and nausea. Because her laboratory data revealed hyponatremia, we performed endocrinological examinations and diagnosed isolated ACTH deficiency. After admission, she went into a delirious state and suffered from takotsubo cardiomyopathy due to adrenal insufficiency. Replacement therapy with hydrocortisone sufficiently improved her delirium and cardiomyopathy. We conclude that her unstable mental state and myocardial dysfunction were closely related to adrenal insufficiency and suggest that adrenal crisis may cause delirium and Takotsubo cardiomyopathy.

1. Introduction

Isolated adrenocorticotropic hormone (ACTH) deficiency causes secondary hypocortisolism. Major symptoms, which include general malaise, fatigability, anorexia, hypotension, and disturbance of consciousness, are due to hypoglycemia or hyponatremia. Isolated ACTH deficiency is suspected when hypocortisolism is present in addition to the major symptoms already listed. A definite diagnosis requires low or absent serum ACTH or cortisol levels under corticotropin-releasing hormone (CRH) challenge. Although depression-like symptoms are common in hypocortisolism [1], only three cases of delirium with isolated ACTH deficiency have been reported [2–4]. In addition, there were some reports of ACTH deficiency associated with Takotsubo cardiomyopathy [5–9], which is characterized by transient left ventricular apical wall motion abnormality with electrocardiographic changes and minimal myocardial enzymatic release mimicking acute myocardial infarction, but without significant coronary artery disease [10–15].

Here, we report a case of delirium and Takotsubo cardiomyopathy during acute adrenal crisis due to isolated ACTH deficiency.

2. Case Report

A 65-year-old woman was admitted to our hospital, complaining of malaise and nausea of one-week duration without preceding infection. She had been in good health until that time except for suffering from Hashimoto's disease,

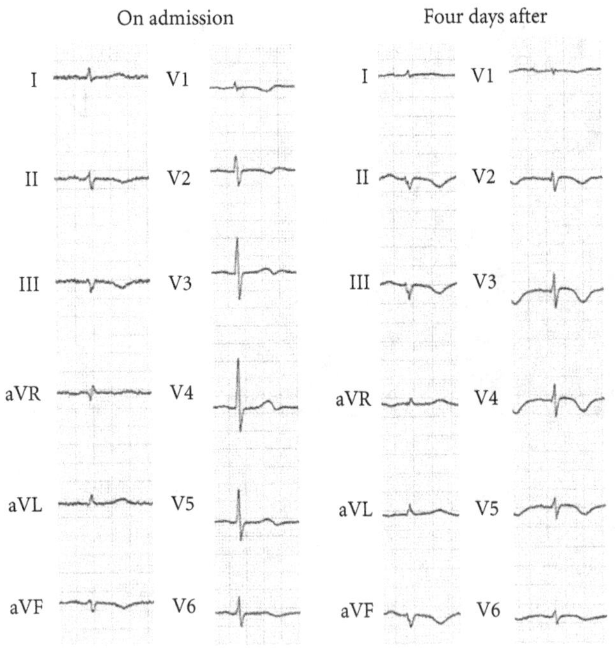

FIGURE 1: Electrocardiogram changes on admission and four days later while suffering from cardiomyopathy. New inverted T waves were present in the V3-4 leads.

which was treated with thyroid hormone, levothyroxine 75 μg/day in another hospital and was well controlled. She was nulligravida and menopausal at 60 years old. In addition, she had no psychiatric history.

On admission, her body temperature was 35.6°C, blood pressure 157/94 mmHg, and pulse rate 75/min. She exhibited obtundation and her Glasgow Coma Scale was 14 (E4V4M6). Physical examination showed no abnormalities. Her skin and mucosa were free of unusual pigmentation and there were no lack of physiological pigmentation and body hair. Laboratory findings showed only low serum levels of sodium (116 mEq/L, Table 1). On electrocardiogram (ECG), T waves were inverted in leads II, III, V1, and V2 as minor abnormalities (Figure 1).

After admission, her consciousness levels were improved for alertness and we tried to treat the hyponatremia by intravenous infusion. However, four days after admission, she presented with paranoia and visual hallucinations. She said, for example, "I was arrested in the hospital," "The pattern on the walls began to spin," and "Grass is growing on the window panes." She was delirious. We consulted psychiatrists who prescribed quetiapine for her delirium. Furthermore, on the same day, she complained of nausea and was pale and sweating. Her blood pressure was 63/48 mmHg, body temperature was 36.0°C, and her SpO_2 index was unstable (70–90%). She was thought to be in a state of acute circulatory failure. Because the electrocardiogram showed new inverted T waves in leads V2-5 (Figure 1), urgent coronary catherization was performed for possible percutaneous intervention. However, coronary angiography demonstrated no significant coronary stenosis. Left ventriculography showed akinesis of the left ventricular apex with

TABLE 1: Laboratory findings on admission.

Peripheral blood	
White blood cells	4600/μL (3300–9500)
Neutrophils	68.5% (37–80)
Lymphocytes	19.7% (11–50)
Monocytes	10.3% (4–11)
Basophils	0.2% (0–2)
Eosinophils	1.3% (0–8)
Red blood cells	386×10^4/μL (389–501)
Hemoglobin	11.7 g/dL (11.3–15.2)
Hematocrit	30.2% (33.4–46.4)
Platelet	16.2×10^4/μL (14–36)
Serum chemistry	
Sodium	116 mEq/L (136–147)
Potassium	4.5 mEq/L (3.5–5.0)
Chloride	84 mEq/L (95–110)
Glucose	132 mg/dL (70–110)
Urea nitrogen	6.4 mg/dL (7.0–22.0)
Creatinine	0.52 mg/dL (0.40–0.90)
Uric acid	3.1 mg/dL (0.0–7.0)
Total protein	6.1 g/dL (6.3–8.5)
Albumin	3.8 g/dL (3.3–5.1)
Aspartate aminotransferase	33 IU/L (10–38)
Alanine aminotransferase	15 IU/L (6–38)
Lactate dehydrogenase	211 IU/L (115–255)
C-reactive protein	0.3 mg/dL (0.0–0.2)

Figures in parentheses indicate the normal range.

ballooning during systole (Figure 2). Blood examination revealed neither significant hypoglycemia nor electrolyte abnormalities other than hyponatremia (118 mEq/L). The serum levels of creatinine kinase (CK) (603 IU/L), CK-MB (24 IU/L), and troponin I (6.80 ng/mL) were slightly elevated. These findings are consistent with Takotsubo cardiomyopathy.

Considering her status of hyponatremia, delirium, and Takotsubo cardiomyopathy, we supposed she could be suffering an acute adrenal crisis and started intravenous administration of 400 mg/day hydrocortisone. On the following day, we confirmed decreased cortisol (2.2 μg/dL, Table 2(a)) and ACTH (8.4 pg/mL) levels and began oral administration of 20 mg/day hydrocortisone. Following the administration of hydrocortisone, the hyponatremia and delirium improved dramatically in 3 days. Her sodium level reached 139 mEq/L and her consciousness level became alert. An echocardiogram showed the left ventricular wall motion abnormalities including apical segment to be also markedly improved by 10 days after steroid administration.

Endocrine studies showed decreases in serum cortisol and ACTH and reduced urinary secretion of free cortisol. The plasma cortisol level responded slightly after a bolus injection of 0.25 mg ACTH (Table 2(b)). In addition, continuous ACTH-Z stimulation (0.5 mg injected daily for 4 days) produced a gradual but clear increase in the urinary excretion of free cortisol (Table 2(d)). Treatment with ACTH-releasing

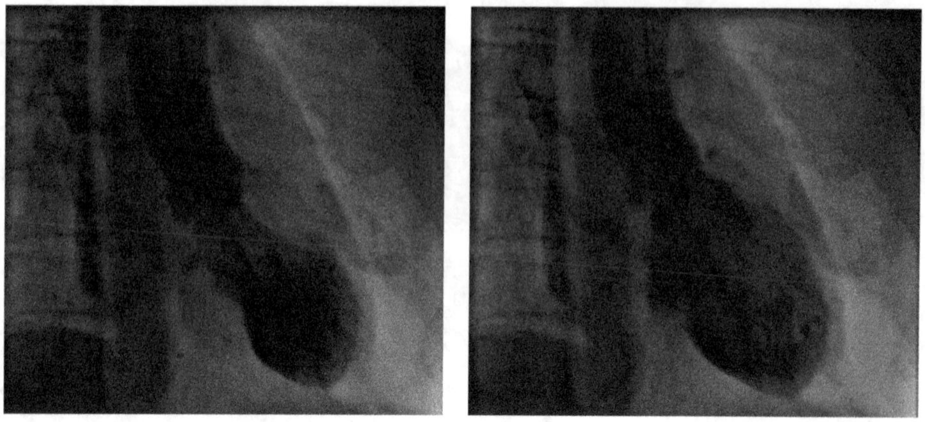

(a) (b)

FIGURE 2: Left ventriculography ((a) systole, (b) diastole) demonstrates akinesis of the apex with systolic ballooning.

TABLE 2: Hormonal data in detailed examination.

(a) Basal levels

ACTH	8.4 pg/mL (7.2–63.3)
Cortisol	2.2 μg/dL (4.0–18.3)
TSH	1.52 μIU/mL (0.55–4.78)
FT3	2.38 pg/mL (2.13–4.07)
FT4	1.89 ng/dL (0.89–1.76)
Plasma renin activity	0.3 ng/mL/hr (0.3–2.9)
Plasma aldosterone	76.8 pg/mL (29.9–159.0)
Urine free cortisol	8.7 μg/day (11.2–80.3)
Urine metanephrine	0.03 mg/day (0.04–0.19)
Urine normetanephrine	0.16 mg/day (0.09–0.33)

Figures in parentheses indicate the normal range.

(b) Rapid ACTH test

Time (min)	0	30	60
Cortisol (μg/dL)	5.4	14.1	16.8

(c) CRH, LHRH, GRH test

Time (min)	0	30	60	90	120
ACTH (pg/mL)	7.8	14.3	11.7	9.2	8.3
Cortisol (μg/dL)	5.7	6.4	5.7	5.4	5.4
LH (mIU/mL)	19.92	64.31	68.04	66.7	62.75
FSH (mIU/mL)	64.50	75.37	79.86	82.44	86.36
GH (ng/mL)	0.64	8.72	12.3	12.1	4.66

(d) Continuous ACTH test

Day	1	2	3	4	5	6	7
Urine free cortisol (μg/day)	5.8	7.0	7.5	99.8	546.0	866.0	2950.0

hormone did not increase the plasma ACTH concentration (Table 2(c)). On the other hand, growth hormone (GH) levels were increased by GH-releasing hormone (Table 2(c)). Although the luteinizing hormone (LH) and follicle stimulating hormone (FSH) levels were slightly increased by LH-releasing hormone, their basal levels were high enough because of her postmenopausal state, and we consider that LH- and FSH-releasing ability was unimpaired (Table 2(c)). We did not perform an infusing TSH-releasing hormone test. Because she was under treatment for Hashimoto's disease involving levothyroxine intake and euthyroid upon admission (Table 2(a)), her hypothalamus function with respect to TSH-releasing ability should not have been impaired. We also did not perform an insulin tolerance test

TABLE 3: Reported cases with isolated ACTH deficiency with delirium.

Case	Age/Sex	Past history	Preceding duration of physical symptoms	Mental symptoms	Normalization of delirium	Steroid hormone therapy	Reference
1	68/M	Stroke	4 months	Disorientation to time and place incontinence	1 day	Cortisone acetate 25 mg/d PO for 10 days 37.5 mg/d PO	[2]
2	74/M	—	1 week	Delirious state	3 days	Hydrocortisone Details unclear	[3]
3	67/M	Cholecystitis	7 weeks	Incoherent speech and conduct incontinence	Details unclear	Hydrocortisone 20 mg/d PO	[4]
4	65/F	Hashimoto's disease	1 week	Paranoia visual hallucinations	3 days	Hydrocortisone 400 mg/d IV for 2 days 20 mg/d PO	Present case

PO: per os, IV: intravenously, and d: day.

(ITT) because she was elderly and the possibility of severe cardiac involvement was present. Plasma renin activity and plasma aldosterone concentration were normal (Table 2(a)). Therefore, the diagnosis of isolated ACTH deficiency was made. Magnetic resonance imaging (MRI) revealed no pituitary lesions or adjacent lesions.

3. Discussion

Adrenal insufficiency was conclusively diagnosed following endocrinological examination based on the markedly decreased plasma cortisol level. The ACTH level was low while the remaining pituitary functions were normal, which led to the diagnosis of isolated ACTH deficiency. Although our patient complained of malaise and nausea for a week prior to admission, the plasma cortisol level responded slightly (<18 μg/mL) after a bolus injection of 0.25 mg ACTH (Table 2(b)). It was considered that she had suffered secondary insufficiency for more than a week.

Three cases of delirium concurrent with isolated ACTH deficiency have been reported [2–4] (Table 3). Administration of hydrocortisone dramatically improved consciousness in all cases including ours, and this immediate improvement suggests significant links between delirium and adrenal insufficiency. Interestingly, the patient in our case showed paranoid thinking and visual hallucinations. In the previous reports, the patients showed symptoms that included incoherent speech, disorientation, and incontinence [2–4]. We believe our case is the first to describe delirium concurrent with isolated ACTH deficiency, presenting paranoid thinking and visual hallucinations. Considering all reports [2–4] (Table 3), most cases developed delirium with preceding unresolved gastrointestinal symptoms in accordance with hyponatremia in geriatric patients. In addition, they did not have any special psychiatric history. Facing delirium patients having these situations, clinicians should pay attention to adrenal insufficiency as a cause of delirium.

Takotsubo cardiomyopathy is now an established syndrome worldwide [16–19], but there are no universally accepted diagnostic criteria for this syndrome. Major clinical characteristics are as follows. First, the symptoms are similar to those of acute myocardial infarction. Second, most cases involve elderly woman. Third, Takotsubo-like left ventricular dysfunction, which extends over more than one coronary artery region, is transient and resolves within several weeks. These findings are consistent with our case. Furthermore, myocardial damage is usually excluded when the CK-MB is <5 or 6% of the total CK activity; in our case, the CK-MB was 4.1% of the total CK activity. The CK elevation may result not from myocardial damage, but rather from the skeletal muscle. Pheochromocytoma can cause myocardial damage unrelated to the coronary arteries [20]. Therefore, although we measured the plasma and urine catecholamine levels, they were within normal limits (Table 2(a)). In addition, computed tomography of the abdomen did not indicate the presence of a mass lesion, which suggests pheochromocytoma; therefore, we ruled out pheochromocytoma.

In our case, immediate replacement therapy with hydrocortisone sufficiently improved her cardiomyopathy. Therefore, we could conclude that her myocardial dysfunction was closely related to adrenal insufficiency. Six cases of reversible left ventricular dysfunction or cardiomyopathy associated with isolated ACTH deficiency have been reported previously [5–9]. Similar to these six cases, intensive stress induced by adrenal insufficiency caused reversible cardiomyopathy in our patient, although the detailed mechanism of left ventricular dysfunction in Takotsubo cardiomyopathy remains unknown [10–17]. According to the report by Ukita et al. [8], they listed all cases of Takotsubo cardiomyopathy with isolated ACTH deficiency [5–7]. Comparing those cases, we found that all cases including ours were female patients although we could not figure out the meanings of the sex difference. Furthermore, though patients with Takotsubo cardiomyopathy often feel chest pain, most of cases with isolated ACTH deficiency did not feel chest pain including ours. Interestingly, Gotyo et al. reported male patient developing Takotsubo cardiomyopathy with idiopathic ACTH deficiency [9]. Their patient also impaired GH secretion, and it was not isolated ACTH deficiency with regard to definition; therefore, they used the word idiopathic ACTH deficiency.

To our knowledge, this case represents the first report of both delirium and Takotsubo cardiomyopathy associated with isolated ACTH deficiency. In summary, the present case of a patient suffering from delirium and Takotsubo cardiomyopathy was subsequently diagnosed with adrenal insufficiency induced by isolated ACTH deficiency secondary to a diagnosis of hyponatremia. Both symptoms resolved immediately after the start of steroid replacement therapy with no subsequent relapse; therefore, the unstable mental status and cardiac dysfunction are considered to have been secondary to adrenal insufficiency. Therefore, patients with delirium or Takotsubo cardiomyopathy with no apparent etiology should be examined for adrenal function and begin immediate steroid replacement, if needed.

References

[1] W. Arlt and B. Allolio, "Adrenal insufficiency," *The Lancet*, vol. 361, no. 9372, pp. 1881–1893, 2003.

[2] V. S. Fang and J. B. Jaspan, "Delirium and neuromuscular symptoms in an elderly man with isolated corticotroph-deficiency syndrome completely reversed with glucocorticoid replacement," *Journal of Clinical Endocrinology and Metabolism*, vol. 69, no. 5, pp. 1073–1077, 1989.

[3] K. Nemoto, Y. Kawanishi, H. Suzuki, K. Mizukami, and T. Asada, "Isolated adrenocorticotropic hormone deficiency presenting with delirium," *American Journal of Psychiatry*, vol. 164, no. 9, p. 1440, 2007.

[4] H. Imai, K. Matsuishi, N. Kitamura et al., "Isolated adrenocorticotropic hormone deficiency accompanied with delirium," *Psychiatry and Clinical Neurosciences*, vol. 63, no. 3, pp. 426–427, 2009.

[5] K. Iga, K. Hori, and H. Gen, "Deep negative T waves associated with reversible left ventricular dysfunction in acute adrenal crisis," *Heart and Vessels*, vol. 7, no. 2, pp. 107–111, 1992.

[6] K. Eto, T. Koga, A. Sakamoto, N. Kawazoe, S. Sadoshima, and K. Onoyama, "Adult reversible cardiomyopathy with pituitary adrenal insufficiency caused by empty sella—a case report," *Angiology*, vol. 51, no. 4, pp. 319–323, 2000.

[7] S. Sakihara, K. Kageyama, T. Nigawara, Y. Kidani, and T. Suda, "Ampulla (takotsubo) cardiomyopathy caused by secondary adrenal insufficiency in ACTH isolated deficiency," *Endocrine Journal*, vol. 54, no. 4, pp. 631–636, 2007.

[8] C. Ukita, H. Miyazaki, N. Toyoda, A. Kosaki, M. Nishikawa, and T. Iwasaka, "Takotsubo cardiomyopathy during acute adrenal crisis due to isolated adrenocorticotropin deficiency," *Internal Medicine*, vol. 48, no. 5, pp. 347–352, 2009.

[9] N. Gotyo, M. Kida, T. Horiuchi, and Y. Hirata, "Torsade de pointes associated with recurrent ampulla cardiomyopathy in a patient with idiopathic ACTH deficiency," *Endocrine Journal*, vol. 56, no. 6, pp. 807–815, 2009.

[10] K. Dote, H. Sato, H. Tateishi, T. Uchida, and M. Ishihara, "Myocardial stunning due to simultaneous multivessel coronary spasms: a review of 5 cases," *Journal of Cardiology*, vol. 21, no. 2, pp. 203–214, 1991.

[11] S. Kawai, H. Suzuki, H. Yamaguchi et al., "Ampulla cardiomyopathy ("Takotusbo" cardiomyopathy) reversible left ventricular dysfunction with ST segment elevation," *Japanese Circulation Journal*, vol. 64, no. 3, pp. 156–159, 2000.

[12] K. Tsuchihashi, K. Ueshima, T. Uchida et al., "Transient left ventricular apical ballooning without coronary artery stenosis: a novel heart syndrome mimicking acute myocardial infarction. Angina Pectoris-Myocardial Infarction Investigations in Japan," *Journal of the American College of Cardiology*, vol. 38, no. 1, pp. 11–18, 2001.

[13] Y. J. Akashi, K. Nakazawa, M. Sakakibara, F. Miyake, H. Koike, and K. Sasaka, "The clinical features of takotsubo cardiomyopathy," *QJM*, vol. 96, no. 8, pp. 563–573, 2003.

[14] S. Kurisu, H. Sato, T. Kawagoe et al., "Tako-tsubo-like left ventricular dysfunction with ST-segment elevation: a novel cardiac syndrome mimicking acute myocardial infarction," *American Heart Journal*, vol. 143, no. 3, pp. 448–455, 2002.

[15] Y. Abe, M. Kondo, R. Matsuoka, M. Araki, K. Dohyama, and H. Tanio, "Assessment of clinical features in transient left ventricular apical ballooning," *Journal of the American College of Cardiology*, vol. 41, no. 5, pp. 737–742, 2003.

[16] K. A. Bybee, T. Kara, A. Prasad et al., "Systematic review: transient left ventricular apical ballooning: a syndrome that mimics ST-segment elevation myocardial infarction," *Annals of Internal Medicine*, vol. 141, no. 11, pp. 858–865, 2004.

[17] S. W. Sharkey, W. Shear, M. Hodges, and C. A. Herzog, "Reversible myocardial contraction abnormalities in patients with an acute noncardiac illness," *Chest*, vol. 114, no. 1, pp. 98–105, 1998.

[18] P. S. Seth, G. P. Aurigemma, J. M. Krasnow, D. A. Tighe, W. J. Untereker, and T. E. Meyer, "A syndrome of transient left ventricular apical wall motion abnormality in the absence of coronary disease: a perspective from the United States," *Cardiology*, vol. 100, no. 2, pp. 61–66, 2003.

[19] W. J. R. Desmet, B. F. M. Adriaenssens, and J. A. Y. Dens, "Apical ballooning of the left ventricle: first series in white patients," *Heart*, vol. 89, no. 9, pp. 1027–1031, 2003.

[20] K. Iga, H. Gen, G. Tomonaga, T. Matsumura, and K. Hori, "Reversible left ventricular wall motion impairment caused by pheochromocytoma. A case report," *Japanese Circulation Journal*, vol. 53, no. 7, pp. 813–818, 1989.

38

Autoimmune Polyendocrine Syndrome 3 Onset with Severe Ketoacidosis in a 74-Year-Old Woman

Stefano Benedini,[1,2,3] **Antonietta Tufano,**[3] **Elena Passeri,**[1,3] **Marco Mendola,**[2,3] **Livio Luzi,**[1,2,3,4] **and Sabrina Corbetta**[1,3]

[1]*Department of Biomedical Sciences for Health, Università degli Studi di Milano, Via Morandi 30, San Donato Milanese, 20097 Milan, Italy*
[2]*Metabolism Research Center, IRCCS Policlinico San Donato, Via Morandi 30, San Donato Milanese, 20097 Milan, Italy*
[3]*Endocrinology Unit, IRCCS Policlinico San Donato, Via Morandi 30, San Donato Milanese, 20097 Milan, Italy*
[4]*Endocrinology and Metabolic Diseases, IRCCS Policlinico San Donato, Via Morandi 30, San Donato Milanese, 20097 Milan, Italy*

Correspondence should be addressed to Stefano Benedini; stefanobenedini@hotmail.com

Academic Editor: Carlo Capella

Type 1 diabetes mellitus (T1D), autoimmune thyroid disease, and autoimmune gastritis often occur together forming the so-called autoimmune polyendocrine syndrome type 3 (APS3). We here report a clinical case of a 74-year-old woman who presented for the first time with severe hyperglycemia and ketoacidosis diagnosed as T1D. Further clinical investigations revealed concomitant severe hypothyroidism with autoimmune thyroid disease and severe cobalamin deficiency due to chronic atrophic gastritis. The diagnosis of type 1 diabetes mellitus was confirmed by the detection of autoantibodies against glutamic acid decarboxylase 65, islet cell antibodies, and anti-insulin autoantibodies. Anti-thyroperoxidase, anti-thyroglobulin, and anti-gastric parietal cell antibodies were also clearly positive. The case emphasized that new onset diabetic ketoacidosis, hypothyroidism, and cobalamin deficiency may simultaneously occur, and one disease can mask the features of the other, thereby making diagnosis difficult. It is noteworthy that an APS3 acute episode occurred in an asymptomatic elder woman for any autoimmune diseases.

1. Introduction

Type 1 diabetes mellitus (T1D), autoimmune thyroid disease (ATD), and autoimmune atrophic gastritis (AAG) often occur together forming the so-called autoimmune polyendocrine syndrome (APS) type 3. Thyroid autoimmunity is evident in up to one-third and gastric autoimmunity in up to a quarter of patients with T1D [1]. T1D has historically been considered a predominant disorder of children and young adults: the disease has been commonly referred to as juvenile diabetes because it shows a peak of occurrence at 10–14 years. However, recent studies support a different model in which the disease may occur at any age. Such patients are best identified by the presence of anti-islet autoantibodies, in particular autoantibodies against glutamic acid decarboxylase 65 (GAD65) [2].

Nonetheless the most common presentation of APS consists in an autoimmune thyroid disease without adrenal insufficiency and another associated autoimmune disease such as T1D, pernicious anemia, vitiligo, or alopecia that usually develops in middle-aged women.

Here a case of APS3 presenting with ketoacidosis in an otherwise healthy elder woman was described.

2. Case Presentation

The female patient, aged 74 years, weighed 45 kg with a BMI of 20.5 Kg/m^2. She was admitted through the Emergency Department at the IRCCS Policlinico San Donato (San Donato Milanese, Italy) for severe drowsiness and unresponsiveness. Symptoms promptly occurred after a flu-like syndrome. Her vital signs were significant for mild hypotension.

TABLE 1: Anthropometrical and clinical characteristics of the patient upon admission to hospital and at discharge.

Variable	Emergency Department	At hospital discharge
Weight (kg)	45	47
Height (cm)	148	148
BMI (kg/m^2)	20.5	21.4
Blood glucose (mmol/L)	61.39	6.83
Insulin (μU/mL)	1.1	0.7
C-peptide (ng/mL)	1.1	0.8
Urinary glucose (mg/dL)	1000	0
Blood K^+ (mEq/L)	4.67	3.93
Blood Na^+ (cm)	141	137
TSH (μUI/mL)	102	10.2
FT3 (pg/mL)	0.6	2.3
FT4 (ng/dL)	0.15	1.01

TABLE 2: Organ specific autoantibodies evaluated during hospitalization.

Organ specific autoantibodies	
GADA (glutamic acid decarboxylase antibodies)	Positive
ICA (islet cell antibodies)	Positive
IAA (insulin autoantibodies)	Positive
IA2 (tyrosine-phosphatase autoantibodies)	Negative
Znt8 (autoantibodies to the islet-specific zinc transporter isoform 8)	Negative
TPO (antibodies anti-peroxidase)	Positive
Ab TG (antibodies anti-thyroglobulin)	Positive
PCA (antibodies anti-parietal cells)	Positive
ACA (adrenal cortex antibodies)	Negative
AGA (anti-gliadin antibodies)	Negative
EMA (anti-endomysium antibody)	Negative

Her physical exam revealed severe dehydration, though the patient was relatively well nourished. Her admission laboratory values were significant for blood glucose level of 61.4 mmol/L and pH of 7.2 with bicarbonate of 19 mmol/L. Urine analysis showed massive glycosuria and ketonuria (Table 1). Brain computed tomography showed no noticeable space occupying cerebral lesion or recent density abnormalities of the white or gray matter. Rehydration and insulin intravenous infusion restored patient's consciousness within 3-4 hours without neuropsychiatric sequelae.

She was admitted to the Endocrine Unit of the IRCCS Policlinico San Donato where metabolic variables were stabilized within 3 days. Endocrine screening unmasked concomitant severe hypothyroidism (serum TSH 102 μU/mL, free T4 0.15 ng/mL). The clinical signs associated with hypothyroidism were elevated total cholesterol (248 mg/dL) and creatine kinase (186 UI/L, n.v <176). Ultrasound imaging of the neck showed a thyroid gland of reduced volume and with hypoechoic features of thyroiditis. L-thyroxine replacement was started following the check of conserved adrenal secretion (ACTH pg/mL, cortisol μg/dL). Further biochemical evaluation revealed mild anemia (haemoglobin 11 g/dL; n.v. 12–16) with macrocytosis (mean red cell volume 100.5 fL) associated with reduced serum folates (5 ng/mL; n.v. 5–19) and vitamin B12 (199 pg/mL; n.v. 191–663). Endoscopy diagnosed severe atrophic gastritis that was histologically confirmed by multiple biopsies. Cobalamin and folates were replaced. The patient significantly improved over a 14-day long hospitalization. She was discharged in good general condition.

An autoimmunity screening was performed: autoantibodies against glutamic acid decarboxylase (GAD) have positive results as well as anti-islet cell autoantibodies (ICA) and anti-insulin autoantibodies (IAA) (Table 2). Moreover, anti-peroxidase (AbTPO) and anti-thyroglobulin (AbTg) autoantibodies (Table 2) as well as anti-parietal cells autoantibodies (APCA) were detected in the patient's serum.

The case here reported emphasizes that new onset diabetic ketoacidosis, hypothyroidism, and cobalamin deficiency may occur, and one disease can mask the features of the other, thereby making diagnosis a clinical challenge. It is noteworthy that an utterly asymptomatic patient to any autoimmune diseases had a APS3 acute episode (i.e., hyperglycemia, severe hypothyroidism, and cobalamin deficiency) in her elder age. Overt diabetes onset with typical signs of polyuria and polydipsia was likely delayed by the concomitant low metabolic basal rate secondary to the severe unrecognized hypothyroidism and malabsorption. In this context, the flu-like episode was sufficient to precipitate the impaired metabolic homeostasis. Indeed, acute infections are known to usually drop myxedematous coma.

Moreover, the present case reminds us that autoimmunity might arise in the elderly. In a previous study on T1D Northern Italian patients, the prevalence of diabetes-related autoantibodies was higher in the 21–40-year-old group compared to the 41–72-year-old group and these antibodies have higher results in females than in males [3]. GAD, ICA, and IAA were clearly detectable in the serum of the reported patient. Autoimmune thyroid disorders are the most prevalent immunological diseases in T1D patients [4]. The prevalence of positive AbTPO has been reported in about 80% of T1D patients with elevated TSH levels and in 10–20% in euthyroid T1D individuals. Most patients have subclinical disease, and the development of diabetes usually precedes the diagnosis of hypothyroidism [5]. Due to the increased prevalence of thyroid dysfunction in T1D subjects, regular screening of TSH is recommended [4]. Atrophic gastritis is present in about 25–40% of patients with T1D, whereas in thyroiditis the prevalence of atrophic gastritis is present in approximately one-third of cases. Therefore, the occurrence of multiorgan autoimmune involvement is not unusual though concomitant related insufficiency, as occurred in the present case, is surprising and, more importantly, might be life-threatening. The present case report supports the inclusion of serum TSH and cobalamin determinations among the hormone tests at admission of diabetic ketoacidotic elder patients.

Consent

Written informed consent was obtained from the patient for publication of this case report and any accompanying images.

References

[1] C. Betterle and R. Zanchetta, "Update on autoimmune polyendocrine syndromes (APS)," *Acta Biomedica de l'Ateneo Parmense*, vol. 74, no. 1, pp. 9–33, 2003.

[2] M. A. Atkinson and G. S. Eisenbarth, "Type 1 diabetes: new perspectives on disease pathogenesis and treatment," *The Lancet*, vol. 358, no. 9277, pp. 221–229, 2001.

[3] C. Betterle, F. Lazzarotto, A. Fusari et al., "Pancreatic autoantibodies in Italian patients with newly diagnosed type 1 diabetes mellitus over the age of 20 years," *Acta Diabetologica*, vol. 43, no. 3, pp. 79–83, 2006.

[4] W. J. Riley, N. K. Maclaren, D. C. Lezotte, R. P. Spillar, and A. L. Rosenbloom, "Thyroid autoimmunity in insulin-dependent diabetes mellitus: the case for routine screening," *The Journal of Pediatrics*, vol. 99, no. 3, pp. 350–354, 1981.

[5] M. Mouradian and N. Abourizk, "Diabetes mellitus and thyroid disease," *Diabetes Care*, vol. 6, no. 5, pp. 512–520, 1983.

Occult Thyroid Carcinoma without Malignant Thyroid Gland Findings during Preoperative Examination: Report of Three Cases

Soji Toda[1] **Hiroyuki Iwasaki**[1] **Nobuyasu Suganuma,**[1] **Yoichiro Okubo**[2] **Hiroyuki Hayashi,**[2] **Katsuhiko Masudo,**[3] **Hirotaka Nakayama**[4] **and Munetaka Masuda**[4]

[1]*Department of Breast and Endocrine Surgery, Kanagawa Cancer Center, Yokohama, Japan*
[2]*Department of Pathology, Kanagawa Cancer Center, Yokohama, Japan*
[3]*Department of Breast and Thyroid Surgery, Yokohama City University Medical Center, Yokohama, Japan*
[4]*Department of Surgery, Yokohama City University School of Medicine, Yokohama, Japan*

Correspondence should be addressed to Soji Toda; s-toda@kcch.jp

Academic Editor: John Broom

Occult thyroid carcinoma preceded by clinical manifestations and findings from extrathyroidal tumors is rare. The lack of malignant findings in the thyroid during the preoperative examination makes diagnosis difficult. We encountered a 71-year-old man with a primary ectopic thyroid carcinoma causing superior vena cava syndrome. Although no malignant findings were found in the thyroid gland, biopsy of bone metastases led to the diagnosis of thyroid cancer. HE staining of bone metastases revealed nuclear features of papillary carcinoma, and immunostaining was positive for thyroglobulin and PAX-8. The second case involved an 84-year-old man with a mediastinal tumor and suspected thyroid cancer because of high thyroglobulin levels in blood. The pathological tumor finding was papillary thyroid cancer. The last case was that of a 56-year-old woman lacking preoperative thyroid examination malignant findings, but with cervical lymph node metastasis. The thyroglobulin level of the lymph node puncture fluid was useful for preoperative diagnosis. We performed total thyroidectomy plus bilateral modified neck dissection. Pathology revealed a 1 mm papillary carcinoma in the left lobe. All of these cases were difficult to diagnose. However, we combined the results of various tests such as radiographic imaging, blood tests, and immunohistological tests to diagnose our patients.

1. Introduction

Papillary thyroid cancer is the most common thyroid cancer and is likely to metastasize to the cervical lymph nodes often found in a thyroid mass. However, some thyroid cancers do not show malignant findings in the thyroid during preoperative examinations. These occult carcinomas are rare, and their diagnosis is difficult. In this paper, we report the cases of three patients with occult thyroid cancer preceded by clinical manifestations and findings from extrathyroidal tumors.

2. Case Presentation

Case 1 is a 71-year-old man who had facial edema for 9 months. He had jugular venous distention and eyelid edema. An enhanced computed tomography (CT) scan showed a 27 mm lump on the right side of the upper mediastinum, stenosis of the superior vena cava, and dilation of surrounding collateral vessels (Figure 1(a)). We diagnosed the patient as presenting superior vena cava syndrome due to superior mediastinal tumor.

Positron emission tomography-computed tomography (PET-CT) showed accumulation in the upper mediastinal tumor (SUVmax = 5.18), the left 1st and 4th ribs (SUVmax = 5.48), and lumbar vertebrae L1 and L2 (SUVmax = 7.64), but no hot spot in the thyroid (Figure 1(b)). A bone biopsy of the lumbar vertebrae revealed atypical epithelial cells with a follicular structure and nuclear groove on HE staining, and immunostaining was positive for thyroglobulin and PAX-8 (Figure 2), indicating the presence of a bone metastasis of papillary thyroid carcinoma.

Cervical ultrasonography showed no obvious malignancy in the thyroid. Tumor markers and thyroid function

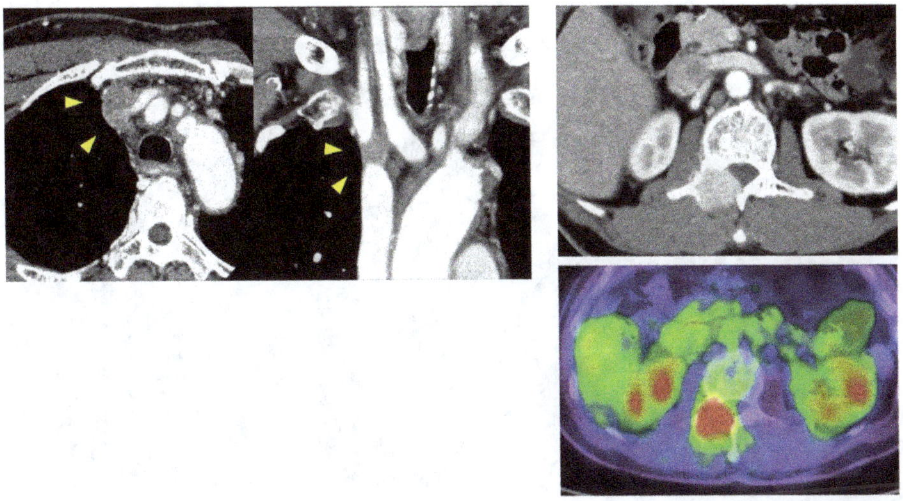

(a) (b)

FIGURE 1: CT and PET-CT findings. (a) Computed tomography showing a 27 mm lump on the right side of the upper mediastinum that is invading the superior vena cava. (b) PET-CT showing metastasis of the lumbar vertebrae.

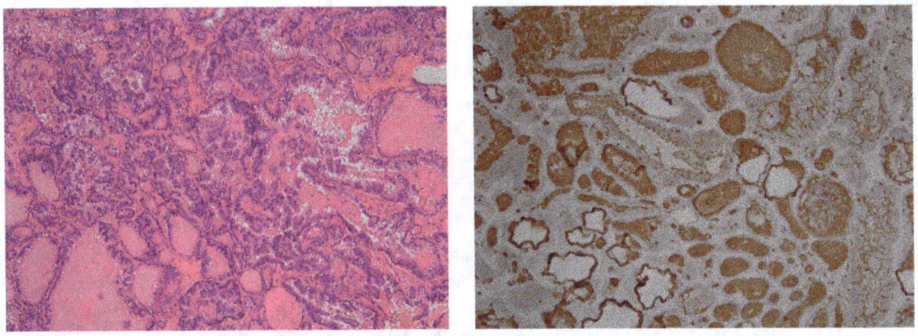

(a) (b)

FIGURE 2: Bone biopsy results of the lumbar vertebrae. HE staining showing a papillary structure and positive immunohistochemistry for thyroglobulin. (a) HE staining ×100. (b) Immunohistochemistry for thyroglobulin ×100.

tests were almost normal without thyroglobulin elevation (103 ng/mL).

We performed total thyroidectomy to administer radioiodine therapy and to reveal any primary tumor present in the thyroid. However, we found no papillary carcinoma in the gland.

The mediastinal tumor seemed to be firmly attached to the superior vena cava, and congestion was strong because of superior vena cava syndrome. Therefore, removing the superior mediastinal tumor or obtaining a biopsy was impossible. However, we suspected that the upper mediastinal tumor was the primary site because we found no other tumors. After surgery, we performed radioactive iodine (RAI) therapy as planned. A dosage of 100 mCi was administered to the patient. Although we observed uptake into the thyroid floor, we found no evidence of uptake into the mediastinum or bone. The thyroglobulin decreased to 26.1 ng/mL after RAI therapy. One year after surgery, there was no tumor growth and the superior vena cava syndrome was improving with the development of collateral circulation.

Case 2 is an 84-year-old man without remarkable medical history other than hyperlipidemia and prostatic hyperplasia. His chief complaint was cough, and an X-ray image showed an abnormal shadow on the upper mediastinum. A CT scan showed a 7.2 cm large mixed mass with a papillary solid component in the anterior mediastinum, and the trachea was compressed to the right and back. We could not confirm continuity with the thyroid; we found no lymph node metastases (Figure 3).

A PET-CT showed accumulation in the upper mediastinal tumor (SUVmax = 46.32) and pale nodules in the left

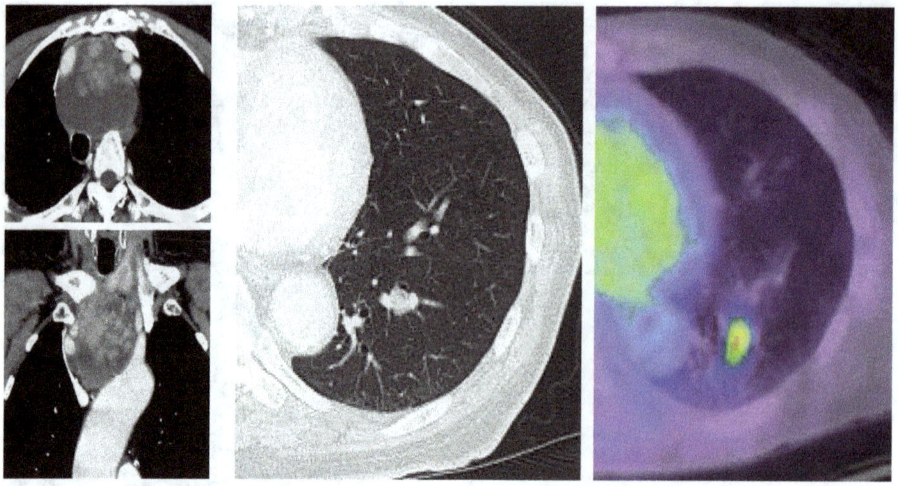

(a) (b)

FIGURE 3: CT images. (a) 7.2 cm mass in the anterior mediastinum. (b) Pulmonary metastasis.

lower lobe (SUVmax = 5.23; Figure 3). Neck ultrasonography revealed multiple nodules reminiscent of an adenomatous goiter in both lobes with no malignant appearance (the mediastinal tumors could not be visualized, and their continuity with the thyroid was unclear).

We performed endobronchial ultrasound-guided transbronchial needle aspiration (EBUS-TBNA) for diagnosis of the mediastinal tumor, but found no tumor cells, and the tumor's origin remained unknown.

In blood tests, the thyroid function was normal, but the thyroglobulin level rose to 2450 ng/mL. No other tumor markers were significant. We suspected that the mediastinal tumor originated from a thyroid cancer, and we decided to resect it.

The patient underwent total thyroidectomy, central neck dissection, and mediastinal tumor resection with sternal incision.

The mediastinal tumor adhered to the brachiocephalic artery and the right recurrent nerve on the right side, with the trachea and esophagus on the dorsal side and with the left recurrent laryngeal nerve on the left side. On the caudal side, a part of the thymus was resected together because the tumor also adhered to it.

Pathological findings included a fibrotic capsule and marked internal necrosis. The pathological report suggested a papillary carcinoma because of the preponderance of papillary growth and the presence of a papillary carcinoma nucleus (nuclear groove; Figure 4). We found no evidence of continuity between the mediastinal tumor and the thyroid. In addition, we noticed a 9 mm nodule in the isthmus of the thyroid and a nuclear finding of papillary carcinoma. We considered the nodule to represent a metastasis to the thyroid. We found no lymph node metastases. The thyroglobulin level decreased to 25.7 ng/mL after surgery. Administration of 131-iodine (100 mCi) resulted in strong accumulation in the thyroid bed and weak accumulation in lung metastasis. Therefore, we plan to follow-up the RAI therapy.

Case 3 is a 56-year-old woman without remarkable medical history. Her chief complaint was a neck mass. We found swelling of the lateral cervical lymph nodes upon examination. Neck ultrasonography showed no thyroid malignancies. Contrast-enhanced CT showed a hepatic hemangioma only, without findings suggesting a primary site (Figure 5). Upper gastrointestinal endoscopy and transvaginal ultrasonography were both normal.

Blood tests showed no tumor marker or thyroid function abnormalities, the thyroglobulin level was 37.9 ng/mL, and anti-thyroglobulin antibody was negative. Fine needle aspiration cytology of the lymph node revealed an adenocarcinoma without nuclear findings of papillary carcinoma. However, the thyroglobulin value of the puncture fluid was high (>500 ng/mL).

Since we suspected a cervical lymph node metastasis of thyroid cancer, we performed total thyroidectomy plus bilateral modified neck dissection to look for the primary tumor and for RAI therapy. A search through the excised thyroid with 4 mm slices revealed 1 mm of papillary carcinoma in the left lobe. We found metastases in 11 of 31 lymph nodes, with a maximum diameter of 23 mm. The metastatic lymph nodes had nuclear findings of papillary thyroid carcinoma (Figure 6).

The patient is considered to be at an ATA intermediate risk as she exhibited clinical N1 within all involved lymph nodes of <3 cm at their largest dimension [1]. She was recommended postoperative RAI, but she refused this procedure. TSH suppression therapy was performed, and TSH was suppressed under 0.1 μU/ml. Thyroglobulin levels decreased to <1 ng/mL following surgery. The patient did not experience recurrences up to 4 postoperative years.

3. Discussion

Occult thyroid carcinoma is a general term indicating clinically different situations that can be classified into five types as described below:

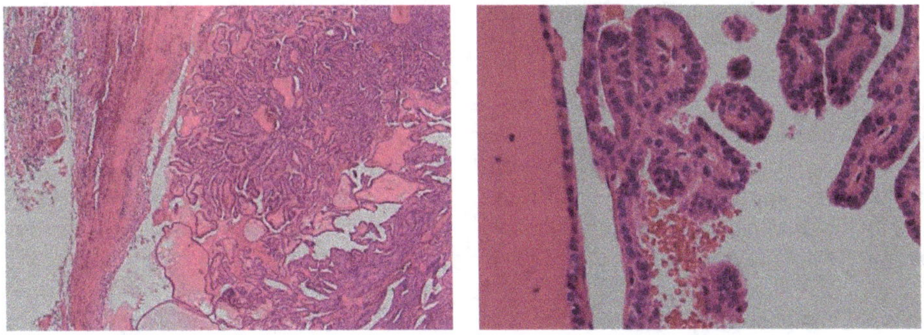

(a) (b)

Figure 4: Pathology results for a tumor. Mediastinal tumor growing in papillary shape with a fibrotic capsule. Tumor cells have nuclear groove and inclusion body (HE staining). (a) ×20. (b) ×400.

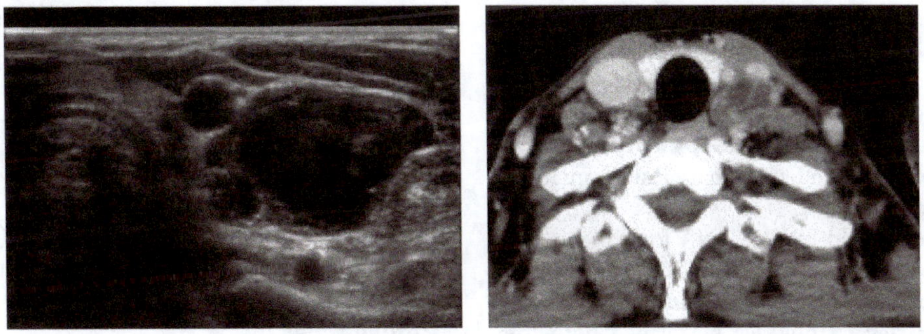

(a) (b)

Figure 5: Left lateral cervical lymph node imaging. Neck ultrasonography (a) and CT scan (b) images showing cervical lymph node swelling.

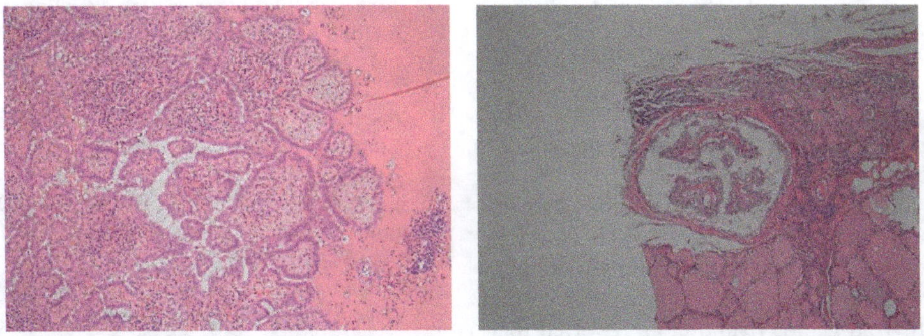

(a) (b)

Figure 6: Microscopic pathology slides of left cervical lymph nodes. (a) Left cervical lymph nodes had nuclear findings of papillary thyroid carcinoma. (b) 1 mm papillary carcinoma tumor in the left lobe (HE staining ×100).

Type 1 is sometimes found by autopsy or surgery for a benign lesion and is sometimes called latent cancer. Type 2 is a papillary thyroid microcarcinoma (PTMC) detected accidentally, mainly by ultrasonography. Type 3 is found with clinically apparent metastases of thyroid carcinoma, where the primary carcinoma is not detectable before surgery but is found in the final histological specimen. Type 4 originates from an ectopic thyroid gland. Type 5 has no carcinoma in the thyroid gland, only metastasis, also known as primary unknown cancer [2, 3].

The frequency of type 2 PTMC has increased because of improvements in diagnostic techniques such as ultrasonography [4], but the frequency of type 3 seems to have decreased. In addition, types 3, 4, and 5 are difficult to diagnose because no preoperative examination shows malignant thyroid findings. Therefore, these three types of occult cancer are clinically problematic. Of the three cases that we have encountered, patients with type 4 (cases 1 and 2) originated from ectopic thyroid gland tissue, and with type 3 (case 3) in an occult thyroid cancer. All of these are very rare cases.

Ultrasonography and fine needle aspiration cytology are useful and recommended for the diagnosis of thyroid cancers [1]. However, these diagnostic procedures are difficult in ectopic thyroid glands in the mediastinum because of anatomical complexity (presence of bones and lungs). We have encountered and reported two cases of patients with mediastinal tumors that were not thyroid cancers and were diagnosed after biopsy by bronchoscopy, immunohistological examination for PAX-8, thyroglobulin, and TTF-1 [5].

In case 1, we detected a papillary thyroid cancer from a bone metastasis biopsy. HE staining revealed an atypical epithelium and nuclear groove with follicular structure, and immunostaining was positive for thyroglobulin and PAX-8. Thus, we diagnosed the patient as having a metastasis of papillary thyroid cancer. The mediastinal tumor had displaced the superior vena cava, and the patient presented a superior vena cava syndrome. We thought that our patient presented a high bleeding risk because of the invasion of the superior vena cava and development of collateral circulation, and we decided not to resect the mediastinal tumor. We considered this ectopic thyroid as the primary tumor site because of the absence of another primary lesion (including in the thyroid gland).

In case 2, we performed EBUS-TBNA for a mediastinal tumor, but were not able to reach a diagnosis. We suspected a thyroid cancer because of the image findings and high blood thyroglobulin level. Thus, we performed both total thyroidectomy and mediastinal tumor resection by sternotomy. The mediastinal tumor pathological findings suggested a papillary thyroid cancer. A small papillary carcinoma was found in the thyroid gland, but the tumor volume was clearly smaller than the mediastinal tumor, and we think that the mediastinal tumor was the primary ectopic thyroid cancer.

Thus, we diagnosed the ectopic thyroid cancer by combining radiographic findings and immunostaining of specimens obtained by biopsy or surgery.

On the other hand, in case 3, we found no papillary thyroid cancer characteristics by cytology of the cervical lymph nodes. However, after measuring the thyroglobulin value of the puncture fluid, we found an adenocarcinoma derived from the thyroid gland. Uruno et al. reported that the measurements of thyroglobulin in the puncture fluid are useful for diagnosing cervical lymph node metastases in differentiated thyroid cancers [6]. Our results with case 3 support this idea. In addition, pathological examination of the thyroid gland after total thyroidectomy revealed a primary tumor in the thyroid gland, but its tumor size was so small that preoperative ultrasonography did not detect it.

Occult thyroid cancers in cervical lymph node metastases are intermediate to high risk, and RAI ablation should be considered [7]. If present in other metastases, RAI is recommended because distant metastases are considered an ATA high risk [1]. In cases where occult thyroid cancer is suspected, the metastasis site should be removed if possible for diagnostic and therapeutic purposes, and total thyroidectomy should be considered to allow for RAI, even if no thyroid gland findings are present.

Although few such cases have been reported, occult carcinoma exhibiting cervical cystic lymph node metastasis as the first manifestation has been reported. Verge et al. described seven papillary thyroid carcinomas that were discovered following a solitary lateral cervical cyst, and reported that ipsilateral modified neck dissection and total thyroidectomy followed by radioactive iodine therapy offered a favorable prognosis [8]. However, pathologic N1 with any metastatic lymph node >3 cm at its largest dimension is described as a high risk for ATA. When a tumor is discovered with cervical lymph node metastasis, the tumor size of lymph node metastasis is expected to be large. In high-risk cases, recurrence should be monitored, just as with regular PTC.

Occult papillary thyroid cancer is rare, and diagnosis is often impossible by ultrasonic examination or puncture aspiration cytology alone. Combining radiographic images, blood tests, immunohistological tests, and clinical signs is necessary. If occult thyroid cancer is suspected, total thyroidectomy should be considered even in the absence of malignant thyroid findings.

Acknowledgments

The authors would like to thank Enago (http://www.enago.jp) for editing a draft of this manuscript.

References

[1] B. R. Haugen, E. K. Alexander, K. C. Bible et al., "American thyroid association management guidelines for adult patients with thyroid nodules and differentiated thyroid cancer: the American thyroid association guidelines task force on thyroid nodules and differentiated thyroid cancer," *Thyroid*, vol. 26, no. 1, pp. 1–133, 2015.

[2] H. Liu, L. Lv, and K. Yang, "Occult thyroid carcinoma: a rare case report and review of literature," *International Journal of Clinical & Experimental Pathology*, vol. 7, no. 8, pp. 5210–5214, 2014.

[3] J. Boucek, J. Kastner, J. Skrivan et al., "Occult thyroid carcinoma," *Acta Otorhinolaryngologica Italica*, vol. 29, no. 6, pp. 296–304, 2009.

[4] L. Enewold, K. Zhu, E. Ron et al., "Rising thyroid cancer incidence in the United States by demographic and tumor characteristics, 1980–2005," *Cancer Epidemiology Biomarkers & Prevention*, vol. 18, no. 3, pp. 784–791, 2009.

[5] H. Yamazaki, H. Iwasaki, Y. Okubo et al., "Two cases of thyroid gland invasion by upper mediastinal carcinoma," *Endocrinology, Diabetes & Metabolism Case Reports*, vol. 2019, 2019.

[6] T. Uruno, A. Miyauchi, K. Shimizu et al., "Usefulness of thyroglobulin measurement in fine-needle aspiration biopsy specimens for diagnosing cervical lymph node metastasis in patients with papillary thyroid cancer," *World Journal of Surgery*, vol. 29, no. 4, pp. 483–485, 2005.

[7] Y. Ito, M. Hirokawa, M. Fukushima et al., "Occult papillary thyroid carcinoma: diagnostic and clinical implications in the era of routine ultrasonography," *World Journal of Surgery*, vol. 32, no. 9, pp. 1955–1960, 2008.

[8] J. Verge, J. Guixa, M. Alejo et al., "Cervical cystic lymph node metastasis as first manifestation of occult papillary thyroid carcinoma: report of seven cases," *Head & Neck*, vol. 21, no. 4, pp. 370–374, 1999.

Disorder of Sexual Development and Congenital Heart Defect in 47XYY: Clinical Disorder or Coincidence?

Hanane Latrech,[1] Imane Skikar,[2] Mohammed El Hassan Gharbi,[3] Abdelmjid Chraïbi,[3] and Ahmed Gaouzi[4]

[1]*Department of Endocrinology, Mohammed VI Hospital, Medical School, Mohammed the First University, 60 000 Oujda, Morocco*
[2]*Department of Radiology, Mohammed VI Hospital, Medical School, Mohammed the First University, 60 000 Oujda, Morocco*
[3]*Department of Endocrinology, Ibn Sina Hospital, Medical School, Mohammed V University, 10 000 Rabat, Morocco*
[4]*Department of Endocrinology Pediatrics, Children Hospital, Medical School, Mohammed V University, 10 000 Rabat, Morocco*

Correspondence should be addressed to Hanane Latrech; hlatrech@hotmail.fr

Academic Editor: Suat Simsek

Background. 47XYY syndrome is a rare sex chromosome variation characterized by an additional Y chromosome. Most patients with 47XYY karyotype have normal phenotype. This disorder seems associated with a higher risk of developing behavioral and cognitive problems, tall stature, and infertility in adulthood. Sexual development disorder is a rare finding. We report a first case with an abnormal left coronary artery originating from the pulmonary artery in a 47XYY patient. *Case.* A one-month-old child was referred for ectopic testis and micropenis. Physical examination revealed facial dysmorphia, micropenis, and curvature of the penis with nonpalpable testis. Laboratory tests showed decreased total testosterone and anti-Mullerian hormone (AMH) levels. Blood karyotyping revealed a 47XYY chromosomal formula. At the age of 3 months, the patient developed dyspnea and tachycardia. Echocardiography revealed an anomalous left coronary artery from pulmonary artery with left ventricular dysfunction requiring surgical revascularization by direct reimplantation of the left coronary artery system. Our second case was a 3-year-old child referred for hypospadias with nonpalpable left testicle. Physical examination showed hypertelorism. Blood karyotyping revealed a 47XYY chromosomal formula. *Conclusion.* To our knowledge, this is the first case of 47XYY syndrome associated with this congenital heart malformation and a sexual development disorder.

1. Introduction

47XYY variation is not an uncommon sex chromosome anomaly estimated in 1/1000 male births [1–3]. It is characterized by an additional Y chromosome secondary to a paternal nondisjunction at meiosis II. In some cases, the failure occurs in the cell division of the postzygotic mitosis in early embryonic development and produces a mosaic 46XY/47XYY karyotype [4–6]. Most patients with 47XYY karyotype have normal phenotype and consequently will have a delayed diagnosis. The child with this abnormality may develop behavioral problems, mild learning disability, delayed speech and language development, and tall stature [3]. We report two cases with 47XYY karyotype associated with micropenis, ectopic testis, and hypospadias rarely described in the literature, one of whom presents congenital heart defect.

2. Case 1

A one-month-old child was referred for ectopic testis and micropenis. In the family history, we found a history of sterility in the father aged 34 years linked to an oligoasthenospermia. There was no family history of consanguinity or similar cases. The patient was born at term with a normal birth weight and height. Physical examination revealed facial dysmorphia including hypertelorism, flat midface, and very marked philtrum. External genitalia examination showed a micropenis (1.5 cm) and curvature of the penis with nonpalpable testis (Figures 1 and 2). The rest of the somatic examination was normal. Laboratory tests showed an LH level at 3.9 UI/L (normal values: 0.55–5.5 mUI/mL), FSH at 7 UI/L (normal values: 1.3–7 mUI/mL), total testosterone level at 1.65 ng/mL (normal values: 1.8–4 ng/mL) and anti-Mullerian hormone (AMH) level at 13.20 ng/mL (normal values: 24–124 ng/mL

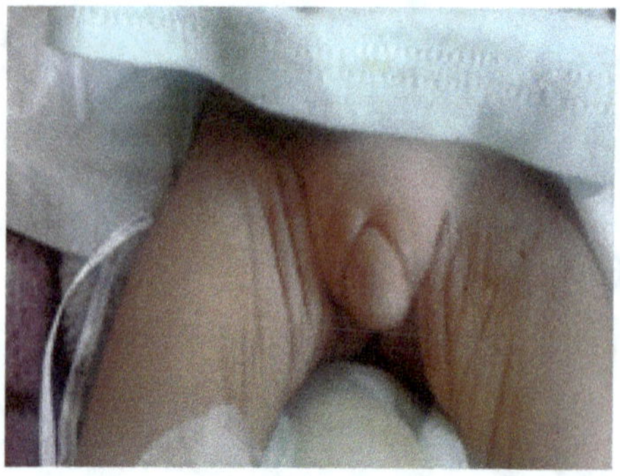

FIGURE 1: Case 1: testis ectopia, micropenis.

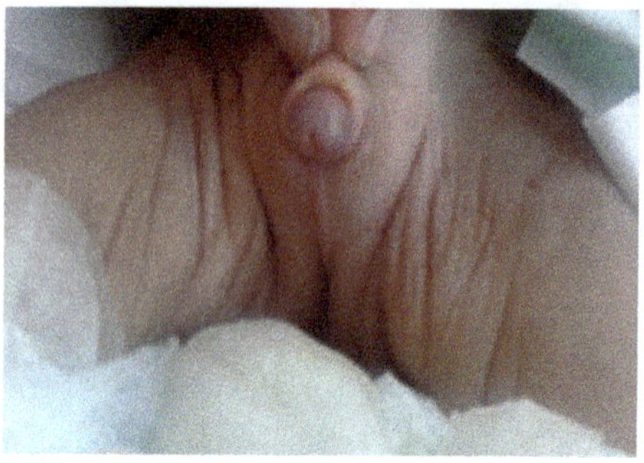

FIGURE 2: Case 1: curvature of the penis.

(EIA Immunotech)). Pelvic ultrasonography showed the testis in inguinal position. Blood karyotyping revealed a 47XYY chromosomal formula. At the age of 3 months, hormonal evaluation showed a total testosterone level at 1.86 ng/mL. Also, the patient developed dyspnea and tachycardia with the presence of cardiomegaly apparent in a chest X-ray. Electrocardiography (ECG) detected q waves in leads DI and aVL with repolarization abnormalities in the left leads. Echocardiography revealed an anomalous left coronary artery originating from the pulmonary artery with left ventricular dysfunction requiring surgical revascularization by direct reimplantation of the left coronary artery system.

3. Case 2

A 3-year-old child was referred to our institution for undescended testes and hypospadias. There was no family history of consanguinity or similar cases. The patient was born at 41 weeks of gestational age with normal birth weight and height. Physical examination revealed normal stature and weight growth for the age, hypertelorism without other facial dysmorphia (Figure 3), and normal psychomotor development. There were no signs of tumor and no other signs of endocrinopathy. Neurological and systemic examinations were unremarkable. External genitalia examination showed anterior hypospadias with nonpalpable left testicle. The right testicle was prepubertal (<3 mL) in scrotal position (Figures 4 and 5). Serum FSH, LH, and testosterone results were age-normal. Both assay of AMH and hCG testing were prescribed. Pelvic ultrasonography showed absence of visible left testis.

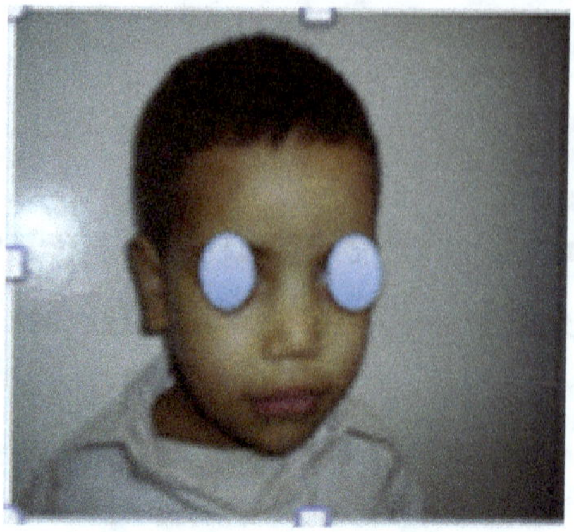

FIGURE 3: Case 2: hypertelorism.

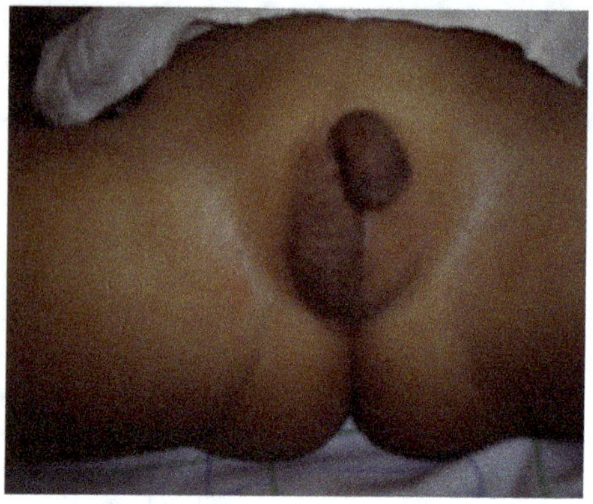

FIGURE 4: Case 2: nonpalpable left testicle and prepubertal right testicle in scrotal position.

Genitography revealed a male urethra without Mullerian ducts (Figure 6).

The karyotype revealed chromosomal formula 47XYY. Surgical treatment for hypospadias and ectopic testis was proposed with medical monitoring of psychomotor and stature development and puberty.

4. Discussion

47XYY variation is the most common sex chromosome anomaly after Klinefelter syndrome (47XXY). The first case with this chromosomal disorder was described in 1961 by Sandberg et al. [7]. This anomaly was the last of the sex chromosome aneuploidies to be discovered. The separation of chromosomes during metaphase II of meiosis called nondisjunction may reveal germ cells with an extra copy of chromosome Y. If one of these atypical sperm cells is involved in fertilization, the child will have an extra Y chromosome in all cells. In some cases, the error occurs in the cell division of the postzygotic mitosis in early embryonic development. This can produce a mosaic 46, XY/47, XYY [3–6]. In 1970, some studies demonstrated that a higher number of persons with 47XYY were in penal and psychiatric institutions [8, 9]. Later, these studies were recognized as having significant methodological flaws [8]. It is currently reported that the patient with

Table 1: Disorder of sexual development in a patient with 47XYY.

	n	Age	DSD
Rivera et al. 1979 [20]	1	5 10/12	Micropenis, hypospadias Right testis regression
Terada et al. 1984 [21]	1	29	Right undescended testis
Okamoto et al. 1988 [22]	2		Hypospadias, cryptorchism
Diego Nunez et al. 1992 [23]	2		Cryptorchism, puberty delay
Suzuki et al. 1999 [24]	1	11 months	Bilateral cryptorchism
Monastirli et al. 2005 [25]	1	72	Cryptorchism, gynecomastia
Bardsley et al. 2013 [26]	1/90 2/90 5/90		Hypospadias Cryptorchism Inguinal hernia
Our cases 2014	2	3 1 month	Hypospadias, ectopic testis Micropenis, ectopic testis (with congenital heart defect)

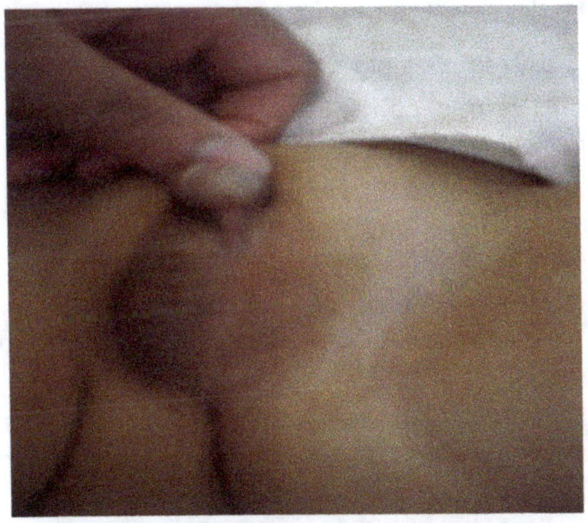

Figure 5: Case 2: hypospadias.

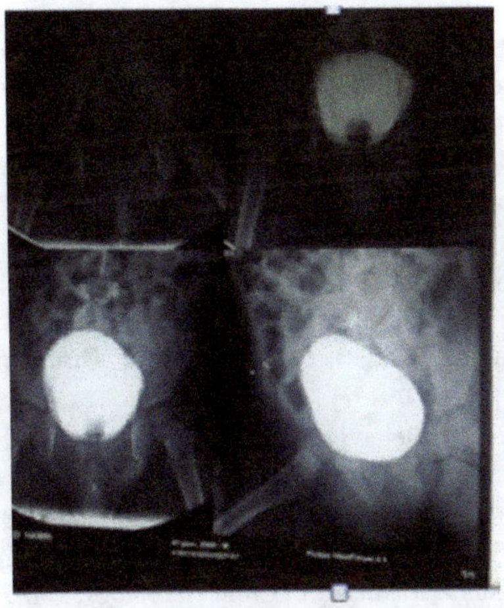

Figure 6: Case 2: male urethra.

47XYY karyotype has cognitive behavioral deficits including delayed language and motor development, impulsivity, poor attention span, and impairment in social interaction with increased risk of autism spectrum disorders [3, 8, 10–15]. In our second case, we did not find these anomalies at this age (3 years). A psychomotor evaluation was proposed with regular monitoring. The study of neuroanatomical variation in 47XYY has shown increased brain matter volumes, a finding putatively related to the increased frequency of autism spectrum disorders. In addition, frontotemporal grey and white matter reductions in XYY syndrome provide a likely neuroanatomical correlate for observed language impairments [10, 16, 17]. It has been reported as an association with 47XYY and migrating partial seizures in infancy, a very rarely reported epilepsy syndrome with unknown etiology. The mechanism of this association is not explained [18]. Most patients with this genetic disorder have no phenotypic abnormalities. Some authors reported tall stature beginning before puberty and increased head circumference [3, 8, 10–12, 19]. In this paper, we report this syndrome recognized at an earlier stage with presence of hypertelorism reported in 59% of cases with 47XYY and disorders of sexual development including hypospadias, micropenis, and ectopic testis. This association has been rarely reported [20–26] (Table 1) and the pathophysiology of the association is not clearly explained. The mechanism by which the excess of genes due to an additional Y chromosome can affect sexual development remains to be fully elucidated. Thus, the external genitalia examination in all patients with 47XYY karyotype may help the clinician to determine whether these disorders of sexual development comprise an incidental finding or are part of the spectrum of XYY syndrome which remains undetected. Some authors have investigated gonadic function in 47XYY children and adolescents and found normal or delayed puberty [26, 27]. Macroorchidism seems to be common with normal testosterone levels [26]. But there have also been reports of a normal or total absence of the testis [20, 28] and increased testosterone levels in institutionalized men with XYY karyotype, with normal [26, 29] or aggressive behavior [27]. In XYY patients with a disorder of sexual development, Rivera et al. reported age-normal basal plasma testosterone levels with an adequate response of the left testicular Leydig cells after hCG stimulation [20]. Our first case revealed a low peak of testosterone secretion (1.86 ng/mL) for a 3-month-old infant. As markers of testicular exocrine functions, inhibin B and anti-Mullerian hormone (AMH) levels were reported as normal in most of the cases. We reported low AMH levels in our first patient. A decrease in the levels of inhibin B has been described in some patients sometimes associated with a high FSH [26, 30]. This may explain some cases of infertility in adults with 47XYY. Indeed, the association with infertility problems was reported with scrotal findings ranging from normal to atrophic testicles, oligospermia, and varying endocrine profiles [3, 8, 10, 31]. It is currently known that some cases with infertility are associated with Yq microdeletions with a significant diagnostic and prognostic value. Therefore, some authors have suggested that, in XYY patients, the excess of copies of genes in the long arm of the Y chromosome could explain this infertility [26, 32]. The offspring of some patients with 47XYY have been studied, yielding reports of abnormal children with gonadal dysgenesis and Down's syndrome [33]. In the child with the extra chromosome, 21 came from the mother. Thus, the necessity of amniocentesis remains to be discussed. In Klinefelter syndrome, the most common genetic disorder characterized by an additional X chromosome, we find tall stature with impairments in language and motor ability similar to those observed in persons with 47XYY karyotype. In addition, Klinefelter syndrome manifests with hypogonadism symptoms including cryptorchidism, small testicles, gynecomastia, impuberism or incomplete pubertal development, sterility in adulthood, and shorter life spans compared with persons with normal karyotype. This shorter lifespan may be due to an increased risk of cancer, pulmonary, neurologic, and unspecified diseases. It has been noted that, for patients with 47XYY, there is significant delay of diagnosis, reduced life expectancy, and an increased overall and cause-specific mortality [3, 34, 35]. The spectra of clinical manifestations of these two different genetic entities vary and seem to produce partially overlapping phenotypes. Thus, multicenter studies are required to further investigate this unusual feature with more evaluation of gonadal function and long-term follow-up in individuals with 47XYY karyotype. In addition, our first patient had a congenital heart defect consisting of an anomalous left coronary artery originating from the pulmonary artery with left ventricular dysfunction requiring surgical reimplantation of the left coronary artery system. It is reported that up to 33% of congenital heart defects are associated with fetal aneuploidy and the majority of fetuses with congenital heart defect and aneuploidy also have extracardiac anomalies [36].

To our knowledge, this is the first case of 47XYY syndrome associated with a disorder of sexual development along with this congenital heart defect. This raises the questions, not only of the mechanism of this association but also of whether this defect is an incidental finding or a new part of the spectrum of XYY syndrome.

5. Conclusion

47XYY syndrome is the most common aneuploidies after Klinefelter syndrome. To date, men with 47XYY have been found to manifest with a characteristic physical phenotype including tall stature and cognitive behavioral deficits with increased risk of autism spectrum disorders and infertility in adulthood. We report a case with this sex chromosome variation associated with disorder of sexual development, an uncommon clinical phenomenon, and with congenital heart malformation. The mechanism of this association remains to be fully elucidated and it remains unclear exactly how an additional Y chromosome could affect testicular and cardiac development in 47XYY syndrome. Thus, multicenter studies are required to carry out more evaluation of gonadal and cardiac function and long-term follow-up in individuals with 47XYY karyotype.

Acknowledgments

The authors would like to thank Dr. Intissar Haddiya for reading the paper and also thank the subjects and their families for their participation.

References

[1] P. A. Jacobs, M. Melville, S. Ratcliffe, A. J. Keay, and J. Syme, "A cytogenetic survey of 11,680 newborn infants," *Annals of Human Genetics*, vol. 37, no. 4, pp. 359–376, 1974.

[2] M. G. Linden and B. G. Bender, "Genetic counseling for sex chromosome abnormalities," *American Journal of Medical Genetics*, vol. 110, no. 1, pp. 3–10, 2002.

[3] I. W. Kim, A. C. Khadilkar, E. Y. Ko, and E. S. Sabanegh Jr., "47,XYY syndrome and male infertility," *Reviews in Urology*, vol. 15, no. 4, pp. 188–196, 2013.

[4] F. El-Dahtory and H. M. Elsheikha, "Male infertility related to an aberrant karyotype, 47,XYY: four case reports," *Cases Journal* vol. 2, no. 1, article 28, 2009.

[5] E. C. Wong, K. A. Ferguson, V. Chow, and S. Ma, "Sperm aneuploidy and meiotic sex chromosome configurations in an infertile XYY male," *Human Reproduction*, vol. 23, no. 2, pp. 374–378, 2008.

[6] E. Moretti, C. Anichini, B. Sartini, and G. Collodel, "Sperm ultrastructure and meiotic segregation in an infertile 47,XYY man," *Andrologia*, vol. 39, no. 6, pp. 229–234, 2007.

[7] A. A. Sandberg, G. F. Koepf, T. Ishihara, and T. S. Hauschka, "An XYY human male," *The Lancet*, vol. 278, no. 7200, pp. 488–489, 1961.

[8] R. K. Lenroot, N. R. Lee, and J. N. Giedd, "Effects of sex chromosome aneuploidies on brain development: evidence from neuroimaging studies," *Developmental Disabilities Research Reviews*, vol. 15, no. 4, pp. 318–327, 2009.

[9] E. B. Hook, "Behavioral implications of the human XYY genotype," *Science*, vol. 179, no. 4069, pp. 139–150, 1973.

[10] D. M. Bryant, F. Hoeft, S. Lai et al., "Sex chromosomes and the brain: a study of neuroanatomy in XYY syndrome," *Developmental Medicine & Child Neurology*, vol. 54, no. 12, pp. 1149–1156, 2012.

[11] M. Geerts, J. Steyaert, and J. P. Fryns, "The XYY syndrome: a follow-up study on 38 boys," *Genetic Counseling*, vol. 14, no. 3, pp. 267–279, 2003.

[12] J. L. Ross, M. P. D. Zeger, H. Kushner, A. R. Zinn, and D. P. Roeltgen, "An extra X or Y chromosome: Contrasting the cognitive and motor phenotypes in childhood in boys with 47,XYY syndrome or 47,XXY Klinefelter syndrome," *Developmental Disabilities Research Reviews*, vol. 15, no. 4, pp. 309–317, 2009.

[13] V. Leggett, P. Jacobs, K. Nation, G. Scerif, and D. V. M. Bishop, "Neurocognitive outcomes of individuals with a sex chromosome trisomy: XXX, XYY, or XXY: A systematic review," *Developmental Medicine and Child Neurology*, vol. 52, no. 2, pp. 119–129, 2010.

[14] D. V. M. Bishop, P. A. Jacobs, K. Lachlan et al., "Autism, language and communication in children with sex chromosome trisomies," *Archives of Disease in Childhood*, vol. 96, no. 10, pp. 954–959, 2011.

[15] N. Tartaglia, S. Davis, R. Hansen et al., "Attention deficit hyperactivity disorder and autism spectrum disorders in males with XXY, XYY, and XXYY syndromes," *Journal of Intellectual Disability Research*, vol. 50, p. 787, 2006.

[16] M. M. Warwick, G. A. Doody, S. M. Lawrie, J. N. Kestelman, J. J. K. Best, and E. C. Johnstone, "Volumetric magnetic resonance imaging study of the brain in subjects with sex chromosome aneuploidies," *Journal of Neurology Neurosurgery and Psychiatry*, vol. 66, no. 5, pp. 628–632, 1999.

[17] D. Shen, D. Liu, H. Liu, L. Clasen, J. Giedd, and C. Davatzikos, "Automated morphometric study of brain variation in XXY males," *NeuroImage*, vol. 23, no. 2, pp. 648–653, 2004.

[18] R. S. Iyer, Thanikasalam, and M. Krishnan, "Migrating partial seizures in infancy and 47XYY syndrome: cause or coincidence?" *Epilepsy & Behavior Case Reports*, vol. 2, no. 1, pp. 43–45, 2014.

[19] S. G. Ratcliffe, N. Masera, H. Pan, and M. McKie, "Head circumference and IQ of children with sex chromosome abnormalities," *Developmental Medicine and Child Neurology*, vol. 36, no. 6, pp. 533–544, 1994.

[20] H. Rivera, A. Hernandez, and R. Martinez, "Malformed genitalia in the 47,XYY genotype," *Annales de Genetique*, vol. 22, no. 4, pp. 225–227, 1979.

[21] T. Terada, S. Yanagi, T. Nakada, and T. Katayama, "A case of XYY syndrome with male infertility and retentio testis," *Hinyokika Kiyo*, vol. 30, no. 5, pp. 701–707, 1984.

[22] E. Okamoto, H. Yabumoto, T. Terakawa et al., "XYY syndrome: report of three cases," *Hinyokika Kiyo*, vol. 34, no. 1, pp. 191–195, 1988.

[23] M. A. Diego Nunez, J. Prieto Veiga, F. Rey Sanchez et al., "The clinical polymorphology of the XYY syndrome," *Anales Espanoles de Pediatria*, vol. 37, no. 2, pp. 140–144, 1992.

[24] Y. Suzuki, I. Sasagawa, T. Kaneko, T. Tateno, Y. Iijima, and T. Nakada, "Bilateral cryptorchidism associated with 47,XYY karyotype," *International Urology and Nephrology*, vol. 31, no. 5, pp. 709–713, 1999.

[25] A. Monastirli, G. Stephanou, S. Georgiou et al., "Short stature, type E brachydactyly, exostoses, gynecomastia, and cryptorchidism in a patient with 47,XYY/45,X/46,XY mosaicism," *The American Journal of the Medical Sciences*, vol. 329, no. 4, pp. 208–210, 2005.

[26] M. Z. Bardsley, K. Kowal, C. Levy et al., "47,XYY syndrome: clinical phenotype and timing of ascertainment," *The Journal of Pediatrics*, vol. 163, no. 4, pp. 1085–1094, 2013.

[27] S. Ratcliffe, "The development of children with sex chromosome abnormalities," *Proceedings of the Royal Society of Medicine*, vol. 69, no. 3, pp. 189–191, 1976.

[28] E. Boisen, "Testicular size and shape of 47,XYY and 47,XXY men in a double-blind, double-matched population survey," *American Journal of Human Genetics*, vol. 31, no. 6, pp. 697–703, 1979.

[29] R. C. Schiavi, A. Theilgaard, D. R. Owen, and D. White, "Sex chromosome anomalies, hormones, and aggressivity," *Archives of General Psychiatry*, vol. 41, no. 1, pp. 93–99, 1984.

[30] L. Aksglaede, R. B. Jensen, E. Carlsen et al., "Increased basal and pulsatile secretion of FSH and LH in young men with 47,XXY or 46,XX karyotypes," *European Journal of Endocrinology*, vol. 158, no. 6, pp. 803–810, 2008.

[31] A. T. Maciel-Guerra, J. De Paulo, A. P. Santos et al., "The use of fluorescence *in situ* hybridization in the diagnosis of hidden mosaicism: apropos of three cases of sex chromosome anomalies," *Arquivos Brasileiros de Endocrinologia & Metabologia*, vol. 56, no. 8, pp. 545–551, 2012.

[32] A. Ferlin, B. Arredi, E. Speltra et al., "Molecular and clinical characterization of Y chromosome microdeletions in infertile men: a 10-year experience in Italy," *Journal of Clinical Endocrinology and Metabolism*, vol. 92, no. 3, pp. 762–770, 2007.

[33] C. Stoll, E. Flori, A. Clavert, D. Beshara, and P. Buck, "Abnormal children of a 47XYY father," *Journal of Medical Genetics*, vol. 16, no. 1, pp. 66–68, 1979.

[34] K. Stochholm, S. Juul, and C. H. Gravholt, "Diagnosis and mortality in 47,XYY persons: a registry study," *Orphanet Journal of Rare Diseases*, vol. 5, no. 1, article 15, 2010.

[35] M. Kielinen, H. Rantala, E. Timonen, S.-L. Linna, and I. Moilanen, "Associated medical disorders and disabilities in children with autistic disorder: a population-based study," *Autism*, vol. 8, no. 1, pp. 49 60, 2004.

[36] R. C. Wimalasundera and H. M. Gardiner, "Congenital heart disease and aneuploidy," *Prenatal Diagnosis*, vol. 24, no. 13, pp. 1116–1122, 2004.

41

Adrenal Mass in a 70-Year-Old Woman

Kiana Karimi,[1,2] Mohsen Nikzad,[3] Sohrab Kulivand,[4] and Shiva Borzouei[5]

[1]*Student Research Committee, Hamadan University of Medical Sciences, Hamadan, Iran*
[2]*Universal Scientific Education and Research Network (USERN), Tehran, Iran*
[3]*Department of Internal Medicine, School of Medicine, Hamadan University of Medical Sciences, Hamadan, Iran*
[4]*Department of Radiology, School of Medicine, Hamadan University of Medical Sciences, Hamadan, Iran*
[5]*Department of Endocrinology, School of Medicine, Hamadan University of Medical Sciences, Hamadan, Iran*

Correspondence should be addressed to Shiva Borzouei; borzooeishiva@yahoo.com

Academic Editor: Osamu Isozaki

Introduction. Adrenocortical carcinoma is a rare endocrine malignancy with a bimodal age distribution pattern that affects women more than men. More than half of the patients present with hormone excess manifestations such as Cushing's syndrome and virilization. Non-functional tumors usually are diagnosed incidentally following imaging studies due to a mass effect or metastatic disease. Surgical resection is considered the best curative treatment for these tumors. *Case Presentation.* A 70-year-old woman presented with a 3-month history of diffuse intermittent abdominal discomfort, weight loss, and additional hair growth. Imaging investigations revealed a large 187 × 85 × 140 mm mass between the liver and upper pole of the right kidney which has displaced the adjacent structures. Hormonal evaluations detected high levels of cortisol and adrenal androgens. She underwent open adrenalectomy and right nephrectomy due to severe adhesion of the mass. Histopathological evaluations revealed adrenocortical carcinoma and the patient received adjuvant radiotherapy. *Conclusion.* Precise physical examination, hormonal evaluation, and imaging studies play a key role in differentiating malignant adrenal masses in all patients, especially in those with vague symptoms. Radical excision of the mass and appropriate adjuvant chemotherapy or radiotherapy improve the outcome for patients.

1. Introduction

Adrenocortical carcinoma (ACC) is a rare endocrine malignancy with an approximate prevalence of 1 to 2 per million. Although this malignancy can develop at any age, it has a bimodal age distribution pattern which commonly affects patients under the age of 5 or in the 4th to 5th decades of life [1]. In addition to genetic predisposition, there is no definite and known risk factor for ACC. However, some studies have shown smoking in men and the use of contraceptives in women as probable risk factors for ACC [2].

Most patients present with signs and symptoms of hormone excess, especially hypercortisolism (50–80%). About one-third of patients have clinical manifestations of local tumor growth, and 20–30% of them are diagnosed incidentally following imaging studies for other reasons [3]. The initial diagnosis of ACC is based on a careful history and physical examination, along with biochemical and endocrinological evaluations. Computed tomography (CT) scanning and magnetic resonance imaging (MRI) are choice imaging modalities for distinguishing ACCs from adrenocortical adenomas, determining local invasion, and distant metastases [4].

In the pathological evaluation of adrenal tumors, size is an important and determining factor in the diagnosis of ACCs [3]. These tumors are typically large, more than 6 cm and diameters of 4–25 cm [5, 6]. Clinical, histological, and immunohistochemical parameters are also conductive in confirming the diagnosis. The Weiss system is the most acceptable histopathological system for assessing malignancy in adrenocortical tumors [7].

Despite the limitation of knowledge about the treatment and prognosis of these patients due to its rarity, some progress has been made in this regard. Surgical resection of the tumor and suspicious lymph nodes is considered a potentially curative treatment. Adjuvant mitotane therapy is recommended for all patients who are at risk for recurrence or have high-grade or incompletely resected tumors. The addition of postoperative radiation therapy (RT) is also suggested for this group of patients [8].

Herein, we present the case of a 70-year-old woman with abdominal discomfort, weight loss, and terminal hair overgrowth that was diagnosed with adrenocortical carcinoma.

2. Case Presentation

A 70-year-old woman, a retired teacher, presented with a 3-month history of abdominal pain. The abdominal discomfort has been intermittent and diffuse without any specific pattern. She has lost her appetite and her body weight decreased about 10 kg over this period. She has complained of malaise and occasional headaches. She denied nausea or vomiting, diaphoresis, palpitation, sleep disturbance, and abnormal uterine bleeding. She has also noted some additional hair growth on her chin, between the breasts, and on the lower abdomen. In her previous medical history, she had controlled hypertension and was on losartan, and she had no history of diabetes. She has also been hospitalized due to COVID-19 one month previously.

On physical examination, she looked cachectic. Her blood pressure was 160/80 mmHg, and other vital signs were normal. On abdominal examination, she had no striae or central obesity. There was mild tenderness over the right upper quadrant and a non-pulsatile 15 cm mass was palpated under the liver. She had excessive terminal hair with a modified Ferriman–Gallwey score of 16. Lower extremities examination showed proximal myopathy in the pelvic girdle. Examination of the cardiovascular and respiratory systems was normal.

The initial laboratory tests revealed an elevation in white blood cell count, fasting glucose concentration, and lactate dehydrogenase level. Other findings were all within the normal limits (Table 1). Contrast-enhanced CT of abdomen indicated a solid retroperitoneal 187 × 85 × 140 mm mass with regular borders and heterogenous enhancement located between the upper pole of the right kidney and VI and VII segments of the liver which has pushed the right kidney down (Figure 1). According to these findings, more hormonal evaluations were performed with the abnormal results shown in Table 2. There was no evidence of bone involvement in the bone scan. Findings suggested adrenal carcinoma, and the patient underwent an exploratory laparotomy after controlling hypertension.

Laparotomy was performed, and the right adrenal mass and kidney were excised due to severe adhesion of the mass to the right renal vein. The inferior vena cava has also been repaired. Macroscopically, the adrenal removed specimen measured 23 × 15 × 9 cm and weighted 1667 g. The tumor was solid, yellowish-gray, and well-defined with an intact capsule. Cross section of the tumor revealed a non-homogenous nodular area with extensive necrosis. There was no evidence of neoplastic invasion to the capsule or external surface of the mass. Microscopic examination revealed polyhedral neoplastic cells in trabecular structures which were arranged in dense cellular sheets. Tumoral cells had giant and pleomorphic nuclei, vesicular chromatin, marked eosinophilic nucleoli, and large amounts of eosinophilic granular to clear cytoplasm. The mitotic activity was more than 6 in 50/high-power fields (HPF), and multifocal coagulation tumoral necrosis was observed. The capsular invasion was identified, but it was not extended beyond it. There was no evidence of tumoral involvement in the right kidney (Figure 2).

Table 1: Initial laboratory workup [9].

Test	Result	Normal range
WBC (white blood cells)	15740/μl	4000–11000
RBC (red blood cells)	5.9 million/μl	4.2–5.4
Hb (hemoglobin)	15.2 g/dl	12.5–16
Platelets	194000/μl	140000–450000
FPG (fasting plasma glucose)	127 mg/dl	60–110
LDH (lactate dehydrogenase)	340 IU/l	140–280
ESR 1h (erythrocyte sedimentation rate)	5 mm/h	0–30
CRP (C-reactive protein)	Negative	
Bun	14 mg/dl	5–23
Cr	1.1 mg/dl	0.6–1.4
Ca	8.6 mg/dl	8.6–11
P	3.4 mg/dl	2.9–5.1
Na	142 mEq/l	135–145
K	3.9 mEq/l	3.9–5.3

The patient was observed in the intensive care unit for a few days after surgery. She was referred to the oncology ward with no surgical complications 9 days after surgery. Since the mass was completely resected and there was no evidence of distant spread of the tumor, she underwent adjuvant radiation therapy without chemotherapy. Follow-up thoracic, abdominal, and pelvic CT 3 months after surgery revealed no recurrence or metastasis, and all hormonal and biochemistry evaluations were within normal limits. 5 months after surgery, she is alive and back to normal in good condition.

3. Discussion

Adrenocortical carcinoma is a rare malignancy in the endocrine system, usually with a poor prognosis [10]. The incidence of these tumors is about 0.7–2.0 cases per million each year, and they are more found in women in the fifth decade of life [11, 12]. They can also affect children, mostly as functional tumors [13]. Most ACC cases appear to be sporadic as in the present case. However, some cases were considered to be associated with several hereditary tumor disorders such as Li-Fraumeni syndrome, multiple endocrine neoplasia type 1, and Beckwith–Wiedemann syndrome [14].

Studies have indicated that more than 60% of ACCs are hormone-producing tumors and they can develop clinical syndromes of hormone excess. These tumors usually induce Cushing's syndrome (45%) in adults and are associated with glucocorticoid excess symptoms, such as weakness, and weight gain, which commonly develop over three to six months. About 25% of patients present with a mixed

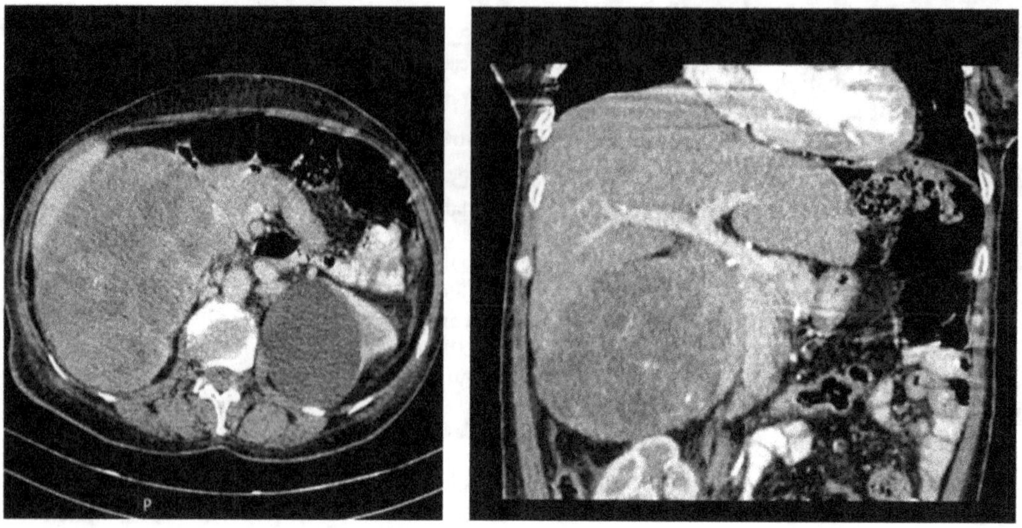

(a) (b)

FIGURE 1: Abdominal CT scan with IV contrast. (a) Axial view of the heterogenous well-defined mass above the right kidney. (b) Coronal view of the adrenal mass effect on the IVC and pancreatic tail.

TABLE 2: Hormonal and tumor marker evaluation [9].

Test	Result	Normal range
Dehydroepiandrosterone sulfate	>1000 μg/dL	Female: 30–400
Testosterone	8.810 ng/ml	>50y: 0.029–0.408
17-OH-progesterone	25.37 ng/ml	Menopause: 0.2–0.9
Estradiol	76 pg/ml	<60
Androstenedione	4.3 ng/ml	0.9–3.2
Cortisol (8 AM)	46.81 micg/dL	6.4–21
24-hour urinary free cortisol	255.1 μg/24 hrs	1.5–63
24-hour urinary metanephrine	30 μg/24 hrs	<350
24-hour urinary normetanephrine	386.9 μg/24 hrs	<600
AFP (alpha-fetoprotein)	3.74 IU/ml	Up to 5.8
CEA (carcinoembryonic antigen)	1.1 ng/ml	Non-smokers: <5.0
CA 125 (carbohydrate antigen 125)	23.48 U/ml	Up to 35

Cushing's and virilization syndrome, due to excessive secretion of both androgens and glucocorticoids and only fewer than 10% of them induce virilization symptoms, implying ACC rather than adenoma [6, 15]. Our patient's main complaint was abdominal discomfort besides recent weight loss which is related to local mass effect. She had no clinical manifestations of Cushing's or virilization syndrome which may be due to the short period from the onset of the tumor growth.

Hormonal estimation including adrenal androgens and glucocorticoids levels may help to determine the adrenal source of the patient's signs and symptoms, providing tumor markers which are useful during patient's follow-up to assess possible tumor recurrence or residual tumor after surgery [8]. In the present case, high adrenal androgens and estradiol levels were detected and made the diagnosis of adrenal carcinomas more probable than adrenal adenomas [16]. Urinary excretion of metanephrines and normetanephrines was measured, and they were within normal range which excluded the possibility of pheochromocytoma.

CT scan and MRI are preferred imaging methods for evaluating the tumor size, local invasion, or distant tumor invasion. These tumors usually have the following features on CT scan: tumor size larger than 4 cm, inhomogeneous but well-defined suprarenal mass, displacing adjacent structure, heterogenous enhancement after IV contrast administration, and less frequent calcification and IVC tumor thrombus, especially in right-sided tumors [4]. As described above, our patient had most of these features in imaging studies.

Fine-needle aspiration biopsy is not usually recommended for distinguishing adrenal carcinoma from a benign adrenal mass. However, it could be performed when there is a high suspicion of distant metastasis in adrenal glands [17]. The Weiss histopathologic system is commonly used for evaluating the probability of malignancy in adrenocortical tumors. The modified Weiss system has the following criteria: abnormal mitoses, >6 mitoses/50 HPF, ≤25% clear tumor cells in the cytoplasm, necrosis, and capsular invasion [7]. The present case had all the features, which led to establishing the diagnosis of malignancy.

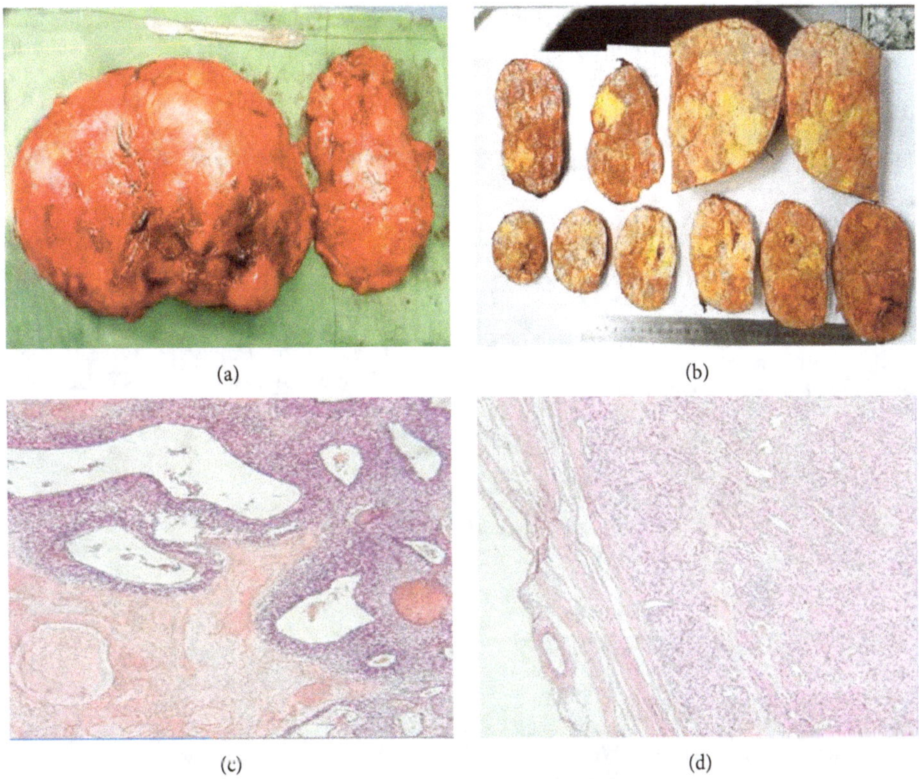

FIGURE 2: (a) Macroscopical view of the adrenal mass and right kidney. (b) The adrenal mass with a nodular and extensive necrotic area at sectioning. (c) High mitotic activity with multifocal necrosis. (d) Extension of the neoplastic cells to the capsule.

TABLE 3: Classification system for staging ACC [9, 20].

ENSAT stage	TNM stage	TNM definition
I	T1, N0, M0	T1, tumor ≤5 cm N0, no positive lymph node M0, no distant metastases
II	T2, N0, M0	T2, tumor >5 cm N0, no positive lymph node M0, no distant metastases
III	T1-T2, N1, M0 T3-T4, N0-N1, M0	N1, positive lymph node(s) M0, no distant metastases T3, tumor infiltration into surrounding tissue T4, tumor invasion into adjacent organs or venous tumor thrombus in vena cava or renal vein
IV	T1-T4, N0-N1, M1	M1, presence of distant metastases

ENSAT, European Network for the Study of Adrenal Tumors; TNM, tumor, node, metastasis.

Complete surgical resection is the only potentially curative treatment for stage I to III ACCs (Table 3). However, due to the presence of occult micrometastases, it may not be curative for many patients [15]. Adjuvant mitotane therapy is recommended for all the patients at high risk of disease recurrence after surgery, including all cases with high-grade disease, intraoperative tumor spillage or fracture, incompletely resected tumor, and vascular or capsular invasion [8, 18]. Previously, ACC was considered to be a relatively radioresistant tumor. However, some studies indicated a benefit in those who are at risk of local recurrence [19]. In the present case, the tumor was in stage III and we decided to perform open surgery rather than laparoscopic resection due to the tumor size, uncertainty about the tumor local invasion, and reducing the risk of spillage or fracture. The mass was successfully resected; after histopathologic evaluation, no invasion beyond the capsule was detected, so we preferred radiotherapy to chemotherapy as adjuvant therapy after surgery.

In conclusion, ACC as a rare neoplasm is a great challenge for diagnosis and treatment. Although most adult patients have functional tumors, precise physical examination, hormonal evaluation, and imaging studies should be conducted for all suspicious patients to diagnose both functional and non-functional tumors and differentiate them from adrenal adenomas. Despite the lack of information about a certain treatment, surgical resection is recommended as a potentially curative treatment. Adjuvant chemotherapy or radiotherapy should be considered based on staging and histopathologic evaluation after surgery.

References

[1] R. Libé, "Adrenocortical carcinoma (ACC): diagnosis, prognosis, and treatment," *Frontiers in Cell and Developmental Biology*, vol. 3, p. 45, 2015.

[2] A. W. Hsing, J. M. Nam, H. T. Co Chien, J. K. McLaughlin, and J. F. Fraumeni Jr., "Risk factors for adrenal cancer: an exploratory study," *International Journal of Cancer*, vol. 65, no. 4, pp. 432–436, 1996.

[3] T. Else, A. C. Kim, A. Sabolch et al., "Adrenocortical carcinoma," *Endocrine Reviews*, vol. 35, no. 2, pp. 282–326, 2014.

[4] N. Bharwani, A. G. Rockall, A. Sahdev et al., "Adrenocortical carcinoma: the range of appearances on CT and MRI," *American Journal of Roentgenology*, vol. 196, no. 6, pp. W706–W714, 2011.

[5] P. M. Copeland, "The incidentally discovered adrenal mass," *The Endocrinologist*, vol. 9, no. 6, pp. 415–423, 1999.

[6] L. Ng and J. M. Libertino, "Adrenocortical carcinoma: diagnosis, evaluation and treatment," *The Journal of Urology* vol. 169, no. 1, pp. 5–11, 2003.

[7] S. Aubert, A. Wacrenier, X. Leroy et al., "Weiss system revisited: a clinicopathologic and immunohistochemical study of 49 adrenocortical tumors," *The American Journal of Surgical Pathology*, vol. 26, no. 12, pp. 1612–1619, 2002.

[8] M. Fassnacht, O. M. Dekkers, T. Else et al., "European society of Endocrinology clinical practice guidelines on the management of adrenocortical carcinoma in adults, in collaboration with the European network for the study of adrenal tumors," *European Journal of Endocrinology*, vol. 179, no. 4, pp. G1–G46, 2018.

[9] V. Chortis, *Developing New Diagnostic and Therapeutic Approaches in Adrenocortical Carcinoma*, University of Birmingham, Edgbaston, UK, 2017.

[10] S. Jasim and M. A. Habra, "Management of adrenocortical carcinoma," *Current Oncology Reports*, vol. 21, no. 3, p. 20, 2019.

[11] J. F. H. Pittaway and L. Guasti, "Pathobiology and genetics of adrenocortical carcinoma," *Journal of Molecular Endocrinology*, vol. 62, no. 2, pp. R105–R119, 2019.

[12] J. P. Luton, S. Cerdas, L. Billaud et al., "Clinical features of adrenocortical carcinoma, prognostic factors, and the effect of mitotane therapy," *New England Journal of Medicine*, vol. 322, no. 17, pp. 1195–1201, 1990.

[13] M. D. Wooten and D. K. King, "Adrenal cortical carcinoma. Epidemiology and treatment with mitotane and a review of the literature," *Cancer*, vol. 72, no. 11, pp. 3145–3155, 1993.

[14] C. A. Koch, K. Pacak, and G. P. Chrousos, "The molecular pathogenesis of hereditary and sporadic adrenocortical and adrenomedullary tumors," *Journal of Clinical Endocrinology and Metabolism*, vol. 87, no. 12, pp. 5367–5384, 2002.

[15] B. Allolio and M. Fassnacht, "Adrenocortical carcinoma: clinical update," *Journal of Clinical Endocrinology and Metabolism*, vol. 91, no. 6, pp. 2027–2037, 2006.

[16] W. Arlt, M. Biehl, A. E. Taylor et al., "Urine steroid metabolomics as a biomarker tool for detecting malignancy in adrenal tumors," *Journal of Clinical Endocrinology and Metabolism*, vol. 96, no. 12, pp. 3775–3784, 2011.

[17] N. C. Jhala, D. Jhala, M. A. Eloubeidi et al., "Endoscopic ultrasound-guided fine-needle aspiration biopsy of the adrenal glands: analysis of 24 patients," *Cancer*, vol. 102, no. 5, pp. 308–314, 2004.

[18] S. Puglisi, A. Calabrese, V. Basile et al., "New perspectives for mitotane treatment of adrenocortical carcinoma," *Best Practice & Research Clinical Endocrinology & Metabolism*, vol. 34, no. 3, Article ID 101415, 2020.

[19] B. Polat, M. Fassnacht, L. Pfreundner et al., "Radiotherapy in adrenocortical carcinoma," *Cancer*, vol. 115, no. 13, pp. 2816–2823, 2009.

[20] D. Kasper, A. Fauci, S. Hauser, D. Longo, J. Jameson, and J. Loscalzo, *Harrison's Principles of Internal Medicine*, McGraw-Hill, New York, NY, USA, 2018.

42

Giant Prolactinoma of Young Onset: A Clue to Diagnosis of MEN-1 Syndrome

Chandrika Jayakanthi Subasinghe,[1] **Noel Somasundaram**,[1] **Pathmanathan Sivatharshya**,[1] **Lalana Devi Ranasinghe**,[1] **and Márta Korbonits**[2]

[1] *Endocrinology Unit, National Hospital of Sri Lanka, Colombo, Sri Lanka*
[2] *Department of Endocrinology, William Harvey Research Institute, Barts and the London School of Medicine and Dentistry, Queen Mary University of London, UK*

Correspondence should be addressed to Chandrika Jayakanthi Subasinghe; chandrika.ucfm@gmail.com

Academic Editor: Eli Hershkovitz

Multiple endocrine neoplasia (MEN) type 1 syndrome is an autosomal dominant disorder caused by germline mutations in *MEN1* gene, characterized by tumours in endocrine and nonendocrine organs. Giant prolactinoma is defined as tumours larger than 40mm with very high prolactin secretion. We report two unrelated Sri Lankan patients (8-year-old boy and a 20-year-old female) who presented with giant prolactinomas with mass effects of the tumours. The female patient showed complete response to medical therapy, while the boy developed recurrent resistant prolactinoma needing surgery and radiotherapy. During follow-up, both developed pancreatic neuroendocrine tumours. Genetic analysis revealed that one was heterozygous for a nonsense mutation and other for missense mutation in *MEN1* gene. Screening confirmed familial MEN-1 syndrome in their families. High clinical suspicion upon unusual clinical presentation prompted genetic evaluation in these patients and detection of *MEN1* gene mutation. Pituitary adenomas in children with MEN-1 syndrome are larger tumours with higher rates of treatment resistance. This report emphasizes importance of screening young patients with giant prolactinoma for MEN-1 syndrome and arranging long-term follow-up for them expecting variable treatment outcomes. Sri Lanka requires further studies to describe the genotypic-phenotypic variability of MEN-1 syndrome in this population.

1. Background

Giant prolactinoma is defined as a pituitary tumour with a largest diameter of 40 mm or more in any direction with massive extrasellar extension and very high prolactin levels (usually above 1000 μg/L) and no concomitant GH or ACTH secretion [1–4]. These are rare, accounting for only 2-3% of prolactinomas with a male to female ratio of 9:1. Prevalence of giant prolactinomas is highest in the fourth to fifth decades, and they often respond to dopamine agonist (DA) therapy [4]. According to a recently published literature review, giant prolactinomas are rare among children and adolescents. In a 2014 review a total of 16 giant prolactinoma cases in children younger than 15 years were found; 15 were boys (age range 6-14 years) with one girl aged 14.5 years [1]. Several authors have recommended genetic testing for aryl hydrocarbon receptor interacting protein (*AIP*) mutation and multiple endocrine neoplasia 1 (*MEN1*) mutation, for isolated sporadic growth hormone (GH) and prolactin (PRL) secreting pituitary tumours in all patients less than 18 years and in patients less than 30 years old with macroadenomas [5, 6]. In a French study, 8.6% of paediatric isolated pituitary macroadenomas were positive for *AIP* mutation, while 3.4% were positive for *MEN1* mutation [6].

MEN-1 syndrome [MEN1; MIM #131100] is an autosomal dominant syndrome characterized by tumours in endocrine and nonendocrine glands with 95% penetrance [7]. According to recently published data from the Dutch MEN-1 study group, 38.1% of MEN-1 syndrome patients harboured a pituitary tumour overall, and in 11% it was the initial presentation [8]. A young (under 21 years) MEN-1 cohort of 160 patients also showed almost similar prevalence (34%) of pituitary tumours [9]. Pituitary tumours in MEN-1 syndrome are usually diagnosed at an earlier age and occur more frequently in females. These are mostly macroadenomas and have a higher degree of aggressiveness and invasiveness according to most of the published data [7, 9–12]. The vast majority of MEN-1 syndrome patients harbour a heterozygous germline mutation in the *MEN1* gene, but a few cases have been identified with a *CDKN1B* mutation and a few have no recognized genetic background. A recent *MEN1* gene mutation update reviewed over 1100 germline and 200 somatic mutations. Among known *MEN1* mutations, 41% are frameshift insertions and deletions, 23% are nonsense mutations, 20% are missense mutations, 9% are splice site defects, and 1% are whole or partial gene gross deletions [13].

Sri Lanka currently lacks facilities for genetic analysis of MEN-1 syndrome, and data on prevalence, phenotype, and genotype variability of MEN-1 syndrome in the country is not known. We report the first two genetically confirmed MEN-1 syndrome cases from Sri Lanka. Both of them presented as isolated sporadic cases of giant prolactinomas at very young age and later are found to have MEN-1 syndrome.

2. Case Presentation

2.1. Case 1. An eight-year-old boy initially presented to us in 2008 with progressive headache and visual disturbances. His imaging revealed a giant pituitary tumour (59 x 45 x 42 mm) with extrasellar extension (Figure 1(a)) with initial prolactin of 91,800 μg/L confirming the diagnosis of giant prolactinoma. Initially, he responded well to high doses of cabergoline (7 mg/week) with normalization of prolactin and total tumour shrinkage. A few years later, he developed recurrence of the tumour, which was resistant to cabergoline therapy (Figure 1(a)), and underwent transcranial excision of the tumour in 2013. During the immediate postoperative period, he developed recurrent hypoglycaemic episodes, which was confirmed to be endogenous insulin dependent hypoglycaemia biochemically (insulin was 15.9 μIU/mL and C-peptide was 3.94 ng/mL when random blood glucose was less than 2.1 mmol/L). Imaging located a well circumscribed lesion (20 x 12 x 10 mm) in the head of pancreas. He underwent enucleation of the tumour, and that was confirmed as an insulinoma histologically with benign characteristics (Ki67<1%). Six months after the pituitary surgery he received three-field radiotherapy (4500 cGy) and continued on cabergoline (3.5 mg/week) resulting in declining prolactin levels. His baseline echocardiography was normal. He had normal calcium at presentation, but currently he is being evaluated for new onset primary hyperparathyroidism (total calcium 2.98 mmol/L [normal range: 2.40-2.55], intact PTH 88.2 pg/L [12-60]).

2.2. Case 2. A Sri Lankan female first presented in 2006 at the age of 20 years to the emergency department with mass effects of a sellar lesion. She gave a history of intermittent galactorrhoea and secondary amenorrhoea since age of 16 years. She was diagnosed to have a giant prolactinoma (40 x 45 x 30 mm, Figure 1(b)) with hyperprolactinaemia (serum prolactin 8930 ng/dL). She responded well to medical therapy with cabergoline (3.5 mg/week) with normalization of prolactin over 1 year and tumour shrinkage over 5 years (Figure 1(b)). Due to the giant prolactinoma she was suspected to have MEN-1 syndrome and testing for other manifestations was initiated. Her calcium levels were normal but pancreas imaging showed a lesion in the pancreas with a cystic (54 x 53 x 49 mm) and a solid (22 x 24 x 20 mm) component. Biochemical evaluation revealed normal serum gastrin, 24 hour urinary 5 HIAA and chromogranin A level, and negative 72 hour fasting test suggesting it to be a nonfunctional pancreatic neuroendocrine tumours (PNET). She underwent distal pancreatectomy with lymphadenectomy. Histological evaluation confirmed PNET with Ki67<1%. Ten years after her first presentation, she was detected to have asymptomatic hyperparathyroidism with corrected ionized calcium of 1.42 mmol/L [normal range: 1.0-1.3], urinary Ca/Cr ratio of 0.32, and intact PTH level of 98.9 pg/L [12-60].

2.3. Genetic Analysis. Following diagnosis of MEN-1 syndrome with the combination of giant prolactinoma and pancreatic neuroendocrine tumour, both patients underwent genetic analysis for *MEN1* gene [14] after genetic counselling and obtaining informed written consent. At the time of genetic testing, none of family members from either families showed any evidence of the disease. Case 1 was heterozygous for nonsense mutation in exon 4 of the *MEN1* gene [NM_130799.2, c.781C>T; p.Gln261Ter]; this change has previously been published in a MEN-1 syndrome family [11]. On family screening, the proband's father and brother were positive for the same mutation, and father was found to have hyperparathyroidism (Figure 2). It is unclear at this stage whether the father received the abnormal gene from one of his parents or it was a *de novo* mutation in him. Proband's brother is being followed up for hyperprolactinaemia (38 ng/dL) with normal pituitary imaging.

Case 2 was heterozygous for missense mutation in exon 10 of the *MEN1* gene [NM_130799.2, c.1736T>C; p.Leu579Pro]; this variant was previously reported in six MEN-1 patients from three Danish families [12]. Same mutation was identified in proband's mother and brother on genetic screening, while her father was found negative. Both the mother and brother had already developed primary hyperparathyroidism of variable severity. Brother had a total calcium of 6.8 mg/dL [normal range: 4.6-5.3], with intact PTH of 240 pg/L [12-60]), and the mother had a corrected ionized calcium of 1.27 mmol/L [normal range: 1.0-1.3] and intact PTH level of 119.4 pg/L). At the time of writing the other hormones are normal and there is no evidence of other endocrine neoplasia in these family members.

Both the families are in the process of undergoing cascade genetic screening (Figure 2). Carriers need endocrine follow-up with screening for clinical, biochemical, and imaging presentation of aspects of the MEN-1 syndrome following available guidelines (Table 1) [7]. Family members with 50% chance to harbour the mutation need genetic testing. Noncarrier family members can be reassured of having

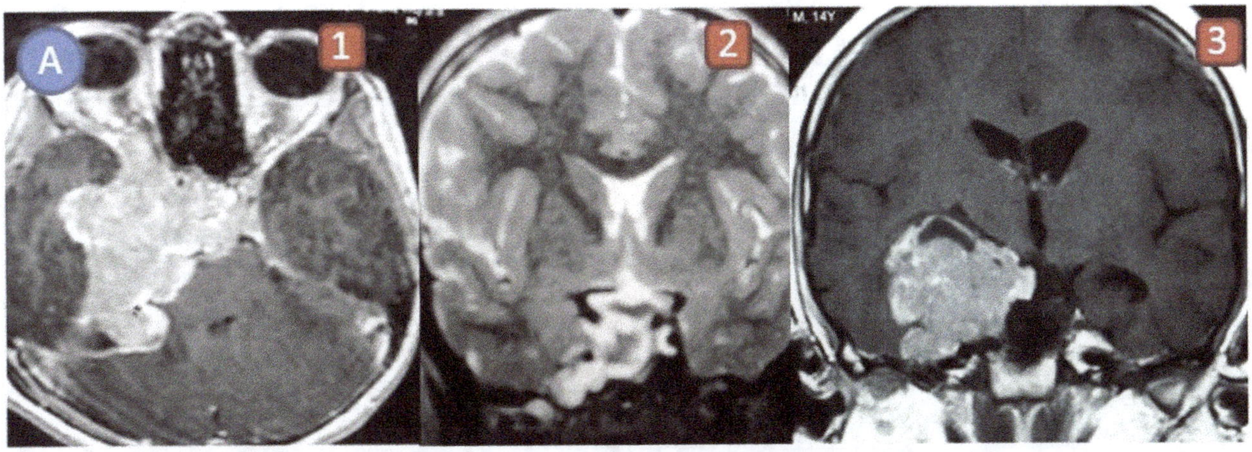

(a)

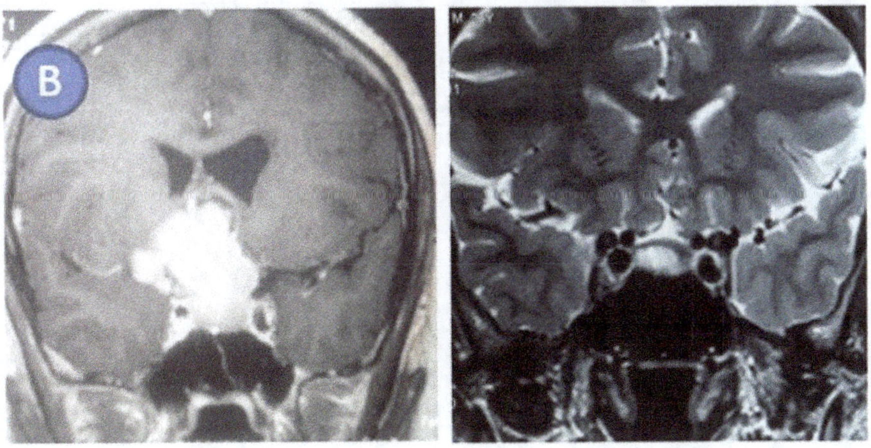

(b)

FIGURE 1: (a) MRI images of Case 1 at diagnosis (1), initial response to dopamine agonist (2), and recurrence of dopamine agonist resistant tumour (3); (b) MRI images of Case 2 at diagnosis and showing tumour shrinkage to subcentimeter level after 5 years of dopamine agonist therapy.

TABLE 1: Suggested biochemical and radiological screening in individuals with *MEN1* mutations [7].

Tumour	Age to begin(y)	Biochemical test annually	Imaging test (Time interval)
Parathyroid	8	Calcium, PTH	None
Pancreas Gastrinoma	20	Gastrin	None
Insulinoma	5	Fasting glucose, Insulin	None
Other pancreatic NET	<10	Chromogranin-A, PP, glucagon, VIP	MRI, CT or endoscopic US
Pituitary	5	Prolactin, IGF-1	MRI (every 3 y)
Adrenal	19	None unless >1cm lesion or symptoms	MRI or CT
Thymic and bronchial carcinoid	15	None	CT or MRI(1-2y)

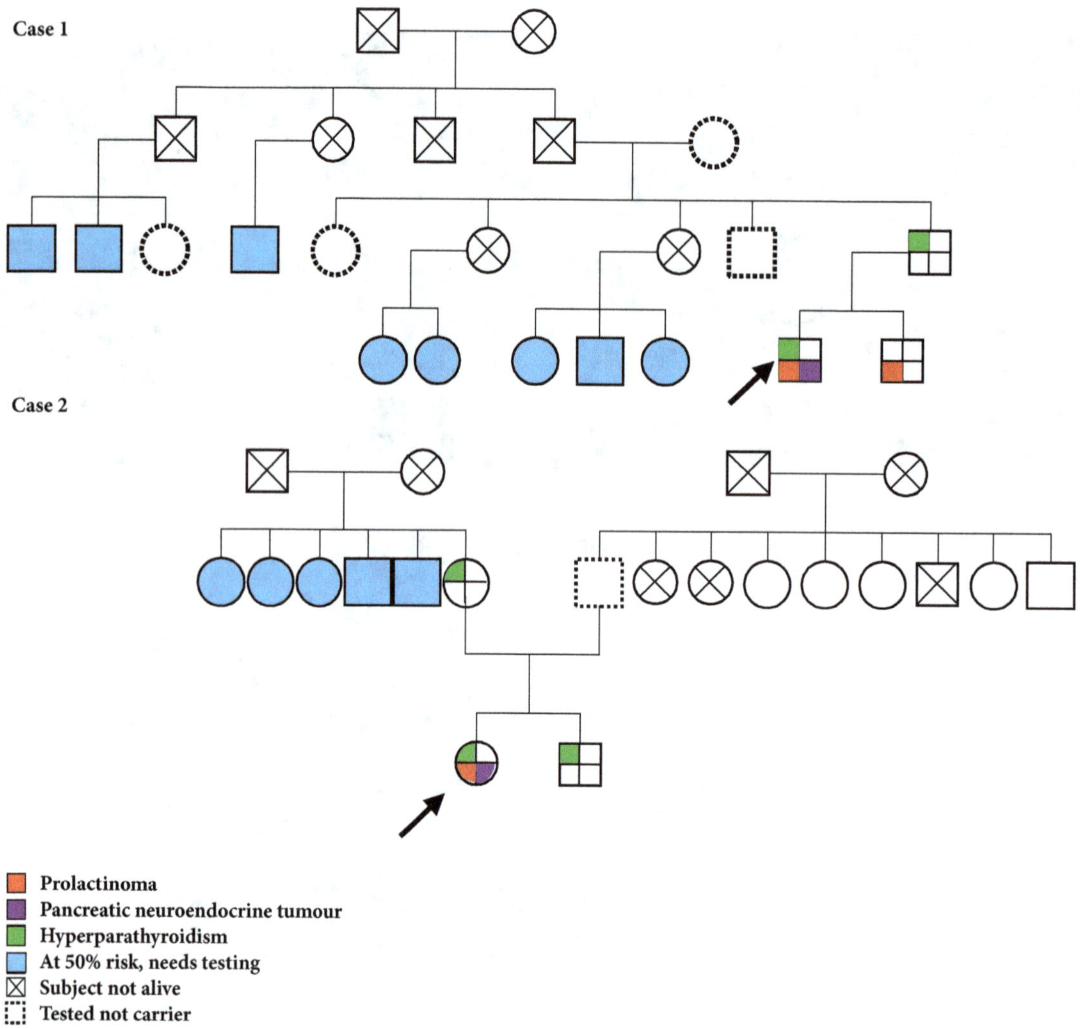

FIGURE 2: Family trees of the two MEN-1 cases. Cascade genetic testing needs to be followed in both families. Carriers need referral to specialist endocrinology clinic for clinical follow-up. Children of carriers need genetic testing.

chance of develop features of the disease not higher than the general population.

3. Discussion

Both of these patients with MEN-1 syndrome presented under the age of 20 years with a giant prolactinoma, in contrast to the usual presentation of such tumours in 4th to 5th decades [1–4]. Early onset of a giant tumour in male patient, in keeping with known literature [1, 2], is thought to be due to rapid growth potential of tumours in males where lower expression of oestrogen receptor alpha may play a role [15]. Young onset giant prolactinomas prompted the evaluation for an underlying genetic syndrome despite apparent absence of positive family history in these two patients.

Treatment response was different in the two patients with a complete response to medical therapy in Case 2 and poor response in Case 1. DA therapy is considered as first-line therapy in giant prolactinoma. According to review of published data from 97 patients, approximately 60% patients had shown complete hormonal response, while 74% had shown tumour shrinkage [1]. No pretreatment predictor of tumour response has been yet identified, but MEN-1 syndrome is reported to be associated with larger tumours (84% versus 24%) and treatment resistance (56% versus 10%) according to most of the published series [2, 8–10, 16, 17]. Prolactinomas in the recently published Dutch series responded well to DA treatment, but many of these were screening-detected microadenomas [8], suggesting a variability in response and a possible difference in responsiveness between small and large MEN-1 syndrome related lesions.

Unusual initial presentation in these patients prompted further evaluation and resulted in diagnosis of MEN-1 syndrome, despite an apparently negative family history. These two cases provide supportive evidence for the importance of genetic evaluation in young patients with giant prolactinomas. Our data also demonstrate the unpredictability of treatment response of these tumours. Vigilance and suspicion in index cases with MEN-1-like features can lead to early diagnosis and better care of these patients and their families.

Abbreviations

MEN: Multiple endocrine neoplasia
DA: Dopamine agonist
AIP: Aryl hydrocarbon receptor interacting protein
GH: Growth hormone
PRL: Prolactin
PNET: Pancreatic neuroendocrine tumour
HPT: Hyperparathyroidism.

Consent

Informed written consent was obtained from the patients to publish details of this case report.

Disclosure

Chandrika Jayakanthi Subasinghe and Lalana Devi Ranasinghe are Senior Registrars in Endocrinology. Pathmanathan Sivatharshya and Noel Somasundaram are Consultant Endocrinologists from Sri Lanka. Márta Korbonits is a Professor of Endocrinology and Metabolism at St. Bartholomew's Hospital, Barts and the London School of Medicine and Dentistry, Queen Mary University of London, UK.

Authors' Contributions

Chandrika Jayakanthi Subasinghe and Pathmanathan Sivatharshya drafted the manuscript. Chandrika Jayakanthi Subasinghe, Pathmanathan Sivatharshya, Lalana Devi Ranasinghe, and Noel Somasundaram clinically evaluated and managed the patients medically. Márta Korbonits contributed to genetic diagnosis. Noel Somasundaram and Márta Korbonits critically revised the final manuscript for important intellectual content and approved it. All authors read and approved the final manuscript.

Acknowledgments

The authors express their gratitude to the patients, who kindly gave consent for their cases to be presented in this paper. Professor Korbonits's familial pituitary adenoma studies are supported by Barts and the London Charity, the Wellcome Trust, the UK's Medical Research Council, and Pfizer Ltd.

References

[1] D. Maiter and E. Delgrange, "Therapy of endocrine disease: the challenges in managing giant prolactinomas," *European Journal of Endocrinology*, vol. 170, no. 6, pp. R213–R227, 2014.

[2] E. Delgrange, G. Raverot, M. Bex et al., "Giant prolactinomas in women," *European Journal of Endocrinology*, vol. 170, no. 1, pp. 31–38, 2014.

[3] I. Shimon, E. Sosa, V. Mendoza et al., "Giant prolactinomas larger than 60 mm in size: a cohort of massive and aggressive prolactin-secreting pituitary adenomas," *The Pituitary Society*, vol. 19, no. 4, pp. 429–436, 2016.

[4] E. Espinosa, E. Sosa, V. Mendoza, C. Ramírez, V. Melgar, and M. Mercado, "Giant prolactinomas: are they really different from ordinary macroprolactinomas?" *Endocrine Journal*, vol. 52, no. 3, pp. 652–659, 2016.

[5] M. Korbonits, H. Storr, and A. V. Kumar, "Familial pituitary adenomas - Who should be tested for AIP mutations?" *Clinical Endocrinology*, vol. 77, no. 3, pp. 351–356, 2012.

[6] T. Cuny, M. Pertuit, M. Sahnoun-Fathallah et al., "Genetic analysis in young patients with sporadic pituitary macroadenomas: besides AIP don't forget MEN1 genetic analysis," *European Journal of Endocrinology*, vol. 168, no. 4, pp. 533–541, 2013.

[7] R. V. Thakker, P. J. Newey, G. V. Walls et al., "Clinical practice guidelines for multiple endocrine neoplasia type 1 (MEN1)," *The Journal of Clinical Endocrinology & Metabolism*, vol. 97, no. 9, pp. 2990–3011, 2012.

[8] J. M. de Laat, O. M. Dekkers, C. R. Pieterman, W. P. Kluijfhout, A. R. Hermus, A. M. Pereira et al., "Long-term natural course of pituitary tumors in patients with MEN1: results from the Dutch-MEN1 study group (DMSG)," *Journal of Clinical Endocrinology and Metabolism*, vol. 100, pp. 3288–3296, 2015.

[9] P. Goudet, A. Dalac, M. Le Bras et al., "MEN1 Disease Occurring Before 21 Years Old: A 160-Patient Cohort Study From the Groupe d'étude des Tumeurs Endocrines," *The Journal of Clinical Endocrinology & Metabolism*, vol. 100, no. 4, pp. 1568–1577, 2015.

[10] B. Vergès, F. Boureille, P. Goudet et al., "Pituitary Disease in MEN Type 1 (MEN1): Data from the France-Belgium MEN1 Multicenter Study," *The Journal of Clinical Endocrinology & Metabolism*, vol. 87, no. 2, pp. 457–465, 2002.

[11] L. V. Syro, B. W. Scheithauer, K. Kovacs et al., "Pituitary tumors in patients with MEN1 syndrome," *Clinics*, vol. 67, Suppl 1, pp. 43–48, 2012.

[12] C. Bulwer, R. Conn, A. Shankar et al., "Cabergoline-related impulse control disorder in an adolescent with a giant prolactinoma," *Clinical Endocrinology*, vol. 86, no. 6, pp. 862–864, 2017.

[13] M. C. Lemos and R. V. Thakker, "Multiple endocrine neoplasia type 1 (MEN1): Analysis of 1336 mutations reported in the first decade following identification of the gene," *Human Mutation*, vol. 29, no. 1, pp. 22–32, 2008.

[14] S. Ellard, A. T. Hattersley, C. M. Brewer, and B. Vaidya, "Detection of an MEN1 gene mutation depends on clinical features and supports current referral criteria for diagnostic molecular genetic testing," *Clinical Endocrinology*, vol. 62, no. 2, pp. 169–175, 2005.

[15] E. Delgrange, A. Vasiljevic, A. Wierinckx et al., "Expression of estrogen receptor alpha is associated with prolactin pituitary tumor prognosis and supports the sex-related difference in tumor growth," *European Journal of Endocrinology*, vol. 172, no. 6, pp. 791–801, 2015.

[16] E. Delgrange, T. Daems, J. Verhelst, R. Abs, and D. Maiter, "Characterization of resistance to the prolactin-lowering effects of cabergoline in macroprolactinomas: a study in 122 patients," *European Journal of Endocrinology*, vol. 160, no. 5, pp. 747–752, 2009.

[17] A. B. Moraes, C. Marques Dos Santos Silva, L. Vieira Neto, and M. R. Gadelha, "Giant prolactinomas: the therapeutic approach," *Clinical Endocrinology*, vol. 79, no. 4, pp. 447–456, 2013.

43

TSH-Secreting Pituitary Macroadenoma in a Girl with Lingual Thyroid

S. Wacharasindhu,[1] S. Shuangshoti,[2] and S. Sunthornyothin[3]

[1] *Department of Pediatrics, Faculty of Medicine, Chulalongkorn University, Bangkok 10330, Thailand*
[2] *Department of Pathology and Chulalongkorn GenePRO Center, Faculty of Medicine, Chulalongkorn University, Bangkok 10330, Thailand*
[3] *Department of Medicine, Faculty of Medicine, Chulalongkorn University, Bangkok 10330, Thailand*

Correspondence should be addressed to S. Wacharasindhu; wacharasindhu@yahoo.com

Academic Editors: G. Aimaretti, J. Broom, W. V. Moore, T. Nagase, and T. Usui

Patients with long-standing hypothyroid are, in some cases, reported to develop pituitary gland hyperplasia due to loss of feedback inhibition of thyroxine in hypothalamus—the condition of which typically regresses after thyroxine replacement. Herein, a 15-year-old girl—with long-standing untreated lingual hypothyroid—presents with a pathologically proven TSH pituitary macroadenoma and bilateral large ovarian cysts. Although MR imaging may differentiate between hyperplasia and macroadenoma of the pituitary gland, pathological examination is still a cornerstone to correct diagnosis.

1. Introduction

Pituitary gland enlargement due to thyrotroph hyperplasia has been well documented in association with long-standing hypothyroidism. The mechanism can be explained by an overstimulation of thyrotrophs by thyrotropin-releasing hormone (TRH) in classic negative feedback loop. Patients with this condition may be asymptomatic or occasionally present with local neurological pressure effect such as visual field defect or squint. The pituitary gland hyperplasia could be reversible after thyroxine replacement and normalisation of serum TSH. We report, herein, an adolescent girl with undiagnosed long-standing congenital hypothyroidism due to lingual thyroid and pituitary gland enlargement which could not be reversible after thyroxine replacement. Histology confirmed the diagnosis of pituitary gland macroadenoma.

2. Case Report

A 15-year-old girl presented with secondary amenorrhea with short stature, abdominal discomfort, and squint. She was born at term with normal birth weight and uneventful post-natal history; nevertheless, growing up, she was considered short compared with girls of the same age. Academically, she was average in class. Her menarche developed when she was 14 years of age; however, secondary amenorrhea had already occurred for 6 months prior to this presentation. On examination, her height and weight were 132 cm and 36 kg, which were on—5 Standard Deviation Score (SDS) and—2 SDS for standard Thai growth chart, respectively. She had breast Tanner III, pubic hair Tanner II. Ophthalmic examination revealed bilateral optic nerve atrophy. Ultrasonography demonstrated bilateral multicystic ovarian masses, 12.8 × 5.6 × 11.3 cm and 12 × 5.9 × 9 cm of the left and right sides, respectively. Free T4 level was 0.08 ng/dL (*N*: 0.8–1.8); TSH >100 mIU/L (*N*: 0.3–4.1); serum prolactin 45.4 ng/mL (*N*: 3–25); FSH 24.5 IU/L; LH <0.1 IU/L; and estradiol 15,469 mmol/L. Ectopic thyroid at sublingual area was detected by technetium thyroid scan.

Because of the optic nerve atrophy, MRI of the pituitary gland was performed and demonstrated a 3.2 × 4.3 × 3.4 cm heterogeneous enhancing sellar/suprasellar mass (Figure 1). The lesion bulged bilaterally into parasellar areas and cavernous sinuses, more on the left side. Four months after replacing Eltroxin (0.1 mg daily), serum free T4 was 1.74 ng/dL; free T3, 4.83; and TSH, 28.25 uIU/L. Serum

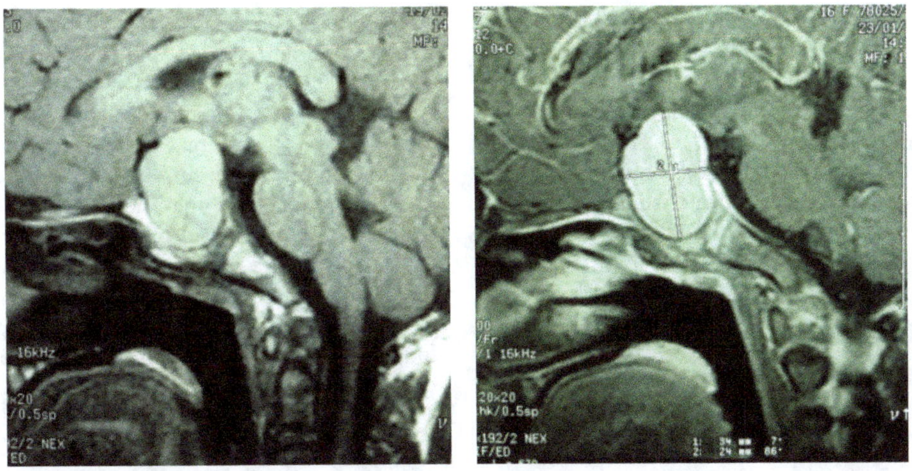

(a) (b)

FIGURE 1: MRI demonstrates a lobulated contour of 3.2 × 4.3 × 3.4 cm mass in sella turcica and suprasellar region (a). After intravenous Gd-DTPA, the mass shows intense enhancement with more intense enhancement in the periphery and central part (b).

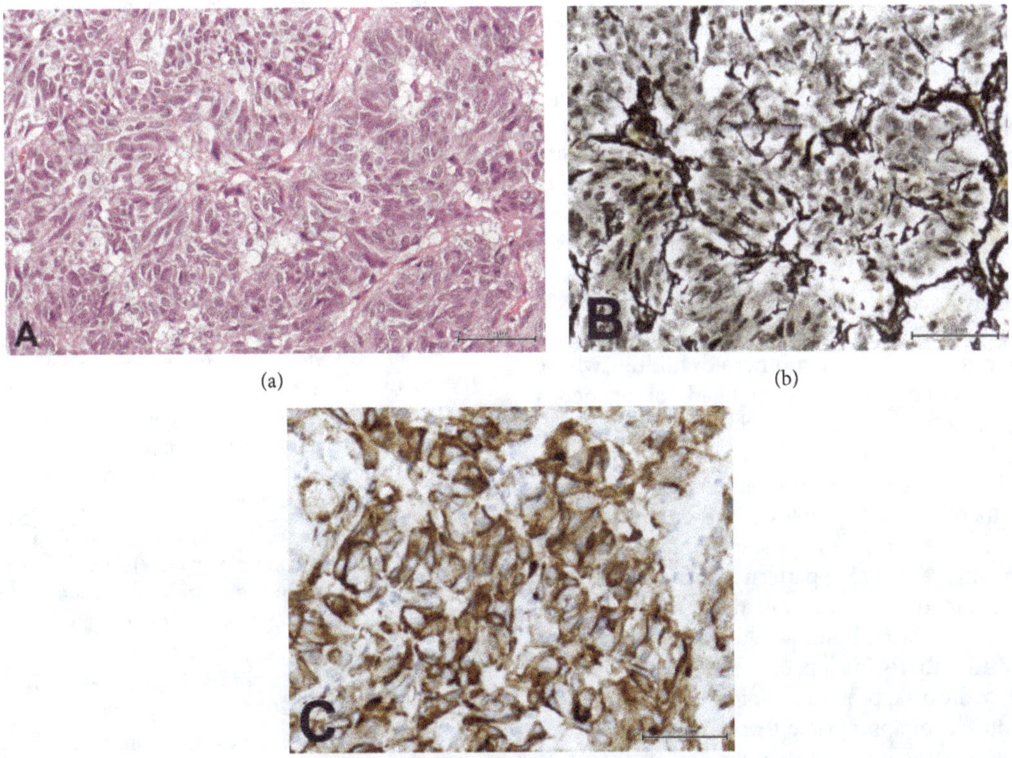

(a) (b) (c)

FIGURE 2: Pathology of TSH pituitary adenoma. Numerous adenoma cells with oval-shaped nuclei are intervened by delicate capillaries (a). Disruption of reticulum framework is depicted (b). Tumor cells are immunoreactive with TSH (c). (A, hematoxylin and eosin; B, reticulin stain; and C, TSH immunostain; each bar = 50 microns).

prolactin was 35 ng/mL. A repeat MRI showed no significant change of sellar and suprasellar tumors.

On a repeat MRI, the mass extended superiorly with pressure effect noted to the optic chiasma and the anterior third ventricle. Due to the compression effect, craniotomy was performed, and the lesion was subtotally removed. Pathologically, monotonous adenoma cells with oval nuclei were found. They were intervened by delicate vasculature (Figure 2(a)). Tumor cells had stippled chromatin pattern, with minute nucleoli and finely granular cytoplasm. Mitotic figures were rarely detected. Disruption of the reticulum architecture, characteristic of pituitary adenoma, was appreciated with reticulin preparation (Figure 2(b)). By immunohistochemical study, tumor cells were diffusely reactive with TSH

(Figure 2(c)), while the remaining adenohypophyseal hormonal immunostains were negative. All of the pathological findings were diagnostic of TSH pituitary adenoma. After the operation, Eltroxin and prednisolone were prescribed. Second craniotomy was performed to remove the residual tumor, and radical radiation was administered. After the second surgery, the patient developed hypopituitarism including diabetic insipidus, adrenal insufficiency, and hypogonadotropic hypogonadism. Eltroxin dosage was gradually increased to 0.2 mg daily, and the serum free T4 and TSH were 1.18 ng/dL and 4.6 mIU/L, respectively. Ten months after the second tumor removal, the patient still had no menstruation. Pelvic ultrasonogram showed small uterus with no ovarian follicular development, suggesting hypogonadotropic hypogonadism.

3. Discussion

Pituitary adenoma is a more common cause of intrasellar lesion in adults than in children and can produce various pituitary hormones. TSH-secreting adenoma is, however, rare as it constitutes only 1% of pituitary adenomas [1]. TSH adenomas typically produce hyperthyroidism but may be asymptomatic. Although the patients generally have high T3 and T4 levels with elevated TSH, peripheral thyroid resistance may occur [2, 3]. Pituitary hyperplasia secondary to primary hypothyroid is well described, probably due to loss of thyroxine feedback mechanism and overproduction of TRH. Up to 81% of patients with primary hypothyroidism had increased volume of the sellar on skull X-ray, and sellar volume was positively correlated with the severity of chemical hypothyroidism but not with the duration of symptoms [4, 5]. Desai et al. report ten congenital hypothyroid children, whose mean age at presentation was 11 years and had homogeneous diffuse enlargement of pituitary gland detected by MRI, and all regressed after restoration of hypothyroid status [6]. Adenoma and hyperplasia of the pituitary glands need to be distinguished. In pituitary hyperplasia, the enlarged gland is homogeneously enhanced on MRI study after gadolinium administration. Such enhancing pattern is indistinguishable from the normal gland [7], and it was not seen in our case. In addition, the hyperplastic gland would either disappear or decrease in size after thyroxine replacement [8, 9]. Wolansky et al. demonstrate the disappearance of pituitary gland hyperplasia after 4 months of appropriate thyroxine dose replacement [9]. For the pathological standpoint, enlargement of pituitary lobules with intact reticulum framework features pituitary hyperplasia while, in adenoma, the framework is disrupted as demonstrated in our case [10].

Occurrence of TSH macroadenoma in a long-standing untreated hypothyroidism is unusual, and has only been rarely reported, mostly in adult subjects [11, 12]. Myers et al. report a 54-year-old woman with primary hypothyroidism who presented with symptoms of increased intracranial pressure and worsening vision due to thyrotropin-secreting adenoma [13]. In a rare instance, concurrent pituitary hyperplasia and thyrotropin-producing microadenoma are found in association with pituitary resistance to thyroid hormone [2, 3].

Multicystic ovarian cyst has been reported in primary hypothyroid and also disappears after thyroid replacement. This association was firstly reported by Wyk and Grumbach [14]. In our patient, hypogonadotropic hypogonadism was detected, which may be due to compression effect of macroadenoma or to surgical damage around the pituitary area. TSH adenomas may need medical treatment such as somatostatin, bromocriptine, or cabergoline. Surgery is indicated if the optic nerve is compressed. Recurrence can be managed with reoperation, radiation, and/or medication.

In conclusion, the study reports an adolescent girl with long-standing, undetected lingual hypothyroidism and TSH-secreting pituitary macroadenoma. It demonstrates that TSH-secreting pituitary adenoma should be considered in patients with persistent high TSH levels in primary hypothyroidism after thyroxine replacement.

References

[1] P. Beck-Peccoz, F. Brucker-Davis, L. Persani, R. C. Smallridge, and B. D. Weintraub, "Thyrotropin-secreting pituitary tumors," *Endocrine Reviews*, vol. 17, no. 6, pp. 610–638, 1996.

[2] K. Watanabe, T. Kameya, A. Yamauchi et al., "Thyrotropin-producing microadenoma associated with pituitary resistance to thyroid hormone," *Journal of Clinical Endocrinology and Metabolism*, vol. 76, no. 4, pp. 1025–1030, 1993.

[3] M. Gurnell, O. Rajanayagam, I. Barbar, M. Keston Jones, and V. K. K. Chatterjee, "Reversible pituitary enlargement in the syndrome of resistance to thyroid hormone," *Thyroid*, vol. 8, no. 8, pp. 679–682, 1998.

[4] S. T. Bigos, E. C. Ridgway, I. A. Kourides, and F. Maloof, "Spectrum of pituitary alterations with mild and severe thyroid impairment," *Journal of Clinical Endocrinology and Metabolism*, vol. 46, no. 2, pp. 317–325, 1978.

[5] T. Yamada, T. Tsukui, K. Ikejiri, and M. Kotani, "Volume of sella turcica in normal subjects and in patients with primary hypothyroidism and hyperthyroidism," *Journal of Clinical Endocrinology and Metabolism*, vol. 42, no. 5, pp. 817–822, 1976.

[6] M. P. Desai, R. U. Mehta, C. S. Choksi, and M. P. Colaco, "Pituitary enlargement on magnetic resonance imaging in congenital hypothyroidism," *Archives of Pediatrics and Adolescent Medicine*, vol. 150, no. 6, pp. 623–628, 1996.

[7] A. G. Osborne, "Pituitary macroadenoma," in *Diagnostic Imaging: Brain*, A. G. Osborn, Ed., pp. II2–II24, Amirsys, Salt Lake City, Utah, USA, 2004.

[8] K. S. Eom, C. See-Sung, J. D. Kim, J. M. Kim, and T. Y. Kim, "Primary hypothyroidism mimicking a pituitary macroadenoma: regression after thyroid hormone replacement therapy," *Pediatric Radiology*, vol. 39, no. 2, pp. 164–167, 2009.

[9] L. J. Wolansky, G. D. Leavitt, B. J. Elias, H. J. Lee, A. Dasmahapatra, and W. Byrne, "MRI of pituitary hyperplasia in hypothyroidism," *Neuroradiology*, vol. 38, no. 1, pp. 50–52, 1996.

[10] S. L. Asa, *Tumors of the Pituitary Gland*, Atlas of Tumor Pathology, 3rd series, Fascicle 22, Armed Forces Institute of Pathology, Washington, DC, USA, 1998.

[11] A. S. Y. Leong, J. C. Chawla, and E. C. Teh, "Pituitary thyrotropic tumour secondary to long standing primary hypothyroidism," *Pathologia Europaea*, vol. 11, no. 1, pp. 49–55, 1976.

[12] B. L. Wajchenberg, A. M. C. Tsanaclis, and R. Marino Jr., "TSH-containing pituitary adenoma associated with primary

hypothyroidism manifested by amenorrhoea and galactorrhoea," *Acta Endocrinologica*, vol. 106, no. 1, pp. 61–66, 1984.

[13] A. Myers, K. Hatanpaa, C. Madden, and I. Lingvay, "Thyrotropin-secreting adenoma in a patient with primary hypothyroidism," *Endocrine Practice*, vol. 17, no. 6, pp. e135–e139, 2011.

[14] J. J. V. Wyk and M. M. Grumbach, "Syndrome of precocious menstruation and galactorrhea in juvenile hypothyroidism: an example of hormonal overlap in pituitary feedback," *The Journal of Pediatrics*, vol. 57, no. 3, pp. 416–435, 1960.

Nephrectomy for Metastatic Kidney Tumor in Patients with Differentiated Thyroid Cancer: A Report of Two Cases

Haruhiko Yamazaki,[1] **Takeshi Kishida**,[2] **Go Noguchi**,[2] **Hiroyuki Iwasaki**,[1] **Nobuyasu Suganuma**,[1] **Katsuhiko Masudo**,[3] **Hirotaka Nakayama**,[4] **Toshinari Yamashita**,[1] **Takashi Yamanaka**,[1] **Yuko Sugawara**,[1] **Yuka Matsubara**,[1] **Kaori Kohagura**,[1] **Yasushi Rino**,[4] **and Munetaka Masuda**[4]

[1]*Department of Breast and Endocrine Surgery, Kanagawa Cancer Center, Yokohama, Japan*
[2]*Department of Urology, Kanagawa Cancer Center, Yokohama, Japan*
[3]*Department of Breast and Thyroid Surgery, Yokohama City University Medical Center, Yokohama, Japan*
[4]*Department of Surgery, Yokohama City University School of Medicine, Yokohama, Japan*

Correspondence should be addressed to Haruhiko Yamazaki; h.yamazaki0413@kcch.jp

Academic Editor: Thomas Grüning

The occurrence of renal tumors originating from thyroid cancer is extremely rare with a few effective treatments for renal metastases. Here, we report the cases of two patients with differentiated thyroid cancer who underwent nephrectomy for a metastatic kidney tumor. Case 1 was a 74-year-old man who was diagnosed with right kidney tumor 10 years after initial surgery for papillary thyroid cancer (PTC). Right nephrectomy was performed, and the pathology was metastatic PTC. Case 2 was a 68-year-old woman who was diagnosed with left kidney tumor 24 years after surgery for follicular thyroid carcinoma (FTC). Left nephrectomy was performed, and the pathology was metastatic FTC. Nephrectomy for single renal metastasis could be considered a treatment option if the patients' general condition is positive.

1. Introduction

The occurrence of renal tumors originating from thyroid cancer is extremely rare with a prevalence of 0.47% [1]. Although radioactive iodine (RAI) therapy has been used to treat metastatic and recurrent differentiated thyroid cancer (DTC), no data establish the efficacy of RAI for the treatment of renal metastases. Thus, to date, effective treatment methods for renal metastasis from thyroid cancer remain unavailable. When a tumor is metastasized to the kidneys, it generally comprises other metastatic lesions or is bilateral [2]. Herein, we report cases of two patients with DTC who underwent nephrectomy for a metastatic kidney tumor.

2. Case Report

2.1. Case 1. A 74 -year-old man was diagnosed with right kidney tumor on routine computed tomography (CT) 10 years after initial surgery. His medical history comprised near total thyroidectomy for papillary thyroid cancer (PTC) 10 years ago and complete thyroidectomy for recurrence 6 years ago. He did not complain of urinary symptoms such as flank pain or hematuria. Blood test results were as follows: creatinine (Cre), 0.78 mg/dL; blood urea nitrogen (BUN), 14.2 mg/dL; thyroid-stimulating hormone (TSH), 0.13 μIU/mL; free thyroxine (F-T4), 1.57 ng/mL; thyroglobulin (Tg), 95.0 ng/dL (Tg doubling time, 0.31 years); and Tg antibody (TgAb), 11 IU/mL. Transabdominal ultrasonography (US) revealed a right kidney tumor measuring 5.3 × 3.7 cm. The tumor blood flow was similar to that of the kidneys. In addition, CT revealed an irregular tumor mass projecting outward from the right kidney with no evidence of other metastatic lesions (Figure 1(a)). Despite a little marginally elevated Tg level, imaging studies of the right kidney raised suspicions of primary renal cell carcinoma (RCC). Following consultations

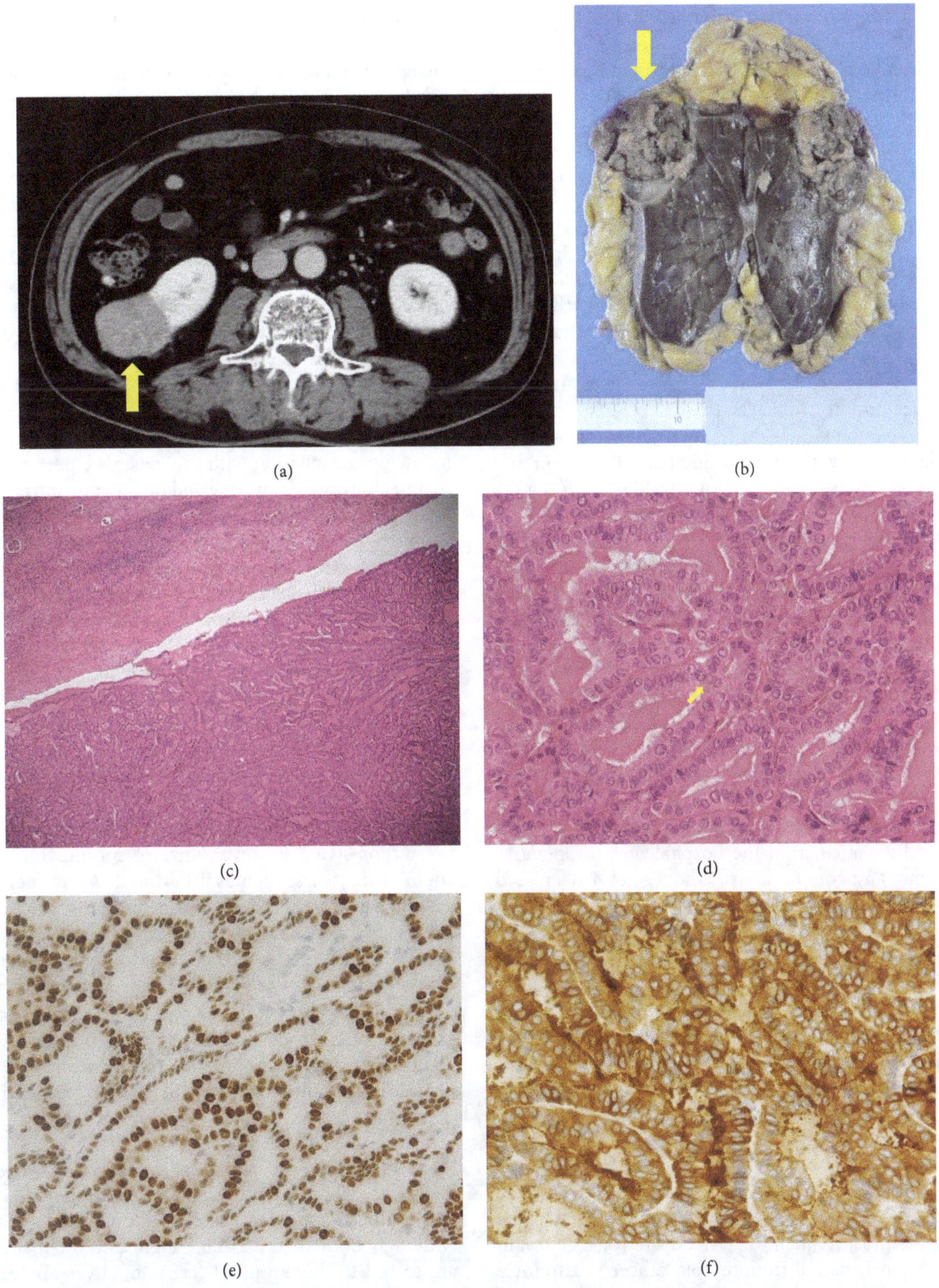

FIGURE 1: (a) Computed tomography showed the right kidney tumor (arrow). (b) The right nephrectomy specimen contained a grayish tumor measuring 5.5cm × 5.0 cm on the upper pole (arrow). (c, d) Histologic sections of the resection specimen showed that the tumor formed a papillary structure, and the lumen was filled with eosinophilic substances considered colloids. Individual cancer cells had nuclear grooves, and findings suggestive of nuclear inclusions were also observed (arrow). (c): Original magnification x200, (d): Original magnification x400. (e, f) Immunohistochemistry revealed positive for thyroid transcription factor 1 (e) and thyroglobulin (f). Original magnification x400.

with urologists, a right laparoscopic radical nephrectomy was performed. The pathology report revealed that the right nephrectomy specimen contained a grayish tumor measuring 5.5 × 5.0 cm on the upper pole (Figure 1(b)). Histological sections of the resected specimen revealed that the tumor formed a papillary structure, and the lumen was filled with eosinophilic substances that were considered colloids. Further, individual cancer cells had nuclear grooves, and findings suggestive of nuclear inclusions were observed (Figures 1(c) and 1(d)). Immunohistochemistry (IHC) results were positive for thyroid transcription factor 1 (TTF-1) and Tg (Figures 1(e) and 1(f)). The patient was discharged from the hospital on postoperative day 7 without any complications. Postoperatively, the Tg level decreased to 3.05 ng/dL and, 3 years after nephrectomy, no recurrence has been reported.

2.2. Case 2. A 68-year-old woman, with medical history of total thyroidectomy for follicular thyroid carcinoma (FTC) 24 years ago, exhibited a high Tg level. However, she did not complain of any urinary symptoms. Her blood test results were as follows: Cre, 0.65 mg/dL; BUN, 14.7 mg/dL; TSH, 0.09 μIU/mL; F-T4, 1.35 ng/mL; Tg, 10500.0 ng/dL (Tg doubling time, 0.31 years); and TgAb, 11 IU/mL. CT revealed a left kidney tumor measuring 4.0 × 3.5 cm (Figure 2(a)). The Tg level was remarkably high; thus, recurrence of FTC was predominantly suspected. However, CT identified no other metastatic lesion, and nephrectomy was performed. The pathology report revealed that the left nephrectomy specimen comprised a light brown tumor measuring 4.5 × 4.4 cm on the lower pole (Figure 2(b)). In addition, histological sections of the resected specimen revealed that the tumor formed a follicular structure and was undergoing infiltration and proliferation (Figures 2(c) and 2(d)). Furthermore, IHC was positive for TTF-1 and Tg (Figures 2(e) and 2(f)). The patient was discharged from the hospital on postoperative day 6 without any complications. The Tg level decreased postoperatively to 298 ng/dL.

3. Discussion

In 2012, approximately 230,000 and 70,000 new cases of thyroid cancer were estimated among females and males, respectively, with an age-standardized (world population) rate of 6.10/100,000 females and 1.90/100,000 males [3]. Both PTC and FTC are called DTC, accounting for >95% of all thyroid carcinoma cases [4]. The prognosis of DTC is good, and the disease-specific survival rate is reportedly >90% [5]. However, some DTCs develop distant metastasis, the frequency of which has been reported to be 4 %-15 %, with the lung being the most frequent metastatic site [6]. The origin of renal tumor originating from thyroid cancer is extremely rare, with a prevalence of 0.47% [1]. Frequently, metastatic renal tumors exhibit poor clinical symptoms, and patients die before developing symptoms. Thus, it is rare for the cancer to be discovered during survival and be treated [7]. The duration from the diagnosis of thyroid cancer to the detection of renal metastasis is long, and cases of >10 years have been reported previously [7, 8]. By the time renal metastasis was diagnosed in cases 1 and 2 of this report, 10 and 24 years had elapsed since initial surgery, respectively. In addition, both patients exhibited no subjective symptoms; however, kidney tumors were detected with whole body CT. The follow-up method following thyroid cancer surgery has recently changed from whole body RAI scanning to US and serum Tg [9]. In our cases, asymptomatic recurrent foci were detected by measuring the serum Tg level. Of note, whole body RAI scanning could also be used to detect recurrent foci after DTC surgery; however, a possibility of false positives exists for the kidneys because of other diseases, necessitating attention for evaluation [10, 11]. Although metastatic renal tumors require differentiation from primary RCC, CT and MRI do not have characteristic findings in metastatic renal tumor originating from thyroid cancer [7]. In our cases, a possibility of renal metastasis of thyroid cancer existed because the serum Tg level had increased. However, a case of thyroid cancer metastasized to RCC has been reported previously [12]. Whether the excision of distant metastasis contributes to the prognosis of thyroid cancer remains unclear. However, following consultation with urologists, we performed radical nephrectomy for diagnostic and therapeutic purposes in both cases. The efficacy of resection of distant metastases has been analyzed in various cancers. In colorectal cancer, hepatic resection is considered a standard treatment option for metastatic colorectal cancer and can result in 10-year survival rates of 20–26%, and potential cure. There is no established evidence in other cancers, but there are cases in which long-term prognosis is obtained by resection of oligometastasis [13]. Therefore, the resection of oligometastasis in thyroid cancer treatment might be considered a treatment option.

The pathology reports revealed characteristic features of DTC. A primary renal tumor that displays similar histology to FTC is known as thyroid-like follicular carcinoma of the kidney (TLFCK). TLFCK is an extremely rare histological variant of RCC; however, thyroid-specific immunohistochemical markers, such as TTF-1 and Tg, are negative [14]. In both cases, TTF-1 and Tg were positive by IHC, and it was feasible to diagnose renal metastasis of thyroid cancer.

RAI is used to treat DTCs that develop recurrence and distant metastasis. The prognosis of patients with the ^{131}I uptake is better than those without the ^{131}I uptake [15]. However, almost all studies reporting the efficacy of RAI comprised lung or bone metastasis cases, with no data demonstrating the efficacy of RAI for the treatment of renal metastases.

To date, radioiodine refractory DTC (RR-DTC) treatment options are very limited. However, sorafenib and lenvatinib, which are tyrosine kinase inhibitors (TKIs), have recently been approved and used to treat RR-DTCs [16, 17]. Although both drugs exhibit high efficacy, many patients are forced to discontinue because of adverse effects (AEs). In the DECISION trial, dose reductions were required in 64.3% of patients in the sorafenib group [16]. Similarly, in the SELECT trial, dose reductions were required in 67.8% of patients in the lenvatinib group and 90% of Japanese patients taking lenvatinib [17, 18]. Moreover, most patients in these trials had lung, lymph node, or bone metastasis, and the efficacy of TKI for renal metastasis remains unknown. In addition, AEs of TKI exhibit a possibility of substantially

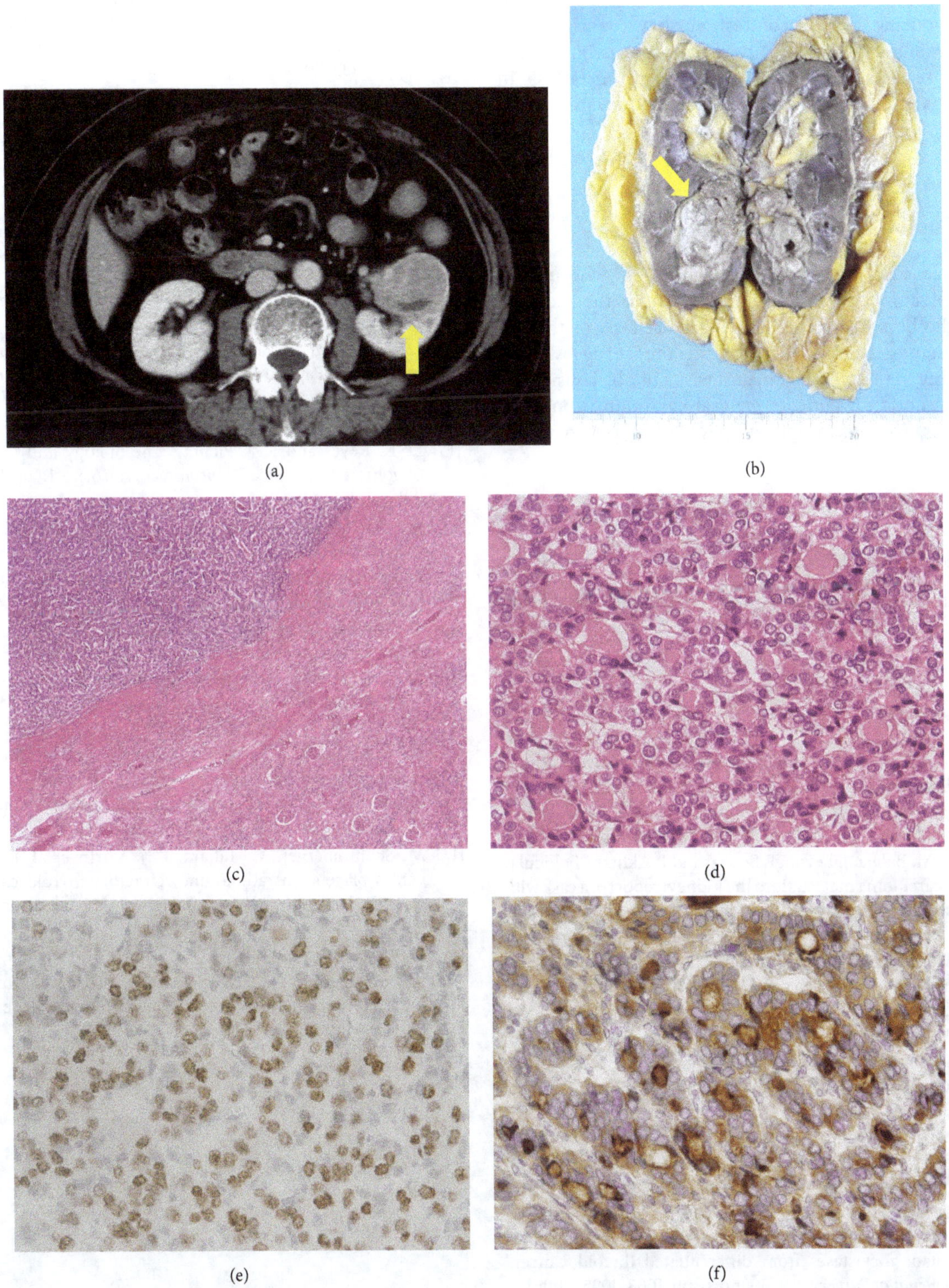

FIGURE 2: (a) Computed tomography showed the left kidney tumor (arrow). (b) The left nephrectomy specimen contained a light brown tumor measuring 4.5cm × 4.4 cm on the lower pole arrow. (c, d) Histologic sections of the resection specimen showed that the tumor formed a follicular structure, and was infiltrating and proliferating. (c): Original magnification x200, (d): Original magnification x400. (e, f) Immunohistochemistry revealed positive for thyroid transcription factor 1 (e) and thyroglobulin (f). Original magnification x400.

decreasing patients' quality of life. In our case, both patients were asymptomatic, and the efficacy of TKI was unknown for these disease conditions, thereby necessitating caution while introducing TKI. In contrast, surgery could result in definitive volume reduction. Overall, radical nephrectomy could be a reasonable treatment if there is no metastasis in other organs and it is not a case of bilateral kidney metastases [2, 7].

4. Conclusions

We reported cases of two patients with DTC who underwent nephrectomy with single metastasis to the kidneys. To date, the best treatment for renal metastasis of thyroid cancer remains debatable. However, this report suggests that nephrectomy for single renal metastasis could be considered a treatment option if patients' general condition is positive. Nevertheless, long-term follow-up is necessary to assess efficacy.

Acknowledgments

The authors thank enago (https://www.enago.jp/) for editing a draft of this manuscript.

References

[1] Z.-L. Qiu, Y.-L. Xue, and Q.-Y. Luo, "Rare renal metastases from differentiated thyroid carcinoma: Early clinical detection and treatment based on radioiodine," *Arquivos Brasileiros de Endocrinologia & Metabologia*, vol. 58, no. 3, pp. 260–269, 2014.

[2] V. Nath, M. Baliga, J. Lewin, F. Souza, and I. Akhtar, "Follicular thyroid carcinoma metastatic to the kidney: report of a case with cytohistologic correlation," *Case Reports in Pathology*, vol. 2015, Article ID 701413, 5 pages, 2015.

[3] C. La Vecchia, M. Malvezzi, C. Bosetti et al., "Thyroid cancer mortality and incidence: a global overview," *International Journal of Cancer*, vol. 136, no. 9, pp. 2187–2195, 2015.

[4] B. Aschebrook-Kilfoy, M. H. Ward, M. M. Sabra, and S. S. Devesa, "Thyroid cancer incidence patterns in the United States by histologic type, 1992–2006," *Thyroid*, vol. 21, no. 2, pp. 125–134, 2011.

[5] K. Matsuzu, K. Sugino, K. Masudo et al., "Thyroid lobectomy for papillary thyroid cancer: Long-term follow-up study of 1,088 cases," *World Journal of Surgery*, vol. 38, no. 1, pp. 68–79, 2014.

[6] C. A. Benbassat, S. Mechlis-Frish, and D. Hirsch, "Clinicopathological characteristics and long-term outcome in patients with distant metastases from differentiated thyroid cancer," *World Journal of Surgery*, vol. 30, no. 6, pp. 1088–1095, 2006.

[7] Y. Inoue, H. Moriyama, H. Mochizuki, M. Nakahara, T. Nishizaka, and T. Fukuhara, "Metastatic renal tumor originating from thyroid cancer : a case report," *Japanese Journal of Clinical Urology*, vol. 55, no. 11, pp. 1049–1051, 2001.

[8] K. Abe, T. Hasegawa, S. Onodera, Y. Oishi, and M. Suzuki, "Renal metastasis of thyroid carcinoma," *International Journal of Urology*, vol. 9, no. 11, pp. 656–658, 2002.

[9] B. R. Haugen, E. K. Alexander, and K. C. Bible, "2015 American thyroid association management guidelines for adult patients with thyroid nodules and differentiated thyroid cancer: the american thyroid association guidelines task force on thyroid nodules and differentiated thyroid cancer," *Thyroid*, vol. 26, no. 1, pp. 1–133, 2016.

[10] A. Claimon, M. Suh, G. J. Cheon, D. S. Lee, E. E. Kim, and J.-K. Chung, "Bilateral Renal Metastasis of Hürthle Cell Thyroid Cancer with Discordant Uptake Between I-131 Sodium Iodide and F-18 FDG," *Nuclear Medicine and Molecular Imaging*, vol. 51, no. 3, pp. 256–260, 2017.

[11] Y.-X. Mi, X. Sui, J.-M. Huang, L.-G. Wei, and P. Xie, "Incidentally polycystic kidney disease identified by SPECT/CT with post-therapy radioiodine scintigraphy in a patient with differentiated thyroid carcinoma," *Medicine*, vol. 96, no. 43, Article ID e8348, 2017.

[12] J. S. A. Song, S. M. Taylor, J. Trites et al., "Tumor-to-tumor metastases: Papillary thyroid carcinoma into a clear cell renal cell carcinoma," *Journal of Otolaryngology - Head and Neck Surgery*, vol. 46, no. 1, article 17, 2017.

[13] D. K. Reyes and K. J. Pienta, "The biology and treatment of oligometastatic cancer," *Oncotarget*, vol. 6, no. 11, pp. 8491–8524, 2015.

[14] M. Ghaouti, L. Roquet, M. Baron, C. Pfister, and J.-C. Sabourin, "Thyroid-like follicular carcinoma of the kidney: a case report and review of the literature," *Diagnostic Pathology*, vol. 9, article 186, 2014.

[15] C. Durante, N. Haddy, E. Baudin et al., "Long-term outcome of 444 patients with distant metastases from papillary and follicular thyroid carcinoma: Benefits and limits of radioiodine therapy," *The Journal of Clinical Endocrinology & Metabolism*, vol. 91, no. 8, pp. 2892–2899, 2006.

[16] M. S. Brose, C. M. Nutting, and B. Jarzab, "Sorafenib in radioactive iodine-refractory, locally advanced or metastatic differentiated thyroid cancer: a randomised, double-blind, phase 3 trial," *The Lancet*, vol. 384, no. 9940, pp. 319–328, 2014.

[17] M. Schlumberger, M. Tahara, L. J. Wirth et al., "Lenvatinib versus placebo in radioiodine-refractory thyroid cancer," *The New England Journal of Medicine*, vol. 372, no. 7, pp. 621–630, 2015.

[18] N. Kiyota, M. Schlumberger, K. Muro et al., "Subgroup analysis of Japanese patients in a phase 3 study of lenvatinib in radioiodine-refractory differentiated thyroid cancer," *Cancer Science*, vol. 106, no. 12, pp. 1714–1721, 2015.

45

Intermittent Fever, Progressive Weight Gain and Personality Changes in a Five-Year-Old Girl: Unusual Praneoplastic Syndrome due to Presacral Ganglioneuroma

Chao Yang, Chang-chun Li, Jun Zhang, Xiang-ru Kong, Zhenzhen Zhao, Xiao-bin Deng, Liang Peng, and Shan Wang

Department of Pediatric Surgical Oncology, Children's Hospital of Chongqing Medical University, 136 Zhongshan 2nd Road, Yuzhong District, Chongqing 400014, China

Correspondence should be addressed to Shan Wang; wangshan778@163.com

Academic Editor: Gianluca Aimaretti

Ganglioneuromas are rare tumors in the neuroblastoma group. Paraneoplastic syndrome (PNS) due to presacral ganglioneuromas was hardly reported in previous literature. Here, we reported that a case of a 5-year-old girl with a presacral ganglioneuroma presented with PNS, who presented with intermittent fever, progressive weight gain, and personality changes. Our report revealed intermittent fever, progressive weight gain, and personality changes may represent rare paraneoplastic syndromes in ganglioneuromas.

1. Introduction

Ganglioneuromas are rare tumors in the neuroblastoma group [1]. They are benign lesions arising from sympathetic ganglion cells and complete surgical excision is considered to be curative [2–4]. Presacral ganglioneuromas are rare and so far less than 20 cases have been reported in the literature [5]. Paraneoplastic syndrome (PNS) due to presacral ganglioneuromas was hardly reported in previous literature. Here, we report a case of a 5-year-old girl with a presacral ganglioneuroma presented with PNS.

2. Case Report

A 5-year-old girl sought medical advice in September 2012 because of a history of progressive weight gain (30 Kg, BMI 29.4), short stature (0.96 m; −2 SDs), obesity, moon face, buffalo hump for more than 1 year, personality changes for 6 months, and intermittent fever for 1 month. She displayed increased weight since she was 4 years old. There was neither hypertension nor headache history observed. Personality changes were noticed 6 months ago and she presented with soliloquy and was annoyed and irritable. Parorexia was also observed. She presented with intermittent fever one month ago with the highest temperature of 40°C, accompanied with convulsions three times and recurrent cough. She was admitted to her local hospital, the diagnosis of pneumonia and obesity was confirmed, and antibiotic and mannitol were administrated; however, the symptoms were not relieved and she was transferred to our hospital for further treatment.

After administration, physical examination and neurologic examination were negative. The blood pressure was 133 over 86. Routine blood tests were made and tumor markers were detected (CEA, CA 19-9, CA 125, AFP, and HCG), but all values were normal. Serum cortisol was 2852 nmol/L, 2201 nmol/L, and 1250 nmol/L, 8/16/24 h, respectively (normal, 138–690 nmol/L). Plasma adrenocorticotropic hormone (ACTH) levels were 162 pg/mL, 108 pg/mL, and 89 pg/mL, 8/16/24 h, respectively (normal, <46 pg/mL). Vanilmandelic acid (VMA) was within the normal range. Karyotype was normal. Pituitary thyroid magnetic resonance imaging (MRI) was negative, and abdomen-thorax computed tomography (CT) scan with contrast enhancement scan revealed a dishomogeneous mass (11.2 mm × 26.9 mm × 11.3 mm) with obvious enhancement located before the sacral vertebra. Pelvic MRI confirmed the origin of the lesion from

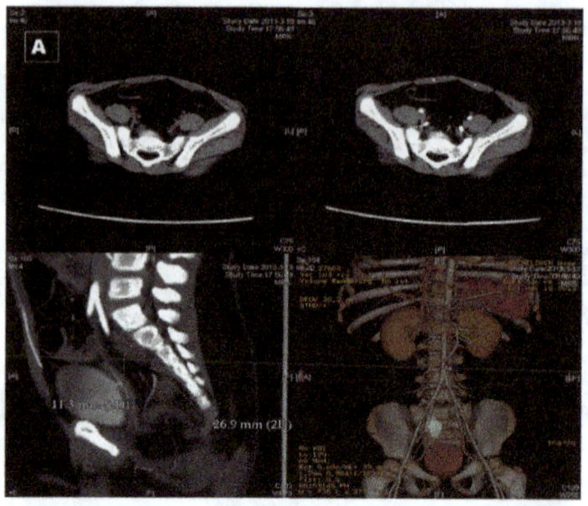

(a)

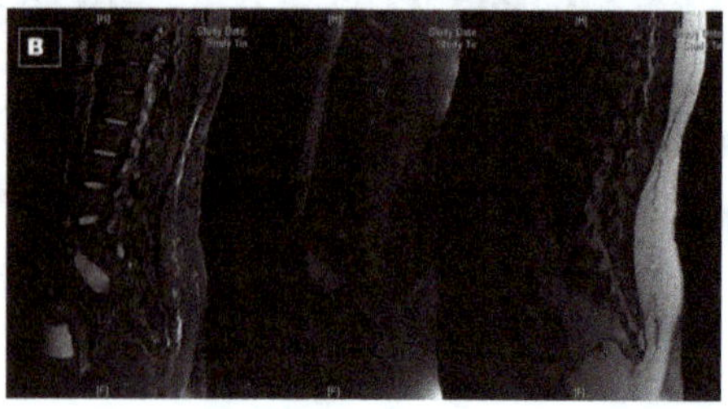

(b)

FIGURE 1: (a) The CT scan abdomen showed a dishomogeneous mass (11.2 mm × 26.9 mm × 11.3 mm) with obvious enhancement located before the sacral vertebra. (b) MR images revealing a presacral ganglioneuroma originated from sacral canal in S1-2.

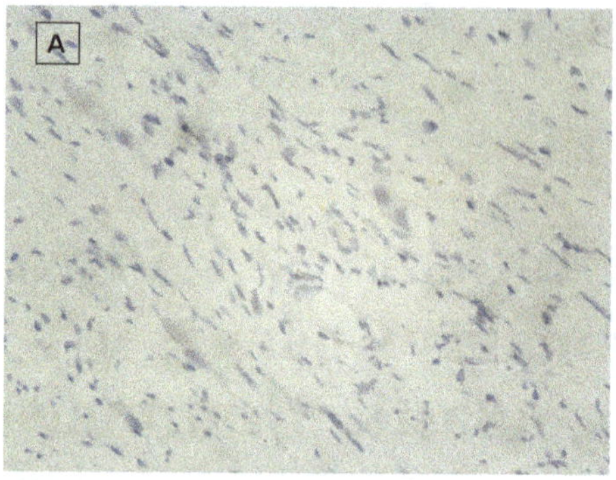

(a)

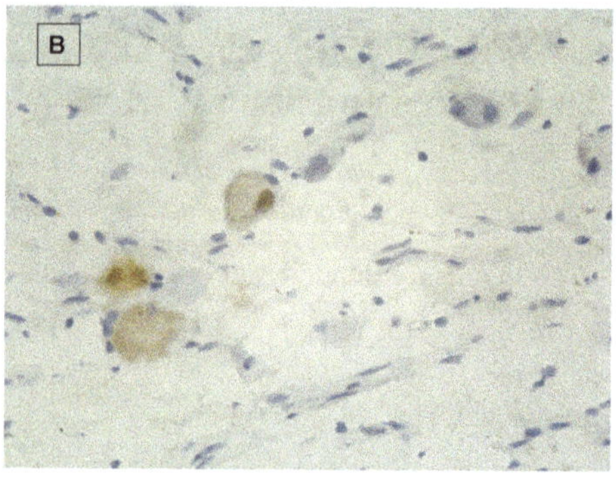

(b)

FIGURE 2: (a) Photomicrograph of a ganglioneuroma showing large mature neurons in a neuromatous proliferation including spindle-shaped Schwann nuclei. (b) Positive immunostaining of neuroganglional cells with anti-ACTH antibodies.

sacral canal in S1-2 (Figure 1) and excluded any sign of sacral or coccygeal metameric infiltration or osteolysis. The diagnosis of Castleman disease was suspected, and PNS due to this mass was also considered. In case of adrenal crisis postoperatively, hydrocortisone was administrated 3 days before and after surgery. The patient was submitted to surgical laparotomy: hypogastrium transverse incision and transperitoneal exposure were performed; small bowel, distal sigmoid, and rectum and their mesenteries were retracted to expose the tumor lesion. A mass measuring 3 cm × 2 cm × 2 cm was revealed and tenaciously stuck to sacral plane. Intraoperative frozen section excluded the malignancy of the lesion. A complete resection was performed. Histopathologic examination confirmed the diagnosis of ganglioneuroma, consisting of a majority of Schwann cells with variable amounts of collagen and some groups of ganglion cells and no neuroblast. Immunostaining for ACTH was focally positive (Figure 2).

After surgery, the patient's serum cortisol returned to the normal range, with values of 380 nmol/L, 320 nmol/L, and 260 nmol/L, 8/16/24 h, respectively, and blood pressure also returned to the normal range, and she had a regular postoperative hospital stay without complications. The temperature returned to normal 4 days after surgery and she was discharged on the 10th postoperative day. After a 6 mo follow-up, her personality changes were improved gradually, and no sign of progressive weight gain was observed. Follow-up of at least 5 years was planned to detect early recurrence if any.

3. Discussion

Histologically ganglioneuromas are considered to be part of the neuroblastoma group together with neuroblastomas and ganglioneuroblastomas [6, 7]; the cell of origin is derived from embryonic neural crest cells, which are destined to form autonomic nerve tissue. Although neuroblastomas are composed of neuroblasts, ganglioneuromas consist of mature ganglion cells and other mature tissues and are considered benign. It is believed that these tumors represent a continuum and that ganglioneuromas are the final stage in the maturation of neuroblastoma cells [6–9].

Arising along the sympathetic chain, ganglioneuromas are commonly localized in the posterior mediastinum followed by retroperitoneum, cervical region, and adrenal gland [7]. The presacral location is very rare. Ganglioneuromas have usually a mean diameter of 7 cm, so our patient is a rare case for both its presacral location and size [1].

These tumors may show hormonal activity. Hypertension, flushing, diarrhea, and virilization may occur as a result of the secretion of catecholamines, vasoactive intestinal polypeptide, or androgenic hormone [10]. Occasional reports of ACTH/CRH-producing ganglioneuromas presenting clinically as Cushing's syndrome were reported.

PNS in children is rare; mature neuroblastomas, that is, ganglioneuroblastomas, are known to produce peptides that may cause PNS, which are mainly neurological, such as cerebellar encephalopathy, opsoclonus-myoclonus, constipation, diarrhoea, and encephalomyelitis/sensory neuronopathy [11]. However, there was little report about PNS due to ganglioneuromas. To our knowledge, ganglioneuromas have been reported to secrete vasointestinal peptide and also can present as Cushing's syndrome [12, 13]. Except ectopic Cushing syndrome, our patient presented a complicated symptom of intermittent fever, progressive weight gain, and personality changes, which was barely observed in ganglioneuroma patients. The body temperature dropped to normal after surgery, which indicated the fever might be due to PNS such as an interleukin secretion by the tumor. After surgery, the serum cortisol and blood pressure returned to the normal range, and her personality changes were improved gradually; also no sign of progressive weight gain was observed at follow-up, which suggested an evidence of these symptoms that were caused by this tumor.

Imaging investigations had not hinted that the etiological diagnosis of these symptoms was a ganglioneuroma. On CT scanning, ganglioneuromas show no or mild heterogeneity, low attenuation and may exhibit calcification [14]. The patient's CT scan showed a dishomogeneous mass with obvious enhancement, which did not support the diagnosis of ganglioneuroma. Combined with her complicated clinical manifestations, Castleman disease was suspected. However, pathological examination confirmed the diagnosis of ganglioneuroma, which suggested ganglioneuroma should be considered in this situation.

4. Conclusion

Presacral ganglioneuromas are rare benign lesions in pediatrics and may present with various symptoms. Surgery is the primary means of diagnosis and treatment. Ganglioneuroma should be considered as a differential diagnosis in patient with presacral tumor accompanied with various clinical manifestations and Cushing syndrome.

Abbreviations

PNS: Paraneoplastic syndrome
VMA: Vanilmandelic acid
CT: Computed tomography
MRI: Magnetic resonance imaging.

Consent

Written informed consent was obtained from the patient for publication of this case report and any accompanying images.

Authors' Contribution

Chao Yang proposed the study and wrote the first draft. All authors contributed to the design and interpretation of the study and to further drafts. Shan Wang is the guarantor.

References

[1] A. Modha, P. Paty, and M. H. Bilsky, "Presacral ganglioneuromas. Report of five cases and review of the literature," *Journal of Neurosurgery Spine*, vol. 2, no. 3, pp. 366–371, 2005.

[2] H. Shimada, I. M. Ambros, L. P. Dehner, J.-I. Hata, V. V. Joshi, and B. Roald, "Terminology and morphologic criteria of neuroblastic tumors: recommendations by the International Neuroblastoma Pathology Committee," *Cancer*, vol. 86, no. 2, pp. 349–363, 1999.

[3] V. V. Joshi, "Peripheral neuroblastic tumors: pathologic classification based on recommendations of international neuroblastoma pathology committee (Modification of shimada classification)," *Pediatric and Developmental Pathology*, vol. 3, no. 2, pp. 184–199, 2000.

[4] E. Marmor, D. R. Fourney, L. D. Rhines, J. M. Skibber, G. N. Fuller, and Z. L. Gokaslan, "Sacrococcygeal ganglioneuroma," *Journal of Spinal Disorders & Techniques*, vol. 15, no. 3, pp. 265–268, 2002.

[5] G. Cerullo, D. Marrelli, B. Rampone et al., "Presacral ganglioneuroma: a case report and review of literature," *World Journal of Gastroenterology*, vol. 13, no. 14, pp. 2129–2131, 2007.

[6] F. A. Hayes, A. A. Green, and B. N. Rao, "Clinical manifestations of ganglioneuroma," *Cancer*, vol. 63, no. 6, pp. 1211–1214, 1989.

[7] V. S. Ghall, J. E. Gold, R. A. Vincent, and J. M. Cosgrove, "Malignant peripheral nerve sheath tumor arising spontaneously from retroperitoneal ganglioneuroma: a case report, review of the literature, and immunohistochemical study," *Human Pathology*, vol. 23, no. 1, pp. 72–75, 1992.

[8] C. H. Lam and M. G. Nagib, "Nonteratomatous tumors in the pediatric sacral region," *Spine*, vol. 27, no. 11, pp. E284–E287, 2002.

[9] G. J. Lonergan, C. M. Schwab, E. S. Suarez, and C. L. Carlson, "From the archives of the AFIP—neuroblastoma, ganglioneuroblastoma, and ganglioneuroma: radiologic-pathologic correlation," *Radiographics*, vol. 22, no. 4, pp. 911–934, 2002.

[10] B. Geoerger, B. Hero, D. Harms, J. Grebe, K. Scheidhauer, and F. Berthold, "Metabolic activity and clinical features of primary ganglioneuromas," *Cancer*, vol. 91, no. 10, pp. 1905–1913, 2001.

[11] B. Wildhaber, F. Niggli, E. Bergsträsser, T. Stallmach, and P. Sacher, "Paraneoplastic syndromes in ganglioneuroblastoma: contrasting symptoms of constipation and diarrhoea," *European Journal of Pediatrics*, vol. 162, no. 7-8, pp. 511–513, 2003.

[12] S. J. R. Reddy, G. Purushottam, K. Pandurangarao, and C. P. T. Ravi, "Para aortic ganglioneuroma presenting as Cushing's syndrome," *Indian Journal of Urology*, vol. 23, no. 4, pp. 471–473, 2007.

[13] J.-B. Corcuff, C. Deminiere, J. Trouillas, O. Puel, Y. Perel, and P. Barat, "Ectopic Cushing's syndrome due to an adrenal ganglioneuroma," *Hormone Research in Paediatrics*, vol. 73, no. 5, pp. 405–408, 2010.

[14] P. Otal, S. Mezghani, S. Hassissene et al., "Imaging of retroperitoneal ganglioneuroma," *European Radiology*, vol. 11, no. 6, pp. 940–945, 2001.

46

Monoballism Associated with Newly Onset Ketotic Hyperglycemia

Dilek Ersil Soysal,[1] Barıs Gelen,[1] Sezin Hızar,[1] Mete Pekdiker,[1] Ebru Tekesin,[1] Yesim Beckmann,[2] and Volkan Karakus[1]

[1] *Department of Internal Medicine, University of Katip Celebi and Ataturk Research and Training Hospital, Basın Sitesi, Izmir 35360, Turkey*
[2] *Department of Neurology, University of Katip Celebi and Ataturk Research and Training Hospital, Basın Sitesi, Izmir 35360, Turkey*

Correspondence should be addressed to Dilek Ersil Soysal, dileksoysal@hotmail.com

Academic Editors: J. P. Frindik, H. Hattori, M. P. Kane, and L. Mastrandrea

Movement disorders as the initial symptoms of diabetes mellitus are rare. Here, we describe one of these rare manifestations of primary diabetes: a case of newly diagnosed diabetes mellitus in an old-age female patient with transient monoballismus during an episode of ketotic hyperglycemia.

1. Introduction

Hemichorea-hemiballismus (HC-HB) constitute a neurological syndrome characterized by violent proximal involuntary movements on one side of the body, involving mainly the upper extremity [1]. Focal epilepsy, transient chorea or ballism provoked by an episode of nonketotic hyperglycemia (NKH) in adults with type 2 diabetes [1–8], and ketotic hyperglycemia in children with type I diabetes mellitus have been reported [9]. Nonketotic hyperglycemia occurs more often in women [1, 3, 6] and usually is associated with very high blood glucose [3]. In these cases, the seizures [7] as well as the choreiform movements have resolved within days to a few weeks after normalization of blood glucose and hence, reversible metabolic derangements within the basal ganglia have often been assumed [1–4, 8, 9]. Most of the cases have MRI changes in the putamen with high signal intensity on T1-weighted images and variable signal characteristics ranging from hyper-, to iso-, to hypointensity on T2-weighted images [1–3, 6, 8].

Movement disorders as the initial symptoms of diabetes mellitus are rare [5, 8]. Here, we describe one of these rare manifestations of primary diabetes: a case of newly diagnosed diabetes mellitus in an old-age female patient with transient monoballismus during an episode of ketotic hyperglycemia.

Ballism can be rapidly controlled by normalization of glycemia. Our patient had monoballism confined to her upper extremity. To our knowledge, this is the first report describing monoballism in a patient with ketotic hyperglycemia. She had a rapid symptomatic remission after correction of the hyperglycemia.

2. Case Presentation

An 84-year-old woman was brought to the emergency department with a complaint of acute onset, rapid, involuntary movements of the left upper limb and she was diagnosed with ketotic hyperglycemia with positive urine ketones. She had no significant past medical history except for essential hypertension. The patient was not exposed to newly onset medications, but was receiving angiotensin receptor blocker (valsartan 160 mg/d, orally) for hypertension. There was no family history of movement disorders, and she had no previous neurological and psychiatric symptoms either. On admission, the general physical examination was normal. Neurological examination showed an alert patient with acute onset involuntary, continuous, jerky movements of the left arm. The rest of the neurologic examination was unremarkable. The random blood glucose concentration was 309 mg/dL with (++) urine ketones and glycosuria. She had normal arterial blood gas analysis of pH, P_{CO_2} and

HCO_3^- concentrations on room air and temperature. Blood count and liver function tests were normal. Her urea was 25 mg/dL and creatinine 1.21 mg/dL. Her glycosylated hemoglobin A1C (HbA1C) was 14.9%. Serum sodium: 130 mEq/L, potassium: 3.9 mEq/L, serum calcium: 8.6 mg/dL, phosphorus: 2.3 mg/dL, magnesium: 1.7 mg/dL, uric acid: 6.1 mg/dL, serum ceruloplasmin: 30.6 mg/dL (N: 20–60), and copper:135 μg/dL (N: 80–155). Estimated blood osmolality was 294 mosm/L (N: 285–295). Antinuclear antibody (ANA) profile, antineutrophilic cytoplasmic antibodies reactive to myeloperoxidase (p-ANCA), and proteinase-3 (c-ANCA), antiphospholipid antibodies (e.g., anticardiolipin antibodies), antismooth muscle antibody (ASMA), anti-liver-kidney-microsome antibody (LKM-1), antimitochondrial antibody (AMA), TSH receptor antibodies (TRab), antithyroid peroxidase (TPO), and antithyroglobulin (anti T) antibodies revealed negative. Chest radiograph and electrocardiograph were normal.

Brain magnetic resonance imaging (MRI) showed hyperintensity in the right striatum on T1-weighted (Figure 1(a)) and low signal intensity on T2-weighted images (Figure 1(b)).

Management for diabetic ketosis was started on intravenous (IV) insulin infusion with hourly blood sugar monitoring. After the patient's glycemic control was achieved and urine ketones were negative, treatment with rapid-acting analog insulin of 8 unit before meals and long-acting analog insulin of 12 unit at night subcutaneously, and quetiapine fumarate 25 mg/d orally were commenced on the second day of her admission.

After achievement of blood glucose levels between 79 and 141 mg/dL, the involuntary movements declined and completely disappeared within 6 days, and quetiapine fumarate was discontinued without any recurrence of the described movements. The patient was discharged on a combination of rapid-and-long acting analog insulin (10 + 10 + 10 + 16 U SC) and advised regular follow up for glycemic profiles.

3. Discussion

"Ballism" refers to violent, irregular flinging limb movements. It constitutes part of the spectrum of chorea and is a result of proximal muscle contraction. There are several types of ballism, depending on the distribution of movements. The most common form is "hemiballism," which involves flinging movements of the upper and lower extremities on one side of the body. Ballism confined to one extremity is referred to as "monoballism." [10]. Chorea or ballismus can be caused by a variety of disorders affecting the basal ganglia such as metabolic diseases (it is possible for a patient with chorea-ballismus to have hyperglycemia at the initial presentation) [1, 6, 8], hypoxic-ischemic events, vascular disorders, structural abnormalities, trauma, drugs and toxins, infections, and inflammatory immunological diseases (rheumatic fever-Sydenham's chorea, systemic lupus erythematosus) [1, 4, 5, 8, 9].

Our patient suffered from monoballismus that was associated with an episode of ketotic hyperglycemia of an undiagnosed diabetes. She recovered quickly after correction of the hyperglycemia and treatment with quetiapine fumarate. Lack of recurrence of the involuntary movements after cessation of the drug suggested that this disorder was related to the metabolic change and that acute chorea-ballismus caused by hyperglycemia was a treatable disorder with a good prognosis [1, 4, 5, 8, 9].

The pathogenesis of ballismus associated with hyperglycemia is poorly understood. In ketoacidosis, ketones are used (an abundant source of acetoacetate from which γ-aminobutyric acid might be resynthesised) as an energy source and γ-aminobutyric acid (GABA) can be produced, but in nonketotic patients GABA will be rapidly depleted [5]. Depletion of GABA may cause a decrease in GABAergic activity, thereby decreasing the inhibition of the thalamus by the medial part of the globus pallidus [1]. As a result, HC-HB or partial seizures rarely occur with diabetic ketoacidosis. In nonketotic hyperglycemia, the brain metabolizes GABA into succinic acid via the succinic acid semialdehyde pathway and thus depletes GABA rapidly [4, 5]. During hyperglycemia, the activity of tricarboxylic acid cycle (Krebs cycle) and glucose utilization are depressed in the brain, so the cerebral metabolism shifts to alternative pathways [4]. In nonketotic hyperglycemia, the shift to anaerobic metabolism causes brain to utilize amino butyric acid which is synthesized from acetoacetate. Unlike in ketoacidosis, acetoacetate is rapidly depleted in nonketotic hyperglycemia causing cellular dysfunction [4, 5, 9].

Most reported cases of hyperglycemia-associated chorea and ballism are elderly, predominantly female diabetic patients with nonketotic hyperglycemia, and of East Asian origin [6] like in our case (except that the patient was ketotic hyperglycemia which was a rare condition), and the presentation is usually acute with the choreic-ballistic movements emerging as hyperglycemia develops. The female predisposition may be related to postmenopausal alterations of GABA or dopamine receptors [1]. Our patient had monoballism confined to her upper extremity. To our knowledge, this is the first report describing monoballism in a patient with ketotic hyperglycemia.

The patient's brain MRI showed a unilateral hyperintense lesion on T1-weighted images, and low signal intensity on T2-weighted images in the right striatum. Unilateral involvement in chorea induced by nonketotic hyperglycemia is more common in the literature than generalized chorea, which is the opposite of what we should expect from a central nervous system disorder provoked by a metabolic abnormality [2, 6]. Also, putamen is the most consistent focus in hyperglycemia-related chorea [2, 8]. A question is raised whether this clinical syndrome is due to selective metabolic vulnerability of the striatum to hyperglycemia and the attendant fluid and electrolyte abnormalities in predisposed individuals [2]. A recent case report on HC-HB assumed that diabetic ketoacidosis could cause this syndrome as a result of osmotic shifts generated by rapid changes in serum glucose levels and the putaminal lesion that was seen on T1-weighted imaging probably resulted from a diverging response to the same hyperglycemia [11].

Chorea-ballism can be rapidly controlled by normalization of glycemia [5, 6]. Resolution of the lesions seen in

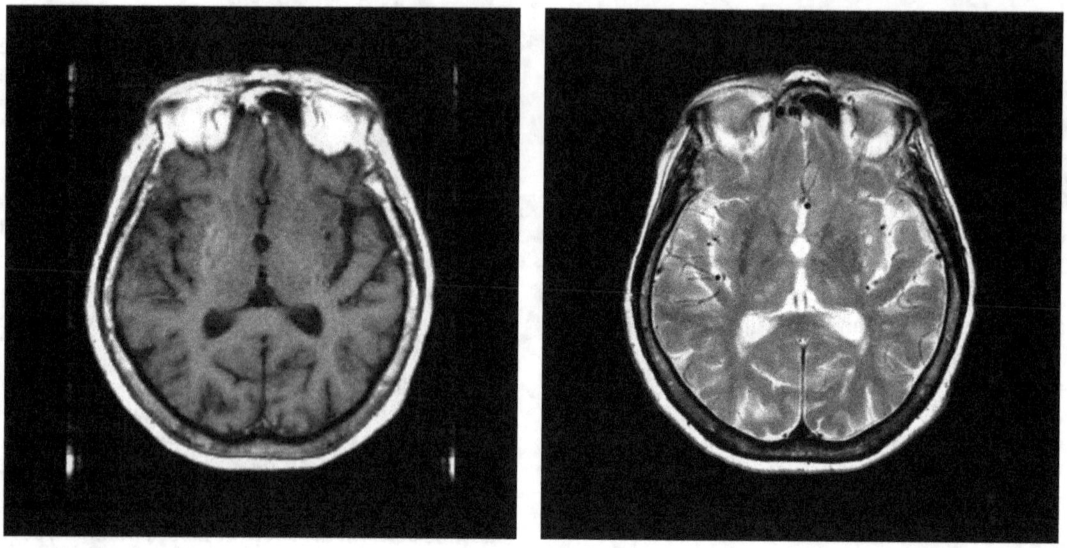

(a) (b)

Figure 1: (a) MRI scan showing a hyperintense lesion on T1-weighted image. Arrow corresponds to the right striatum. (b) MRI scan showing a low signal intensity on T2-weighted image.

imaging studies was found to be slower than the clinical course [6, 8, 11]. Our patient had a rapid symptomatic remission after correction of hyperglycemia. In some cases, involuntary movements can persist for a longer period despite correction of hyperglycemia [2, 6], and these patients may respond to conventional neuroleptics, particularly haloperidol, perphenazine, and chlorpromazine; risperidone and anticonvulsants may also be useful [6].

4. Conclusion

Even though numerous cases of hyperglycemia-provoked chorea-ballism have been described since its first report in 1960, it is uncommon in clinical practice [6].

Ballism is rarely caused by a dysfunction of glucose metabolism. Checking blood glucose in patients with this type of hyperkinesia, particularly in older women, is advised as the condition may rapidly resolve with hydration and resolution of the hyperglycemia. It is also advisable to keep in mind that this movement disorder may be the initial presenting symptom of diabetes mellitus [5].

Consent

Written informed consent was obtained from the patient for the publication of this case report and any accompanying images.

Authors' Contribution

B. Gelen, S. Hızar and M. Pekdiker acquired the data, D. E. Soysal wrote the paper, E. Tekesin and V. Karakus performed the clinical followup of the patient, and Y. Beckmann performed the neurologic evaluation.

References

[1] G. Ifergane, R. Masalha, and Y. O. Herishanu, "Transient hemichorea/hemiballismus associated with new onset hyperglycemia," *Canadian Journal of Neurological Sciences*, vol. 28, no. 4, pp. 365–368, 2001.

[2] J. E. Ahlskog, H. Nishino, V. G. H. Evidente et al., "Persistent chorea triggered by hyperglycemic crisis in diabetics," *Movement Disorders*, vol. 16, no. 5, pp. 890–898, 2001.

[3] B. Barton, S. E. Zauber, and C. G. Goetz, "Movement disorders caused by medical disease," *Seminars in Neurology*, vol. 29, no. 2, pp. 97–110, 2009.

[4] C. M. Mihai, D. Catrinoiu, and R. M. Stoicescu, "Atypical onset of diabetes in a teenage girl: a case report," *Cases Journal*, vol. 1, no. 1, p. 425, 2008.

[5] J.-J. Lin and M.-K. Chang, "Hemiballism—hemichorea and non-ketotic hyperglycaemia," *Journal of Neurology Neurosurgery and Psychiatry*, vol. 57, no. 6, pp. 748–750, 1994.

[6] C. V. Chang, A. C. Felicio, C. O. Godeiro Jr. et al., "Chorea-ballism as a manifestation of decompensated type 2 diabetes mellitus," *American Journal of the Medical Sciences*, vol. 333, no. 3, pp. 175–177, 2007.

[7] C. Grant and C. Warlow, "Focal epilepsy in diabetic non-ketotic hyperglycaemia," *British Medical Journal*, vol. 290, no. 6476, pp. 1204–1205, 1985.

[8] P.-H. Lai, R. D. Tien, M.-H. Chang et al., "Chorea-ballismus with nonketotic hyperglycemia in primary diabetes mellitus," *American Journal of Neuroradiology*, vol. 17, no. 6, pp. 1057–1064, 1996.

[9] D. Awasthi, A. K. Tiwari, A. Upadhyaya, B. Singh, and G. S. Tomar, "Ketotic hyperglycemia with movement disorder," *Journal of Emergencies, Trauma and Shock*, vol. 5, pp. 90–91, 2012.

[10] Y. Yetimalar, M. Seçkin, Y. Seçil, and M. Başoglu, "Lamotrigine-induced bilateral ballism," *Movement Disorders*, vol. 22, no. 12, pp. 1832–1833, 2007.

[11] A. P. Duker and A. J. Espay, "Hemichorea—hemiballism after diabetic ketoacidosis," *The New England Journal of Medicine*, vol. 363, no. 17, p. e27, 2010.

47

A Case of Growth Hormone use in Dyggve–Melchior–Clausen Syndrome

Ravi Upadhyay,[1] **Claire Ruane**,[1] **Rachel Umans**,[1] **Beth A. Pletcher**,[2] **Aditi Khokhar**,[2] **and Kristin Wong**[1]

[1]*Departments of Medicine and Pediatrics, Rutgers University New Jersey Medical School, Newark, NJ, USA*
[2]*Department of Pediatrics, Rutgers University New Jersey Medical School, Newark, NJ, USA*

Correspondence should be addressed to Kristin Wong; kgw22@njms.rutgers.edu

Academic Editor: Michaël R. Laurent

Short stature has many causes including genetic disease, skeletal dysplasias, endocrinopathies, familial short stature, and nutritional deficiencies. Recombinant growth hormone (rGH) therapy may be employed to improve stature based on the underlying etiology and growth velocity. Skeletal dysplasia in Dyggve–Melchior–Clausen (DMC) syndrome tends to be progressive, typically with hip involvement, and ultimately leads to bilateral dislocation of the hip joints. Here, we present a pediatric patient with short stature treated with rGH therapy, complicated by the development of debilitating, bilateral hip pain, and found to have DMC syndrome. Our patient had limited range of motion at several joints including the hips after receiving 6 months of rGH therapy. Given the timing of the patient's rGH therapy and the progression of her disease, it is difficult to determine if there were any benefits and instead, is concerning for worsening of her skeletal dysplasia with rGH therapy use. Consequently, patients with severe short stature should have a thorough workup for genetic causes like DMC syndrome, before initiating rGH therapy to determine any potential benefits or harms of treatment.

1. Introduction

Short stature is defined as a height of 2 standard deviations (SDs) or more below the mean height for children of that age and sex in a given population. Extreme cases of short stature, such as height standard deviations below 2.5 or 3, account for approximately 0.6 and 0.1% of the general population, respectively, and are usually associated with syndromic conditions such as skeletal dysplasias [1]. After a thorough workup, she was diagnosed with Dyggve–Melchior–Clausen (DMC) syndrome, a rare autosomal recessive genetic disorder. This syndrome is associated with short stature, intellectual disability, and a host of skeletal abnormalities which can affect the hips, vertebrae, and extremities [2]. Short stature is a universal feature of the disease with presentation typically after 5 years of age [3]. Recombinant growth hormone (rGH) therapy may be considered in patients with certain genetic diseases and idiopathic short stature, but in patients with severe short statures, especially those with skeletal disproportion and other developmental abnormalities, a thorough workup, including investigation of possible endocrine and genetic causes, is warranted to identify any underlying condition that should preclude treatment. In this case report, we present a pediatric patient who had progressive, severe bilateral hip pain after treatment of her short stature with rGH.

2. Case Presentation

A 12-year-old Hispanic girl, with a past medical history of short stature and microcephaly, presented to the ambulatory clinic to establish care. Physically, her mother reported that the patient had always been "small for her age." She was noted to have growth delays and was followed by pediatric endocrinology beginning at 7 years of age in Honduras. At age 10.5 years, she was started on rGH therapy (dose unknown). Therapy was discontinued after 6 months on noting a disproportionate growth of limbs relative to the torso. She

Table 1: Laboratory analysis.

Laboratory results on presentation	
Thyroid stimulating hormone	3.4 uu/ml
Free T4	1.0 ng/dl
Parathyroid hormone	31 pg/ml
Calcitriol	54.7 pg/ml
ESR	17 mm/hr
CRP	<1 mg/l
Lead	<1 ug/dl
HIV antibody/antigen screen	Nonreactive
Phosphorus	4.3 mg/dl
Alkaline phosphatase	233 u/l
Complete blood count	
White blood cell count	8.4×10^3/ul
Hemoglobin	13.7 g/dl
Hematocrit	41.1%
Platelet count	298×10^3/ul
Creatinine kinase	126 u/l

also reported that the patient had severe pain in the bilateral thighs, knees, and posterior calves with inability to walk. The pain gradually worsened over the prior four months and was also associated with a regression in her gross motor skills, including her ability to jump and ride a bike. The patient's gross motor milestones were otherwise appropriate until her recent difficulties ambulating.

Developmentally, the patient began to exhibit speech and language delays beginning at the age of 18 months. She was not able to use 2-word phrases until 4 or 5 years of age. She also reported a history of fine motor delays, being unable to tie her shoes or print her name. Her emotional and cognitive abilities were also delayed and the patient had never learned to name colors, recite the alphabet, or participate in elaborate play.

Birth history revealed that the patient was born full-term via a repeat cesarean section to nonconsanguineous Honduran parents after an uneventful pregnancy. There were no complications during delivery; the patient was noted to have microcephaly at birth, but no other abnormalities were identified. The mother was only able to reproduce a viral test report showing Rubeola IgG+ and IgM−. Upon social history, the patient had immigrated from Honduras 5 months prior to presentation and had no other significant exposures or risks. Her family history was also noncontributory to the patient's condition, and she had two healthy siblings. There was no family history of learning or intellectual disabilities nor neurological, growth, or genetic disorders.

Physical examination on presentation revealed a short (height 121.9 cm, <1%, $Z = -3.80$; weight 30.8 kg, 5%, $Z = -1.63$; BMI 20.75 kg/m^2, 80%, $Z = 0.83$; head circumference 49.5 cm, < 1%; midparental height 160 cm, 6%) and an alert, social, and friendly girl who looked younger than the stated age. Her vital signs were within normal limits for age. At 12 years, she was able to speak in simple phrases and name some objects but was unable to name letters or numbers, count fingers, or write her name. She was unable to answer simple questions and could follow only very simple commands. She had a short neck, broad chest, kyphosis with no scoliosis, brachydactyly with broad feet and hands, and

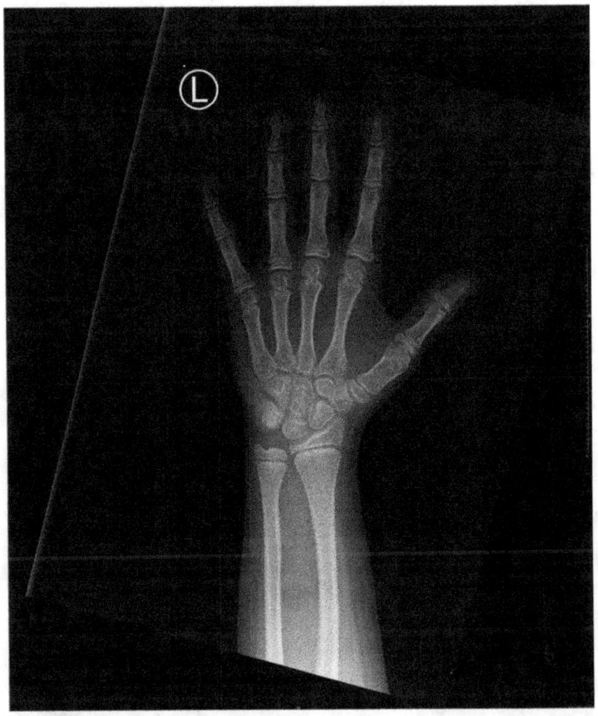

Figure 1: PA radiograph of the left hand for bone age evaluation. A radiograph of the left hand is depicted. The patient's chronological age at the time of the evaluation was 12 years and 2 months. According to the second edition of Greulich and Pyle, the patient's bone age is 11 years. Also noted is a short first metacarpal bone. The remaining bones have normal morphology. There is normal bone mineral density.

Tanner 2 breast development. Lower extremity exam revealed severe genu valgum, tenderness over bilateral posteromedial knees, and generalized, diffuse lower extremity tenderness, with a limited active range of motion due to pain; no pain elicited on passive movement. Bilateral hip flexor strength was 4/5 (limited by pain), while it was 5/5 in all the other major muscle groups. Clumsy fine motor movements were noted in the upper extremities with normal tone, intact sensation, and normal reflexes. No spasticity, atrophy, tremors, ataxia, or dysmetria were found. Her gait was notable for genu valgum, intoeing, and asymmetric step with limping greater on the right than the left side. She was able to take only a few steps without support.

The patient was referred to genetics, endocrinology, neurology, developmental pediatrics, and orthopedics. Laboratory workup including thyroid-stimulating hormone, lead level, hepatitis panel, and human immunodeficiency virus testing was all normal (Table 1). Her bone age was consistent with her chronological age. Her chromosomal microarray, however, showed normal dosage with a single large region of homozygosity on the long arm of chromosome 18, which increased concerns for an autosomal recessive condition. Radiographic imaging revealed a shortened 1st metacarpal bone of the left hand, diminished height of the cervical vertebrae along with a dysmorphic appearance (Figures 1 and 2), exaggerated lumbar lordosis, severe subluxation of bilateral femoral heads with

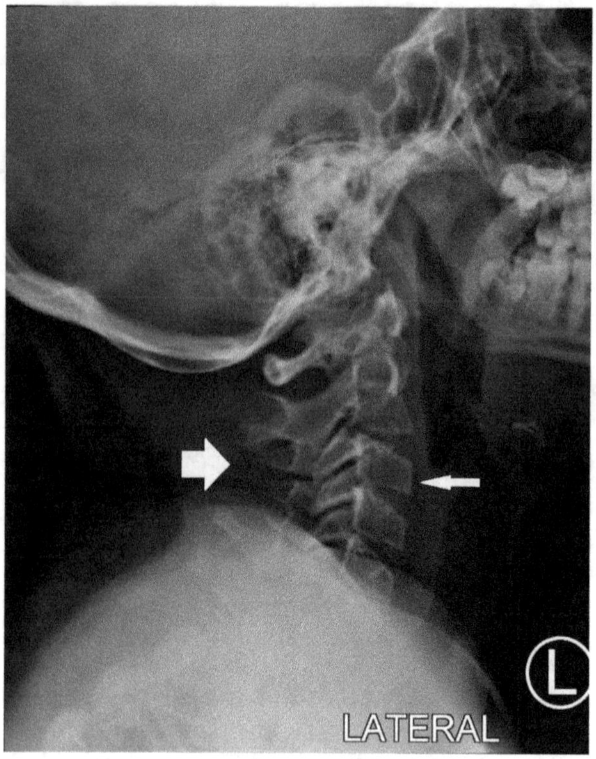

Figure 2: The cervical spine visualized to the C5 level. The vertebrae are diminished in height and dysmorphic in appearance (thick arrow). There is anterior wedging (thin arrow).

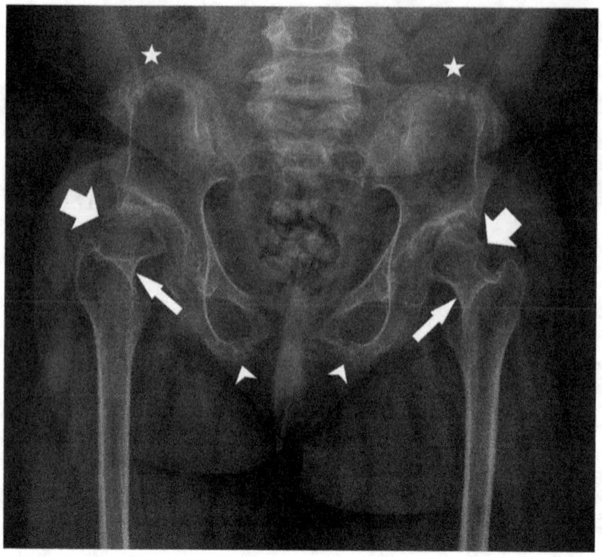

Figure 3: Pelvic and hip abnormalities associated with DMC syndrome. The pelvis with both hips is depicted. Both femoral heads are essentially dislocated/severely subluxated from the shallow, dysplastic acetabulum with resultant formation of a pseudoacetabulum superior and lateral to the native acetabulum bilaterally (thick arrow). Both femoral heads are deformed and small in size (thick arrow). There is premature growth plate fusion at the proximal femoral epiphyses (thin arrow). The iliac rest margins appear deformed (star). The ischial bones and inferior pubic rami are hypoplastic as well (arrowhead). There is decreased bone mineral density throughout, and the bones appear gracile.

dysplastic acetabulae and pseudoacetabulum formation (Figure 3), deformed iliac crests with hypoplasia of inferior pubic rami (Figure 3), and bowing of the right femur. Magnetic resonance imaging of the brain depicted partial agenesis of the corpus callosum and distal body of the splenium but was otherwise unremarkable. Subsequent genetic testing included an Invitae Skeletal Dysplasia Panel which revealed a homozygous missense mutation in a highly conserved region of the DYM gene (c 1244A⟶T, p.His415Leu in exon 11), with algorithms predicting this to be a pathogenic mutation. This particular mutation has not been seen in population databases but has been seen in patients with DMC syndrome. Written informed consent for publication of this case report was provided by the parent.

3. Discussion

Our case revolves around a 12-year-old girl with short stature, developmental delays, and skeletal dysplasia who was eventually diagnosed with DMC syndrome and had bilateral femoral head subluxation which was preceded by a 6-month course of rGH therapy in Honduras. DMC syndrome is a rare progressive genetic disorder which is characterized by intellectual disability, microcephaly, short stature, and progressive spondyloepimetaphyseal dysplasia, with skeletal deformities such as shallow acetabular roofs, lace-like iliac crests, and small femoral heads [3]. Approximately 100 cases have been described in the literature to date. The genetic syndrome is caused by mutations in the dymeclin (DYM) gene on the long arm of chromosome 18 which encodes a protein that is necessary for normal skeletal development and brain function [4]. The exact mechanism of the osteochondrodysplasia requires further elucidation, but DYM deficient murine models suggest that disorganized chondrocyte ossification is the result of impaired vesicular trafficking to and from the Golgi complex [5].

According to one study, age at presentation can vary with a reported range of 3 to 17 years, although delays in motor and intellectual development tend to be identified in the first few years of life [3]. The very specific lace-like appearance of the iliac crests and double-humped vertebral bodies become evident by 3-4 years of age [6]. Interestingly, one study found that subluxation of the hips is not a universal feature of the disease [3]. When present, progressive hip deformities in patients with DMC syndrome invariably lead to bilateral hip subluxation and eventual bilateral dislocation of the hip joint. The pain associated with changes at the hip is ultimately managed surgically although this can be delayed until late adolescence in some cases [7]. At the time of our initial evaluation, our patient already had limited range of motion at several joints including the hips. Radiographic studies revealed severe subluxation at the hips bilaterally along with bowing of the right femur. Our patient falls within the reported age range for skeletal dysplasia progression described in patients with DMC syndrome, but it is not known if prior rGH therapy could have precipitated or worsened hip subluxation in this case given the close timing of events.

Histochemical analysis of iliac crest growth plates in patients with DMC syndrome has revealed that a defect in endochondral ossification may cause skeletal dysplasia [8, 9]. Studies thus far have not evaluated the GH axis in patients with this syndrome, and the role of rGH therapy in this disorder has not been studied either. Our patient received daily rGH injections for six months before it was self-discontinued by the family on noting disproportionate limb growth, and she presented within a year of treatment with debilitating hip pain and gait abnormalities. To the best of our knowledge, this is the first reported case of rGH therapy use in a patient with DMC syndrome.

It is interesting to note that rGH therapy in other syndromes with skeletal dysplasias have had mixed results. On occasion, DMC syndrome can be misdiagnosed as a mucopolysaccharidosis (MPS) due to similar radiologic and clinical features [10]. Recombinant growth hormone therapy has shown some benefit in patients with MPS with reversion of growth deceleration, although controlled clinical trials are lacking [11, 12]. One clinical trial demonstrated efficacy of rGH therapy in patients with achondroplasia with only modest clinical impact, but not in patients with endochondral ossification abnormalities, such as spondyloepiphyseal dysplasia congenita, a disorder that shares features of skeletal dysplasia with DMC disease [13]. Therefore, it is difficult to ascertain whether rGH treatment was of any benefit to our patient, or if it accentuated the patient's skeletal dysplasia or precipitated her hip subluxation. Recombinant growth hormone therapy has indeed been associated with several orthopedic complications including scoliosis and slipped capital femoral epiphysis [14]. Adult height is severely reduced in DMC syndrome with a height range of 115–127 cm [15]. It will be interesting to see what the postpubertal height of this patient will be and whether it will be outside of the range of final height typically seen in this disorder. In our patient with severe short stature, skeletal disproportion, and developmental abnormalities, a thorough genetic workup was likely indicated prior to initiation of rGH therapy. Further studies are needed involving patients with DMC in order to determine the indications of use and possible adverse effects of rGH therapy in this rare genetic disorder.

Authors' Contributions

All authors have provided substantial contributions to the conception and design, acquisition and interpretation of data, and/or the drafting and revisions for intellectual content. All authors have provided final approval for publication and agree to be accountable for all aspects of the work.

References

[1] M. Grunauer and A. A. L. Jorge, "Genetic short stature," *Growth Hormone & IGF Research*, vol. 38, pp. 29–33, 2018.

[2] Rare Disease Database, "Dyggve Melchior Clausen syndrome," 2021, https://rarediseases.org/rare-diseases/dyggve-melchior-clausen-syndrome/.

[3] M. S. Aglan, S. A. Temtamy, E. Fateen, A. M. Ashour, K. Eldeeb, and G. A. Hosny, "Dyggve-Melchior-Clausen syndrome: clinical, genetic, and radiological study of 15 Egyptian patients from nine unrelated families," *Journal of Children's Orthopaedics*, vol. 3, no. 6, pp. 451–458, 2009.

[4] N. E. A. Gaboon, A. Parveen, K. A. Ahmad et al., "A novel homozygous frameshift variant in DYM causing dyggve-melchior-clausen syndrome in Pakistani patients," *Frontiers in Pediatrics*, vol. 8, p. 383, 2020.

[5] A. B. Osipovich, J. L. Jennings, Q. Lin, A. J. Link, H. E. Ruley, and H. Earl Ruley, "Dyggve-Melchior-Clausen syndrome: chondrodysplasia resulting from defects in intracellular vesicle traffic," *Proceedings of the National Academy of Sciences*, vol. 105, no. 42, pp. 16171–16176, 2008.

[6] V. Paupe, T. Gilbert, M. Le Merrer, A. Munnich, V. Cormier-Daire, and V. El Ghouzzi, "Recent advances in Dyggve-Melchior-Clausen syndrome," *Molecular Genetics and Metabolism*, vol. 83, no. 1-2, pp. 51–59, 2004.

[7] E. Nectoux, B. Hocquet, D. Fron, A. Mezel, A. Paris, and B. Herbaux, "Unpredictability of hip behavior in Dyggve-Melchior-Clausen syndrome: a mid-term assessment of siblings," *Orthopaedics and Traumatology: Surgery & Research*, vol. 99, no. 6, pp. 745–748, 2013.

[8] W. A. Horton and C. I. Scott, "Dyggve-Melchior-Clausen syndrome. A histochemical study of the growth plate," *The Journal of Bone and Joint Surgery*, vol. 64, no. 3, pp. 408–415, 1982.

[9] B. Engfeldt, T.-H. Bui, O. Eklöf et al., "Dyggve-melchior-clausen dysplasia," *Acta Paediatrica*, vol. 72, no. 2, pp. 269–274, 1983.

[10] A. Coëslier, O. Boute-Bénéjean, A. Moerman, D. Fron, and S. Manouvrier-Hanu, "Dyggve-Melchior-Clausen syndrome: differential diagnosis of mucopolysaccharidosis type IV or Morquio disease," *Archives of Pediatrics*, vol. 8, no. 8, pp. 838–842, 2001.

[11] L. E. Polgreen and B. S. Miller, "Growth patterns and the use of growth hormone in the mucopolysaccharidoses," *Journal of Pediatric Rehabilitation Medicine*, vol. 3, no. 1, pp. 25–38, 2010.

[12] A. Cattoni, S. Motta, N. Masera, S. Gasperini, A. Rovelli, and R. Parini, "The use of recombinant human growth hormone in patients with Mucopolysaccharidoses and growth hormone deficiency: a case series," *Italian Journal of Pediatrics*, vol. 45, no. 1, p. 93, 2019.

[13] H. Kanazawa, H. Tanaka, M. Inoue, Y. Yamanaka, N. Namba, and Y. Seino, "Efficacy of growth hormone therapy for patients with skeletal dysplasia," *Journal of Bone and Mineral Metabolism*, vol. 21, no. 5, pp. 307–310, 2003.

[14] R. K. Haidar, M. P. Nasrallah, A. H. Der-Boghossian, and I. B. Ghanem, "Orthopedic complications related to growth hormone therapy in a pediatric population," *Journal of Pediatric Orthopaedics B*, vol. 20, no. 1, pp. 57–61, 2011.

[15] V. Kenis, A. Baindurashvili, E. Melchenko, F. Grill, and A. Al Kaissi, "Management of progressive genu varum in a patient with Dyggve-Melchior-Clausen syndrome," *GMS German Medical Science*, vol. 9, 2011.

Permissions

All chapters in this book were first published by Hindawi Publishing Corporation; hereby published with permission under the Creative Commons Attribution License or equivalent. Every chapter published in this book has been scrutinized by our experts. Their significance has been extensively debated. The topics covered herein carry significant findings which will fuel the growth of the discipline. They may even be implemented as practical applications or may be referred to as a beginning point for another development.

The contributors of this book come from diverse backgrounds, making this book a truly international effort. This book will bring forth new frontiers with its revolutionizing research information and detailed analysis of the nascent developments around the world.

We would like to thank all the contributing authors for lending their expertise to make the book truly unique. They have played a crucial role in the development of this book. Without their invaluable contributions this book wouldn't have been possible. They have made vital efforts to compile up to date information on the varied aspects of this subject to make this book a valuable addition to the collection of many professionals and students.

This book was conceptualized with the vision of imparting up-to-date information and advanced data in this field. To ensure the same, a matchless editorial board was set up. Every individual on the board went through rigorous rounds of assessment to prove their worth. After which they invested a large part of their time researching and compiling the most relevant data for our readers.

The editorial board has been involved in producing this book since its inception. They have spent rigorous hours researching and exploring the diverse topics which have resulted in the successful publishing of this book. They have passed on their knowledge of decades through this book. To expedite this challenging task, the publisher supported the team at every step. A small team of assistant editors was also appointed to further simplify the editing procedure and attain best results for the readers.

Apart from the editorial board, the designing team has also invested a significant amount of their time in understanding the subject and creating the most relevant covers. They scrutinized every image to scout for the most suitable representation of the subject and create an appropriate cover for the book.

The publishing team has been an ardent support to the editorial, designing and production team. Their endless efforts to recruit the best for this project, has resulted in the accomplishment of this book. They are a veteran in the field of academics and their pool of knowledge is as vast as their experience in printing. Their expertise and guidance has proved useful at every step. Their uncompromising quality standards have made this book an exceptional effort. Their encouragement from time to time has been an inspiration for everyone.

The publisher and the editorial board hope that this book will prove to be a valuable piece of knowledge for researchers, students, practitioners and scholars across the globe.

List of Contributors

Meghan E. Fredette and Lisa Swartz Topor
Pediatric Endocrinology, Rhode Island Hospital/The Warren Alpert Medical School of Brown University, 111 Plain Street, 3rd Floor, Providence, RI 02903, USA

Valeria Calcaterra, Mauro Bozzola and Daniela Larizza
Department of Internal Medicine, University of Pavia, 27100 Pavia, Italy
Department of Pediatrics, IRCCS Policlinico S. Matteo Foundation, 27100 Pavia, Italy

Annachiara Malvezzi and Rossana Toglia
Department of Pediatrics, IRCCS Policlinico S. Matteo Foundation, 27100 Pavia, Italy

Angela Berardinelli
IRCCS C. Mondino Foundation and University of Pavia, 27100 Pavia, Italy

Elena Bozzola
Pediatric and Infectious Disease Unit, Department of Pediatrics, Bambino Gesù Children's Hospital, 00165 Rome, Italy

Rosa Maria Paragliola, Pietro Locantore, Alfredo Pontecorvi and Salvatore Maria Corsello
Endocrinology Unit, Catholic University School of Medicine, Largo Gemelli No. 8, 00168 Rome, Italy

Heather Choat and Kerri Derrevere
Department of Pediatrics, University of South Carolina School of Medicine, Columbia, SC 29203, USA

Lisa Knight and Whitney Brown
Division of Pediatric Endocrinology,Department of Pediatrics,University of South Carolina School ofMedicine, 9Medical ParkDrive, Suite 230A, Columbia, SC 29203, USA

Elizabeth H. Mack
Division of Pediatric Critical Care, Palmetto Health Children's Hospital, Columbia, SC 29203, USA

Jacqueline Chan, Fabiola D'Ambrosio Rodriguez, Deepank Sahni and Claudia Boucher-Berry
Department of Pediatric, Children's Hospital of the University of Illinois, Chicago, IL, USA

Ramin Alemzadeh
Division of Pediatric Endocrinology, University of Illinois College ofMedicine at Chicago, 1853W. Polk Street, Chicago, IL 60612, USA

Elizabeth Isaacoff and Sogol Mostoufi-Moab
Department of Pediatrics,The Children's Hospital of Philadelphia, 34th Street and Civic Center Boulevard, 3535 Market Street, Room 1562, Philadelphia, PA 19104, USA

Filippina Filia Dimitriadi
Division of Pediatric Endocrinology, St. Christopher's Hospital for Children, 3601 A. Street, Philadelphia, PA 19134, USA

Frank Barrows
Division of Pediatric Endocrinology, Monmouth Medical Children's Hospital, 180 Avenue at the Commons, Suite 7B, Shrewsbury, NJ 07702, USA

Bruce Pawel
Department of Pathology, The Children's Hospital of Philadelphia, 34th Street and Civic Center Boulevard, Philadelphia, PA 19104, USA

Peter Mattei
Department of General Surgery, The Children's Hospital of Philadelphia, 34th Street and Civic Center Boulevard, Philadelphia, PA 19104, USA

Ambreen Sonawalla
Pediatric Residency Program, University of Arkansas for Medical Sciences, Little Rock, AR, USA

Manish Raisingani
Department of Pediatrics, Division of Endocrinology and Diabetes, University of Arkansas for Medical Sciences, Little Rock, AR, USA

Emir Tas
Department of Pediatrics, University of Arkansas for Medical Sciences, Little Rock, AR, USA
Department of Pediatrics, Division of Endocrinology and Diabetes, University of Arkansas for Medical Sciences, Little Rock, AR, USA

Gerdi Tuli, Jessica Munarin, Daniele Tessaris, Raffaele Buganza, Patrizia Matarazzo and Luisa De Sanctis
Department of Pediatric Endocrinology, Regina Margherita Children's Hospital of Turin, Turin, Italy
Department of Sciences of Public Health and Pediatrics, University of Turin, Turin, Italy

M. Aabdi, O. Es-Saad, K. Malki, H. Bkiyar and B. Housni
Anesthesiology and Intensive Care Unit Department, MOHAMMED VI University Hospital Center, Oujda, Morocco

A. Aarab
Laboratory Unit Department, MOHAMMED VI University Hospital Center, Oujda, Morocco

Muhammad Rajib Hossain and Mahzabin Kibria
Department of Medicine, Shaheed Suhrawardy Medical College Hospital, Sher-e-Bangla Nagar, Dhaka 1207, Bangladesh

Md. Mashiul Alam
Department of Pediatrics, Dhaka Medical College Hospital, 100 Ramna, Dhaka 1000, Bangladesh

Junaid Nabi
Department of Surgery, Shaheed Suhrawardy Medical College Hospital, Sher-e-Bangla Nagar, Dhaka 1207, Bangladesh

Dhrubajyoti Sharma, Devi Dayal and Anju Gupta
Departments of Pediatrics, Advanced Pediatrics Center, Postgraduate Institute of Medical Education and Research, Chandigarh-160012, India

Akshay Saxena
Departments of Radiodiagnosis, Advanced Pediatrics Center, Postgraduate Institute of Medical Education and Research, Chandigarh-160012, India

Pooja E. Mishra
St John's Medical College, Bangalore, India

Betsy L. Schwartz
Pediatric Endocrinology, Park Nicollet, Minneapolis, MN, USA

Kyriakie Sarafoglou and Anna Petryk
Pediatric Endocrinology, University of Minnesota, Minneapolis, MN, USA

Kristen Hook
Pediatric Dermatology, University of Minnesota, Minneapolis, MN, USA

Youngki Kim
Pediatric Nephrology, University of Minnesota, Minneapolis, MN, USA

Rita Ann Kubicky and Francesco De Luca
Section of Endocrinology and Diabetes, St. Christopher's Hospital for Children, Drexel University College of Medicine, Philadelphia, PA 19134, USA
Department of Pediatrics, Drexel University College of Medicine, Philadelphia, PA 19102, USA

Evan Weiner
Department of Pediatrics, Drexel University College of Medicine, Philadelphia, PA 19102, USA
Department of Emergency Medicine, St. Christopher's Hospital for Children, Drexel University College of Medicine, Philadelphia, PA 19134, USA

Bronwyn Carlson
Department of Pediatrics, Drexel University College of Medicine, Philadelphia, PA 19102, USA

Nthabiseng Ellen Mothata and Moshawa Calvin Khaba
Department of Anatomical Pathology, Dr George Mukhari Academic Laboratory, National Health Laboratory Services, Sefako Makgatho Health Sciences University, Ga-Rankuwa, South Africa

Takalani Gidion Morulana and Nyaweleni Tshifularo
Department of Paediatric Surgery, Dr George Mukhari Academic Hospital, Sefako Makgatho Health Sciences University, Ga-Rankuwa, South Africa

Phumudzo Bridgett Nemutaduni and Nozipho Elizabeth Nyakale
Department of Nuclear Medicine, Dr George Mukhari Academic Hospital, Sefako Makgatho Health Sciences University, Ga-Rankuwa, South Africa

Pratibha Rana and Patria Alba Aponte
Children's Mercy Hospital, 3101 Broadway Blvd., Kansas City, MO 64111, USA

Ghufran Babar
Department of Pediatric Endocrinology, Children's Mercy Hospital, 3101 Broadway Blvd., Kansas City, MO 64111, USA

Somayyeh Hashemian, Siroos Karimdadi, Nosrat Ghaemi, Peyman Eshraghi and Rahim Vakili
Department of Pediatric Diseases, Akbar Hospital, Faculty of Medicine, Mashhad University of Medical Sciences, Mashhad, Iran

Reza Jafarzadeh Esfehani
Department of Medical Genetics, Faculty of Medicine, Mashhad University of Medical Sciences, Mashhad, Iran

Najmeh Malekzadeh Gonabadi
Faculty of Sciences, Sistan and Baluchestan University, Zahedan, Iran

Amirhossein Sahebkar
Biotechnology Research Center, Pharmaceutical Technology Institute, Mashhad University of Medical Sciences, Mashhad, Iran
Applied Biomedical Research Center, Mashhad University of Medical Sciences, Mashhad, Iran
School of Pharmacy, Mashhad University of Medical Sciences, Mashhad, Iran

Mohammad Reza Abbaszadegan
Medical Genetic Research Center, Medical School, Mashhad University of Medical Sciences, Mashhad, Iran

Arpita Kalla Vyas and Neil H. White
Division of Pediatric Endocrinology and Diabetes, Department of Pediatrics, Washington University in Saint Louis and Saint Louis Children's Hospital, Saint Louis, MO 63110, USA

Tansit Saengkaew, Taninee Sahakitrungruang, Suttipong Wacharasindhu and Vichit Supornsilchai
Division of Endocrinology, Department of Pediatrics, Faculty of Medicine, Chulalongkorn University, Bangkok 10330, Thailand

Rohan K. Henry
Division of Endocrinology, Department of Pediatrics, Nationwide Children's Hospital, The Ohio State University College of Medicine, Columbus, OH 43205, USA

Ram K. Menon
Division of Endocrinology, Department of Pediatrics, C.S. Mott Children's Hospital, Michigan Medicine, University of Michigan Medical School, Ann Arbor, MI 48109, USA

Patrizia Del Monte, Carla Micaela Cuttica and Alessandro Marugo
Endocrine Unit, Galliera Hospital, Genoa, Italy

Luca Foppiani
Internal Medicine Unit, Galliera Hospital, Genoa, Italy

Daniela Audenino
Neurology Unit, Galliera Hospital, Genoa, Italy

Tomasz Tadeusz Godowicz
Neurosurgery Unit, Galliera Hospital, Genoa, Italy

Francesca Marta Elli and Giovanna Mantovani
Fondazione IRCCS Ca' Granda OspedaleMaggiore Policlinico, Endocrinology and Diabetology Unit, Department of Clinical Sciences and Community Health, University of Milan,Milan, Italy

Emilio DiMaria
Department of Health Sciences, University of Genoa; Medical Genetics Unit, Galliera Hospital, Genoa, Italy

Chandan Shaw
Department of Pediatrics, Sri Manakula Vinayagar Medical College and Hospital, Kalitheerthalkuppam, Madagadipet, Pondicherry 605 107, India

Prachi Shaw
Department of Microbiology, Sri Manakula Vinayagar Medical College and Hospital, Kalitheerthalkuppam, Madagadipet, Pondicherry 605 107, India

Elizabeth Jasola Omoniyi and Richard J. Robbins
From the Division of Endocrinology, Diabetes and Metabolism, Department of Medicine, Houston Methodist Hospital, Houston, TX, USA
Weill Cornell Medical College, New York, NY, USA

Jennifer Apsan and Zoltan Antal
Department of Pediatrics, Division of Endocrinology Weill Cornell Medicine, New York Presbyterian Hospital, New York, NY, USA

Peter N. Taylor and Onyebuchi Okosieme
Endocrinology andDiabetesDepartment, Prince CharlesHospital, CwmTaf University Health Board, MerthyrTydfil CF47 9DT, UK
Thyroid Research Group, Institute of Molecular and Experimental Medicine, Cardiff University School of Medicine, Cardiff CF144XN, UK

Gina Sanki and Brian P. Tennant
Biochemistry Department, Prince Charles Hospital, Cwm Taf University Health Board, Merthyr Tydfil CF47 9DT, UK

James White
Department of Medicine of the Elderly, Prince Charles Hospital, Cwm Taf University Health Board, Merthyr Tydfil CF47 9DT, UK

Andrew Aldridge
Pharmacy, Prince CharlesHospital, CwmTaf University Health Board, Merthyr Tydfil CF47 9DT, UK

Arshiya Tabasum, David Burberry and Gautam Das
Endocrinology andDiabetesDepartment, Prince CharlesHospital, CwmTaf University Health Board, MerthyrTydfil CF47 9DT, UK

Kenneth Sluis, Hyon Kim, Yuling He, Beatrice Wong and Xiangbing Wang
Division of Endocrinology, Metabolism, and Nutrition, Department of Medicine, Rutgers University-Robert Wood Johnson Medical School, New Jersey, NJ 08903, USA

Mathilde Sollier, Marine Halbron, Olivier Bourron, Marie Bastin, Héléna Mosbah, Agnès Hartemann, Fabrizio Andreelli and Chloé Amouyal
Diabetology-Metabolism Dpt, Sorbonne Université, APHP, Institut Hospitalo-Universitaire de Cardiometabolisme et Nutrition (ICAN), Pitié-Salpêtrière-Charles Foix Hospital, 75013 Paris, France

Jean Donadieu
Hemato-Oncology Dpt, Trousseau Hospital, APHP, 75012 Paris, France

Ahmed Idbaih
Sorbonne Université, Inserm, CNRS, UMRS 1127, Institut du Cerveau et de la Moelle épinière, ICM, AP-HP, Hôpitaux Universitaires La Pitié Salpêtrière -Charles Foix, Service de Neurologie 2, Mazarin, 75013 Paris, France

Fleur Cohen Aubart
Department of Internal Medicine 2, Sorbonne Université, APHP, Institut Hospitalo-Universitaire de Cardiometabolisme et Nutrition (ICAN), Pitié-Salpêtrière-Charles Foix Hospital, 75013 Paris, France

Corinne Vigouroux and Martine Auclair
Inserm UMRS 938, Centre de Recherche Saint-Antoine, Sorbonne Université, Reference Center for Rare Diseases of Insulin Secretion and Insulin Sensitivity, Institut Hospitalo-Universitaire de Cardiometabolisme et Nutrition (ICAN), Paris, APHP, Saint Antoine Hospital, Paris, France

Géraldine Béra
Nuclear Medicine Dpt, Sorbonne Université, APHP, Pitié-Salpêtrière-Charles Foix Hospital, 75013

Philippe Touraine
Department of Endocrinology and Reproductive Medicine, Pitié-Salpêtrière Hospital, APHP, Reference Center for Rare Endocrine Diseases of Growth, Reference Center for Rare Gynecological Pathologies, Institut Hospitalo-Universitaire de Cardiometabolisme et Nutrition (ICAN), Sorbonne University, 75013 Paris, France
Pitié-Salpêtrière-Charles Foix Hospital, 75013 Paris, France

Jacques Young
Reproductive Endocrinology Department, Paris Sud University, APHP, Le Kremlin-Bicêtre, 94275, France

Meliha Demiral, Ciğdem Binay and Enver Simsek
Department of Pediatric Endocrinology, School of Medicine, Eskişehir Osmangazi University, Eskişehir, Turkey

Hüseyin Ilhan
Department of Pediatric Surgery, School of Medicine, Eskişehir Osmangazi University, Eskişehir, Turkey

Ichiro Abe
Department of Medicine and Bioregulatory Science, Graduate School of Medical Science, Kyushu University, Maidashi 3-1-1, HigashiWard, Fukuoka 812-8582, Japan
Department of Endocrinology and Diabetes Mellitus, Fukuoka University Chikushi Hospital, 1-1-1 Zokumyoin, Chikushino, Fukuoka 818-8502, Japan

Satoko Karasaki, Yayoi Matsuda, Shohei Sakamoto, Hisaya Kawate, Keizo Ohnaka, Masatoshi Nomura and Ryoichi Takayanagi
Department of Medicine and Bioregulatory Science, Graduate School of Medical Science, Kyushu University, Maidashi 3-1-1, HigashiWard, Fukuoka 812-8582, Japan

Kunihisa Kobayashi
Department of Endocrinology and Diabetes Mellitus, Fukuoka University Chikushi Hospital, 1-1-1 Zokumyoin, Chikushino, Fukuoka 818-8502, Japan

Torahiko Nakashima
Department of Otorhinolaryngology, Graduate School of Medical Science, Kyushu University, Maidashi 3-1-1, HigashiWard, Fukuoka 812-8582, Japan

Hidetaka Yamamoto and Yoshinao Oda
Department of Anatomic Pathology, Graduate School of Medical Science, Kyushu University, Maidashi 3-1-1, HigashiWard, Fukuoka 812-8582, Japan

Hisashi Nakashima
Department of Internal Medicine, Haradoi Hospital, Aoba 6-40-8, HigashiWard, Fukuoka 813-8588, Japan

Niranjan Tachamo
Department of Internal Medicine, Reading Health System,West Reading, PA 19611, USA

Brian Le
Department of Pathology, Reading Health System,West Reading, PA 19611, USA

Jeffrey Driben
ENT Head & Neck Specialists,Wyomissing, PA 19610, USA

Vasudev Magaji
Department of Endocrinology, Reading Health System,West Reading, PA 19611, USA

Gerry Samantha Eichelberger
Florida State University College of Medicine, 1115 W. Call Street, Tallahassee, FL, USA 32304

Jordan Carbono and Zachary Field
Department of Internal Medicine, Orlando Regional Healthcare, 21 W. Columbia St., Orlando, FL, USA 32806

KanwarAnoop Kainaur
Department of Pathology, Orlando Regional Healthcare, 52 W. Underwood St., Orlando, FL, USA 32806

Federico Montalvo
Florida State University College of Medicine, 1115 W. Call Street, Tallahassee, FL, USA 32304
Department of Internal Medicine, Orlando Regional Healthcare, 21 W. Columbia St., Orlando, FL, USA 32806

Vildan Tas and Juan D. Mejia-Otero
Department of Pediatrics, University of Arkansas for Medical Sciences, Little Rock, AR, USA

Serife E. Uzun
College of Osteopathic Medicine, New York Institute of Technology, Glen Head, Long Island, NY, USA

Murat Atmaca, Rıfkı Üçler and Murat Alay
Department of Endocrinology and Metabolism, Yuzuncu Yil University Faculty of Medicine, 65100 Van, Turkey

Esmet Seven, Veysi Barut, Yaren Dirik and Yasin Sezgin
Department of Internal Medicine, Yuzuncu Yil University Faculty of Medicine, 65100 Van, Turkey

Marco Ciacciarelli, Carmen Misurale, Eleonora D'Armiento, Alessandro Polidoro, Cristina Napoli, Alberto Lombardini, Umberto Ceratti, Ruben Manuel Luciano Colunga Biancatelli, Leonardo Calvosa, Romina Milanese, Sonia Ferri, Teresa Massaro, Andrea Lorusso and Luigi Iuliano
Department of Medico-Surgical Sciences and Biotechnologies, Internal Medicine Unit, ICOT Hospital, "Sapienza" University of Rome, Via Franco Faggiana 1668, Latina 04100, Italy

Gianluca Caruso, Veronica Sorrentino and Vincenzo Petrozza
Department of Medico-Surgical Sciences and Biotechnologies, Pathology Unit, ICOT Hospital, "Sapienza" University of Rome, Via Franco Faggiana 1668, Latina 04100, Italy

Marco Rengo and Piero Maceroni
Department of Radiological Sciences, Oncology and Pathology, ICOT Hospital, "Sapienza" University of Rome, Via Franco Faggiana 1668, Latina 04100, Italy

Valérie Spalart
AZ Turnhout, Department of Internal Medicine, Turnhout, Belgium

Barbara Legius and Lynn Decoster
AZ Turnhout, Department of Pulmonology/ Respiratory Oncology, Turnhout, Belgium

Kurt Segers
AZ Turnhout, Department of Pathology, Turnhout, Belgium

Johan Coolen
University Hospitals Leuven, Department of Radiology, Leuven, Belgium

Brigitte Maes
Jessa Hospital Hasselt, Laboratory for Molecular Diagnostics, Department of Clinical Biology, Hasselt, Belgium

Nelly Capetillo-Ventura
Department of Psychiatry, "Dr. José Eleuterio González" University Hospital, UANL, Avenida Francisco I. Madero and Avenida Gonzalitos, Mitras Centro, 64460 Monterrey, NL, Mexico

Inmaculada Baeza
Department of Child and Adolescent Psychiatry and Psychology, Institut Clínic de Neurociencies, Hospital Clínic, IDIBAPS, CIBERSAM, Barcelona, Spain

Masanori Murakami, Naohiro Takahashi, Sayaka Suzuki, Sachio Takekawa, Fumiko Iwashima and Toshiyuki Horiuchi
Department of Endocrinology and Metabolism, Tokyo Metropolitan Health Medical Treatment Corporation Toshima Hospital, 33-1 Sakae-cho, Itabashi-ku, Tokyo 173-0015, Japan

Noriko Matsushita, Ryuki Kawamura, Takashi Shibui and Akihiro Hata
Department of Cardiology, Tokyo Metropolitan Health Medical Treatment Corporation Toshima Hospital, 33-1 Sakae-cho, Itabashi-ku, Tokyo 173-0015, Japan

Rie Arai
Department of Psychiatry, Tokyo Metropolitan Health Medical Treatment Corporation Toshima Hospital, 33-1 Sakae-cho, Itabashi-ku, Tokyo 173-0015, Japan

Yoshihiro Ogawa
Department of Molecular Endocrinology and Metabolism, Graduate School of Medical and Dental Sciences, Tokyo Medical and Dental University, 1-5-45 Yushima, Bunkyo-ku, Tokyo 113-8510, Japan

Livio Luzi
Department of Biomedical Sciences for Health, Universit`a degli Studi di Milano, Via Morandi 30, San Donato Milanese, 20097 Milan, Italy
Metabolism Research Center, IRCCS Policlinico San Donato, Via Morandi 30, San Donato Milanese, 20097 Milan, Italy
Endocrinology Unit, IRCCS Policlinico San Donato, Via Morandi 30, San Donato Milanese, 20097 Milan, Italy
Endocrinology and Metabolic Diseases, IRCCS Policlinico San Donato, Via Morandi 30, San Donato Milanese, 20097 Milan, Italy

Stefano Benedini
Department of Biomedical Sciences for Health, Universit`a degli Studi di Milano, Via Morandi 30, San Donato Milanese, 20097 Milan, Italy
Metabolism Research Center, IRCCS Policlinico San Donato, Via Morandi 30, San Donato Milanese, 20097 Milan, Italy
Endocrinology Unit, IRCCS Policlinico San Donato, Via Morandi 30, San Donato Milanese, 20097 Milan, Italy

Antonietta Tufano
Endocrinology Unit, IRCCS Policlinico San Donato, Via Morandi 30, San Donato Milanese, 20097 Milan, Italy

Marco Mendola
Metabolism Research Center, IRCCS Policlinico San Donato, Via Morandi 30, San Donato Milanese, 20097 Milan, Italy
Endocrinology Unit, IRCCS Policlinico San Donato, Via Morandi 30, San Donato Milanese, 20097 Milan, Italy

Elena Passeri and Sabrina Corbetta
Department of Biomedical Sciences for Health, Universit`a degli Studi di Milano, Via Morandi 30, San Donato Milanese, 20097 Milan, Italy
Endocrinology Unit, IRCCS Policlinico San Donato, Via Morandi 30, San Donato Milanese, 20097 Milan, Italy

Yoichiro Okubo and Hiroyuki Hayashi
Department of Pathology, Kanagawa Cancer Center, Yokohama, Japan

Katsuhiko Masudo
Department of Breast and #yroid Surgery, Yokohama City University Medical Center, Yokohama, Japan

Hirotaka Nakayama, Yasushi Rino and Munetaka Masuda
Department of Surgery, Yokohama City University School of Medicine, Yokohama, Japan

Hanane Latrech
Department of Endocrinology, Mohammed VI Hospital, Medical School, Mohammed the First University, 60 000 Oujda, Morocco

Imane Skikar
Department of Radiology, Mohammed VI Hospital, Medical School, Mohammed the First University, 60 000 Oujda, Morocco

Mohammed El Hassan Gharbi and Abdelmjid Chraïbi
Department of Endocrinology, Ibn Sina Hospital, Medical School, Mohammed V University, 10 000 Rabat, Morocco

Ahmed Gaouzi
Department of Endocrinology Pediatrics, Children Hospital, Medical School, Mohammed V University, 10 000 Rabat, Morocco

Kiana Karimi
Student Research Committee, Hamadan University of Medical Sciences, Hamadan, Iran
Universal Scientific Education and Research Network (USERN), Tehran, Iran

Mohsen Nikzad
Department of Internal Medicine, School of Medicine, Hamadan University of Medical Sciences, Hamadan, Iran

Sohrab Kulivand
Department of Radiology, School of Medicine, Hamadan University of Medical Sciences, Hamadan, Iran

Shiva Borzouei
Department of Endocrinology, School of Medicine, Hamadan University of Medical Sciences, Hamadan, Iran

Chandrika Jayakanthi Subasinghe, Noel Somasundaram, Pathmanathan Sivatharshya, Lalana Devi Ranasinghe
Endocrinology Unit, National Hospital of Sri Lanka, Colombo, Sri Lanka

Márta Korbonits
Department of Endocrinology, William Harvey Research Institute, Barts and the London School of Medicine and Dentistry, Queen Mary University of London, UK

S. Wacharasindhu
Department of Pediatrics, Faculty of Medicine, Chulalongkorn University, Bangkok 10330, Thailand

S. Shuangshoti
Department of Pathology and Chulalongkorn GenePRO Center, Faculty of Medicine, Chulalongkorn University, Bangkok 10330, Thailand

S. Sunthornyothin
Department of Medicine, Faculty of Medicine, Chulalongkorn University, Bangkok 10330, Thailand

Haruhiko Yamazaki, Hiroyuki Iwasaki, Nobuyasu Suganuma, Toshinari Yamashita, Takashi Yamanaka, Soji Toda, Yuko Sugawara, Yuka Matsubara and Kaori Kohagura
Department of Breast and Endocrine Surgery, Kanagawa Cancer Center, Yokohama, Japan

Takeshi Kishida and Go Noguchi
Department of Urology, Kanagawa Cancer Center, Yokohama, Japan

Katsuhiko Masudo
Department of Breast andThyroid Surgery, Yokohama City University Medical Center, Yokohama, Japan

Chao Yang, Chang-chun Li, Jun Zhang, Xiang-ru Kong, Zhenzhen Zhao, Xiao-bin Deng, Liang Peng and Shan Wang
Department of Pediatric Surgical Oncology, Children's Hospital of Chongqing Medical University, 136 Zhongshan 2nd Road, Yuzhong District, Chongqing 400014, China

Dilek Ersil Soysal, Barıs Gelen, Sezin Hızar, Mete Pekdiker, Ebru Tekesin and Volkan Karakus
Department of Internal Medicine, University of Katip Celebi and Ataturk Research and Training Hospital, Basın Sitesi, Izmir 35360, Turkey

Yesim Beckmann
Department of Neurology, University of Katip Celebi and Ataturk Research and Training Hospital, Basın Sitesi, Izmir 35360, Turkey

Ravi Upadhyay, Claire Ruane, Rachel Umans and Kristin Wong
Departments of Medicine and Pediatrics, Rutgers University New Jersey Medical School, Newark, NJ, USA

Beth A. Pletcher and Aditi Khokhar
Department of Pediatrics, Rutgers University New Jersey Medical School, Newark, NJ, USA

Index

www.ingramcontent.com/pod-product-compliance
Lightning Source LLC
LaVergne TN
LVHW060059220926
848484LV00008BA/2294